Transcatheter Embolization and Therapy

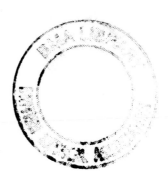

Techniques in Interventional Radiology

Series Editors

Michael J. Lee

Anthony F. Watkinson

Other titles in this Series:

Handbook of Angioplasty and Stenting Procedures

Interventional Radiology Procedures in Biopsy and Drainage (forthcoming)

Interventional Radiology Techniques in Ablation (forthcoming)

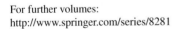

For further volumes:

http://www.springer.com/series/8281

David O. Kessel · Charles E. Ray
Editors

Transcatheter Embolization and Therapy

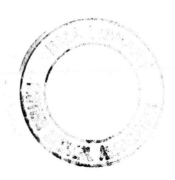

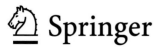

Series Editors
Michael J. Lee, MD
Professor of Interventional Radiology
Beaumont Hospital and Royal College
  of Surgeons in Ireland
Dublin
Ireland

Anthony F. Watkinson, BSc MSc(Oxon)
  MBBS FRCS FRCR
Professor of Interventional Radiology
The Royal Devon and Exeter Hospital and
  Peninsula Medical School
Exeter
UK

Editors
David O. Kessel, MA MRCP FRCR
Leeds Teaching Hospitals
Dept. Radiology
Leeds
United Kingdom

Charles E. Ray, MD
University of Colorado
Health Sciences Center
Dept. Radiology
Aurora CO
USA

ISBN 978-1-84800-896-0   e-ISBN 978-1-84800-897-7
DOI 10.1007/978-1-84800-897-7
Springer London Dordrecht Heidelberg New York

British Library Cataloguing in Publication Data
A catalogue record for this book is available from the British Library

Library of Congress Control Number: 2009940451

Printed on acid-free paper

Springer is part of Springer Science+Business Media (www.springer.com)

Thanks to Jamie, Ross, Anna, and Debbie Kessel for maintaining a sense of humour and supporting us through the process of writing and editing

To Kris, who supported much and gained little during this project, and others.

Foreword

Embolization is a powerful technique that is now making a significant contribution to the treatment of a very large number of patients. Since it was first used in the 1960s, physicians have been attracted by its power to occlude a vessel without the need to use much more invasive, and usually less effective, open surgical techniques to achieve the same purpose. Recent advances in materials technology, and great improvements in methods of imaging guidance, have greatly increased the effectiveness of this attractive technique, enabling the occlusion of vessels in a large variety of organs.

This textbook is being published at exactly the right time, as it brings together in a single volume all aspects of embolization and allows the reader to appreciate the power and scope of this attractive method of treatment. It is edited by two of the world's greatest authorities in this field, and the list of authors includes many of the leading exponents of embolization on both sides of the Atlantic.

The first section of the book covers the relevant technology, discussing the characteristics of catheters and embolization materials, as well as the underlying principles of the technique. The second and larger section deals with all the important applications of embolization in a variety of organ systems and clinical situations.

The reader of this book will gain a clear understanding of how to use embolization effectively and safely. Interventional radiologists in training will find it an invaluable guide to all aspects of the technique; and experienced operators will use it to update their knowledge and to obtain advice on the use of embolization in vascular territories that are not part of their routine practice.

David O. Kessel and Chuck Ray deserve our thanks and our congratulations on producing a magnificent book.

Andy Adam, MBBS (Hons), FRCP, FRCS,
FRCR, FFRRCSI (Hon)
Professor of Interventional Radiology
Department of Radiology
St Thomas' Hospital
King's College London
London, UK

Preface from the Series Editors

Interventional radiology treatments now play a major role in many disease processes and continue to mushroom with novel procedures appearing almost, on a yearly basis. Indeed, it is becoming more and more difficult to be an expert in all facets of interventional radiology. The interventional trainee and practising interventional radiologist will have to attend meetings and read extensively to keep up to date. There are many IR textbooks which are disease specific, but incorporate interventional radiology techniques. These books are important to understand the natural history, epidemiology, pathophysiology and diagnosis of disease processes. However, a detailed handbook that is technique based is a useful addition to have in the Cath Lab, office or at home where information can be accessed quickly, before or even during a case. With this in mind we have embarked on a series of books which will provide technique specific information on IR procedures. Initialy, technique handbooks on Angioplasty and Stenting, Transcatheter Embolization, Biopsy and Drainage and Ablative techniques will comprise the series. In the future we hope to add books on Pediatric and Neuro intervention.

We have chosen two editors, who are expert in their fields, for each book. One editor is European and one is American so that the knowledge of IR techniques detailed is balanced and representative. We have tried to make the information easy to access using a consistent bullet point format with sections on clinical features, anatomy, tools, patient preparation, technique, aftercare, complications and key points at the end of each chapter.

These technique-specific books will be of benefit to those Residents and Fellows who are training in interventional radiology and who may be taking subspeciality certificate examinations in interventional radiology. In addition, these books will be of help to most practicing interventional radiologists in academic or private practice. We hope that these books will be left in the interventional lab where they should also be of benefit to ancillary staff, such as radiology technicians/radiographers or nurses who are specialising in the care of patients referred to interventional radiology.

We hope that you will use these books extensively and that they will be of help during you working IR career.

Anthony F. Watkinson   Michael J. Lee
Exeter, UK   Dublin, Ireland

Preface from the Editors

Charles Dotter originally described the use of embolization therapy to deliberately occlude blood vessels in 1966. The ingenuity and expertise of interventional radiologists have seen embolotherapy as the embodiment of Dotter's remark "that an angiographic catheter ... if used with imagination ... can become an important surgical instrument."

Embolotherapy started gaining clinical acceptance in the early 1970s for stopping bleeding in the context of gastric hemorrhage and pelvic trauma. In keeping with a preference for minimally invasive therapy, embolization is becoming the primary treatment of choice for the management of a diverse range of clinical conditions.

Interventional Radiologists are uniquely equipped to deal with technical and intellectual challenges of contemporary embolization therapy. Safe and successful embolization requires understanding of the pre-procedure imaging, advanced catheter and wire skills plus knowledge of a wide variety of techniques, tools, agents, and pathologies in different organ systems. The possibility of horrific outcomes if performed incorrectly means that embolization therapy must remain in the realm of interventional radiology. We can ensure this by embracing pre-procedure assessment, post-procedure care, and 24/7 availability.

This book is a practical guide to the performance of embolization procedures. The first section introduces the general concepts of embolization procedures and materials used. The second section provides details of organ- or disease-specific procedures. Each of these chapters is a stand-alone guide to the subject. Contributors were sought from Europe and North America in order to a balanced and comprehensive view of the topic. We are indebted to our authors for their expertise, patience, and understanding. It is our hope that the reader will find this enjoyable, informative, and educational.

Charles E. Ray   David O. Kessel
Aurora, CO, USA   Leeds, UK

Contents

Contributors

Hamed Aryafar MD Department of Radiology (Interventional), University of California San Diego, San Diego, CA, USA

Sriharsha Athreya FRCS FRCR McMaster University Faculty of Health Sciences and St Joseph's Healthcare, Hamilton, ON, Canada

George Behrens MD Department of Interventional Radiology, Rush University Medical Center, Chicago, IL, USA

Mark Brinckman MD Department of Radiology, University of Colorado, Aurora, CO, USA

Jess Campagna MD BS Department of Radiology, University of Colorado Denver, Aurora, CO, USA

Nicholas Chalmers MA MB ChB FRCR Radiology Department, Manchester Royal Infirmary, Manchester, UK

Trevor Cleveland BMedSci BM BS FRCS FRCR Sheffield Vascular Institute, Sheffield Teaching Hospitals, Sheffield, UK

Douglas Coldwell PhD MD, Department of Radiology, Jane Phillips Medical Center, Bartlesville, OK, USA

Erik Cressman PhD MD Department of Radiology, University of Minnesota Medical Center, Minneapolis, MN, USA

Benjamin English MD Department of Diagnostic Radiology, University of Colorado Health Sciences, Aurora, CO, USA

Audrey Fohlen MD Department of Radiology, Centre Hospitalier Universitaire de Caen, Caen, France

Jennifer Fraser BA Department of Radiology, University of Colorado, Centennial, CO, USA

Brian Funaki MD, Department of Radiology, University of Chicago Medical Center, Chicago, IL, USA

Peter Gaines MBChB FRCP FRCR, Sheffield Vascular Institute, Northern General Hospital, Sheffield, UK

Ian Gillespie MB ChB DMRD FRCSEd FRCR Department of Radiology, Edinburgh Royal Infirmary, Edinburgh, UK

Rajan Gupta MD BSE Department of Interventional Radiology, University of Colorado Denver, Aurora, CO, USA

Eric J. Hohenwalter MD Department of Radiology/Vascular and Interventional Radiology, Medical College of Wisconsin, Froedtert Memorial Lutheran Hospital, Milwaukee, WI, USA

Hamish Ireland MB ChB MRCP FRCR Department of Radiology, Edinburgh Royal Infirmary, Edinburgh UK

James Jackson MRCP FRCR Department of Imaging, Hammersmith Hospital, London, UK

Raj Jain MD Department of Radiology, University of Colorado Denver, Aurora, CO, USA

Stephen Johnson MD, DOVT, CPMG Medical Group, Golden, CO, USA

John A. Kaufman MD Dotter Interventional Institute, Oregon Health and Science University, Portland, OR, USA

Aoife N. Keeling FFR RCSI MRCPI MSc Department of Radiology, Northwestern Memorial Hospital, Chicago, IL USA

David O. Kessel MA MRCP FRCR Department of Imaging, Leeds Teaching Hospitals NHS Trust, Leeds, UK

David M. King MD Department of Orthopedic Surgery, Medical College of Wisconsin, Froedtert Memorial Lutheran Hospital, Milwaukee, WI, USA

Thomas Kinney MD MSME FSIR Department of Radiology, UCSD Medical Center, San Diego, CA, USA

Kenneth J. Kolbeck MD PhD Dotter Interventional Institute, Oregon Health and Science University, Portland, OR, USA

Kimi Kondo DO Department of Radiology, Division of Interventional Radiology, University of Colorado Denver, Aurora, CO, USA

Michael J. Lee MD Department of Radiology, Beaumont Hospital, Dublin, Ireland

Peter Littler MRCP FRCR Department of Radiology, Royal Liverpool University Hospital, Liverpool, UK

Louis Lucas MD Department of Radiology, University of Colorado Health Sciences Center, Aurora, CO, USA

Lindsay Machan MD Department of Radiology, University of British Colombia Hospital, Vancouver, Canada

Hegoda L.D. Makalanda MBBS BSc MRCS FRCR, Department of Radiology, The Royal Free Hospital, London, UK

Simon McPherson BSc MBBS MRCR FRCR Department of Radiology, Leeds Teaching Hospitals NHS Trust, Leeds, UK

Richard McWilliams Department of Radiology, Royal Liverpool University Hospital, Liverpool, UK

Robert Morgan MB ChB MRCP FRCR Department of Radiology, St Georges NHS Trust, London, UK

Jon Moss FRCS FRCR Department of Radiology, Gartnavel General Hospital, Glasgow, UK

Tony Nicholson BSc MSc MB ChB FRCR, Department of Radiology, Leeds Teaching Hospitals, Leeds, UK

Kevin O'Reagan MB BCh BAO BMedSci MRCPI FFRRSCI, Department of Radiology, Cork University Hospital, Cork, Ireland

Richard J.T. Owen MB BCh Department of Diagnostic Imaging, University of Alberta, Edmonton, AB, Canada

Anthie M. Papadopoulou BSc MBBS FRCR Department of Radiology, Royal Free Hospital NHS Trust, London, UK

Jai Patel MB ChB MRCP FRCR Department of Radiology, The Leeds Teaching Hospitals NHS Trust, St James' University Hospital, Leeds, UK

Nilesh H. Patel MD FSIR Vascular and Instrumental Program, Central DuPage Hospital, Winfield, IL, USA

Jean-Pierre Pelage MD PhD Department of Radiology, Hôpital Ambroise Paré, Université Paris Ouest, Boulogne, France

Andrew Platts MB BS FRCS FRCR Department of RadiologyRoyal Free Hospital NHS Trust, London, UK

Sapna Puppala MBBS MRCS FRCSEd FRCR CBCCT Department of Radiology, Leeds Teaching Hospital NHS Trust, Leeds, UK

Lakshmi A. Ratnam MBChB MRCP FRCR Department of Radiology, St George's Hospital, London, UK

Ahsun Riaz MD Department of Interventional Radiology, Northwestern Memorial Hospital, Chicago, IL, USA

William S. Rilling MD Department of Radiology, Medical College of Wisconsin, Froedtert Memorial Lutheran Hospital, Milwaukee, WI, USA

Iain Robertson MBChB MRCP FRCR Department of Imaging, Gartnavel General Hospital, Glasgow, UK

Graham Robinson MA BM BCh FRCS FRCR, Department of Radiology, Hull Royal Infirmary, Hull, UK

Robert Rosen MD Department of Interventional Cardiology, Lenox Hill Heart and Vascular Institute, New York, NY, USA

Peter Rowlands FRCP FRCR Department of Radiology, Royal Liverpool University Hospital, Liverpool, UK

Riad Salem MD MBA Department of Interventional Radiology, Northwestern Memorial Hospital, Chicago, IL, USA

P. Anondo Stangl MD Department of Radiology, Mount Sinai School of Medicine, New York, NY, USA

Tanya Tivorsak MD Department of Radiology, University of Colorado Denver Health Sciences Center, Aurora, CO, USA

Clayton Trimmer DO Department of Radiology, University of Texas Southwestern Medical Center, Dallas, TX, USA

David Tuite FFRRCSI MB BCh BAO BA Department of Radiology, Cork University Hospital, Cork, Ireland

Otto Van Delden MD PhD Department of Radiology, Academic Medical Center of the University of Amsterdam, Amsterdam, The Netherlands

Catherine Vu MD Department of Radiology, University of Colorado Denver, Aurora CO, USA

David West MB ChB FRCR Department of Imaging, University Hospital of North Staffordshire, Newcastle-under-Lyme, UK

Kimberley Wright MD Department of Radiology, University of Colorado Denver, Aurora, CO, USA

Stan Zipser MD JD Department of Diagnostic Imaging, Santa Clara Valley Medical Center, San Jose, CA, USA

Section I

Chapter 1
Basic Principles of Embolization

Iain Robertson

Introduction

Embolization therapy covers an enormous spectrum of procedures, from simple varicocoele embolization to occlusion of complex arteriovenous malformations. Both procedures aim to provide vascular occlusion, but the techniques, equipment, approach, outcomes, and hazards are very different. This chapter aims to set the scene for the rest of the book by covering some of the "philosophy" of embolotherapy. Later chapters in this section will deal with specifics of embolic agents and imaging. The second section covers individual indications.

Underlying Principles

There is no "one size fits all" solution to embolization, and success is dependent on adapting the procedure to account for the unique problems presented by each patient. Embolization is often technically demanding and mistakes can have serious consequences. It is often impossible to recanalize a vessel or vascular bed accidentally occluded during treatment.

The aim of every embolization treatment is to deliver effective treatment while minimizing damage to adjacent structures. This will only occur with careful *planning* and *execution*. The remainder of this chapter will cover concepts which can be applied across the entire range of embolotherapy.

Knowledge: Before starting any embolization procedure, it is essential to have a thorough understanding of the following:

- The pathophysiology of the underlying condition
- The role of alternative therapies
- The likely therapeutic outcomes of the various therapies
- The vascular anatomy relevant to the clinical scenario
- The different types of embolic agents and how to use them
- The likelihood of success and recurrence

Transcatheter Embolization and Therapy,
Techniques in Interventional Radiology, DOI 10.1007/978-1-84800-897-7_1,
© Springer-Verlag London Limited 2010

- The potential to cause and manage adverse events
  - target organ dysfunction
  - collateral (non-target) embolization
  - post-embolization syndrome

Planning the Procedure

Planning, understanding, good technique, and a high level of vigilance can avoid many of the complications associated with embolization. Careful planning should start well in advance of the procedure and has been made easier by the advent of computed tomography (CT) and magnetic resonance (MR) angiography. The key elements in planning are as follows:

Understanding the Underlying Pathological Process

The conditions treated by embolization have very different pathophysiological driving processes and have different treatment objectives, and therefore require different treatment strategies. Broadly speaking

- If the pathology has an ongoing tissue-based process (e.g., inflammatory/neoplastic), then occlusion is required at small vessel/capillary level to achieve a durable result.
- When there is a single stimulus to vessel injury (e.g., post-renal biopsy), then occlusion at arterial level will be enough to produce a durable result, though reperfusion via collateral pathways needs to be considered.

Understanding the Role of Alternative Therapies

Embolotherapy may be the only one of several therapeutic options for a particular scenario. It is important to understand the pros and cons of all of the alternative therapies and for these to be discussed with the referring clinicians and the patient. As always, there are a range of possibilities as follows:

- Embolization may be complementary to other therapies.
- Embolization may be a vital prelude to other therapy (e.g., surgery).
- Embolization may be the only viable therapy.
- Embolization may not be the optimal therapy.

Which of these is true will depend on the circumstances of the case and the local expertise. Be flexible, honest, and pragmatic.

Identifying the Target

Clearly it is impossible to treat anything unless you know the location, the local blood supply, and any other tissues that may be affected by vascular occlusion.

- Often common sense will direct you to the appropriate vascular distribution. In the example above, bleeding following renal biopsy will originate from the corresponding renal arterial branches.
- When the situation is not so obvious (e.g., gastrointestinal hemorrhage), then cross-sectional imaging will commonly identify the site of bleeding. This will often direct angiographic interrogation.
- Most proximal arterial variations can be identified by careful interpretation of CT angiography.
- CT will not always identify the vessel of origin. For example, bleeding into the retroperitoneum can come from a large number of adjacent vessels—and some work will still be required at angiography!

Knowing the Arterial Anatomy and Collateral Pathways

Understanding the arterial and venous anatomy of the target lesion is essential to permit safe and effective embolization. Embolization requires both meticulous angiographic technique and patience to carefully unravel the pathway to the target lesion.

Normal Anatomy and Anatomic Variations

Arterial and venous variants are a common trap for the unwary, and knowledge of the common patterns can prevent an easy case going far astray.

- In general, even with the advent of CT and MR angiography, it is always better to start by establishing the arterial anatomy with overview (non-selective) angiography.
- In some vascular territories (e.g., the visceral circulation), variant anatomy will be present in over a quarter of cases. Subtle arterial variations are still best appreciated at selective angiography. Only after the anatomy has been established should the operator proceed to more selective catheterization of the target vessel.

Collateral Perfusion

- Collateral pathways are a mixed blessing for embolization therapy. While in some circumstances the existence of a collateral pathway can prevent tissue ischemia after embolization, the same network of pathways may continue to perfuse a target lesion beyond embolization coils.

Fig. 1.1 Gastroduodenal
artery pseudoeneurysm;
a lesion here can be supplied
by both celiac axis and
superior mesenteric artery

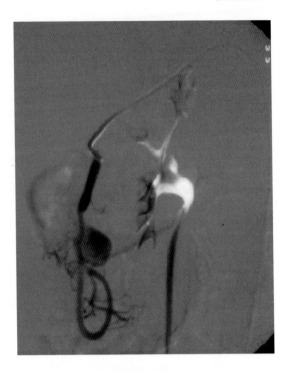

- The classic collateral pathway of the gastroduodenal artery (Fig. 1.1) is a perfect illustration. A lesion in the mid gastroduodenal artery cannot be successfully treated by proximal embolization of the common hepatic artery or even the gastroduodenal artery alone. The lesion will continue to be supplied via the superior mesenteric artery/inferior pancreaticoduodenal arcade.

This introduces the concept of closing both the "front and back doors." In other words, successful embolization of this lesion requires occlusion of both the inflow and outflow arteries. This is usually achieved by starting embolization distal to the lesion and working backward.

- It is important to remember that collateral pathways are not solely limited to major vessels and exist within the parenchyma of some solid organs (e.g., the liver).

End Arterial Supply

End arteries are vessels that provide the sole supply to an organ or vascular territory.

- Occlusion of an end artery will lead to ischemia throughout the territory it supplies. This can have vital implications for embolotherapy, as without care it is possible to cause more harm than good.

- Obvious examples are the coronary arteries, renal arteries, splenic artery, and the brachial artery. When dealing with an end artery, the embolization is normally performed as distally as possible to minimize the ischemic consequences. In some cases, however, even this might be unacceptable. For example, there would be no prizes for occluding a left main stem coronary artery to treat a false aneurysm.

Choosing the Correct Embolic Material

The choice of embolic material is dictated by two principal factors: is permanent or temporary occlusion required and what is the level of vascular occlusion necessary for effective treatment.

Temporary occlusion is useful when the aim is to stop bleeding which is from a lesion that will undergo spontaneous healing.

- A good clinical example is the trauma patient with bleeding from a pelvic fracture; temporary embolization of the entire internal iliac artery can be a rapid and life-saving maneuver.
- Recanalization of the temporary occlusion will not cause rebleeding, as healing and fracture immobilization will have occurred.
- The choice of temporary embolic agents is fairly limited. Gelfoam and now increasingly rarely autologous blood clot are the temporary agents in use.

Level of vascular occlusion. The effectiveness of an embolization treatment will depend on controlling the level of vascular occlusion appropriate for the underlying pathological processes.

- If there is an ongoing angiogenic stimulus, then proximal occlusion will simply result in the lesion rapidly re-establishing collateral circulation which will be much more difficult if not impossible to treat.
- In the treatment of chronic inflammatory and most neoplastic processes, more distal occlusion with particulate, or less often liquid embolic agents, is required to obtain a more durable result.
- Particulate agents come in a range of sizes; the smaller the particles, the more distal the level of embolization down to capillary level. The more distal the embolization, the greater the risk of tissue necrosis.

The over-riding principle is always to use the safest, most readily controlled, effective agent.

Understanding the Likely Outcomes/Consequences of Embolization

There is no single answer to this, as it depends on the territory, nature of the pathology, and extent of embolization. The following questions should be considered:

- How much non-target tissue is likely to be affected and what will be the consequence of this?
- Can supply be preserved to vital structures? It might, for example, be possible to occlude a carotid artery, if there was good collateral supply to the brain around the Circle of Willis.
- Whether arteries are end arteries which if occluded will lead to important distal ischemia.
- If tumor embolization is being performed, then think how much target tissue will need to be infarcted. Sometimes it is better to stage the procedure than to have the patient sustain a massive physiological assault from post-embolization syndrome.
- Remember that all these issues are relative in the context of a life-threatening situation.

Performing the Procedure

Following planning comes the technical part of the procedure; much of this should be thought out in advance. Before starting ask yourself the following questions:

- Do I understand the procedure to be performed?
- Do I have the technical ability to perform the procedure?

If the answer to either of these is no, then seek assistance if there is time. In an emergency ask yourself for instance, if a temporizing measure such as balloon occlusion might act as a bridge to more definitive therapy. If this is not possible, then there may have to be a decision about "the lesser evil" as long as the patient's interests are put first, e.g., it is better to have a less selective embolization than to bleed to death.

Informing Others: The Patient and Clinicians

The scope for discussion will obviously relate to the urgency of the clinical scenario. Elective embolization procedures should always be discussed in advance with the patient and clinician. In a life-threatening emergency, there is no time for this and the patient's survival comes first.

- Consent should reflect the likely outcomes and risks of this treatment and this should be clearly recorded in the patient's records.
- At a practical level, always give the patient a clear idea about the likely duration of the treatment.
- The patient will want to know if the procedure is palliative or curative, especially in the context of cancer therapy.
- Most embolization procedures are performed under conscious sedation and the patient must be co-operative during the procedure.

- Whether it will be painful? For long or particularly painful procedures, it may be best to consider general anesthesia. The same applies in children. This should remind you to ensure that you prescribe appropriate analgesia for the peri- and post-procedural period.
- Finally, make sure that senior referring clinicians have a very clear picture of the risks, success rate for the procedure and that a collaborative management plan has been discussed.

Planning Vascular Access

The shortest straightest route is usually best and is considered on the basis of the likely target and associated anatomy. Most cases will be approached from the femoral artery.

- If imaging is available, review the whole access route on the CTA or MRA.
- Elderly patients frequently have diseased iliac vessels that can require treatment to achieve access.
- Very tortuous iliac vessels can make alternative access sites such as the brachial arteries more appropriate.

Selective Catheterization

Embolization often requires selective catheterization of a small branch vessel to deliver effective treatment and to minimize damage to non-target tissue. A high level of technical catheter and wire skill is essential and is only acquired with practice. The following outlines some key concepts which will help.

Achieving a stable catheter position. This is a vital component to successful embolization and is analogous to ensuring a firm footing when working up a high ladder!

- A stable position will permit the deployment of coils or injection of liquid embolic materials.
- In general, the deeper the catheter is within the target arterial circulation, the more stable the catheter position.
- A more difficult position occurs when the target vessel or lesion lies close to the origin of a major vessel. In this position, it is all too easy for the delivery catheter to "back off" during delivery of the embolic agent with loss of embolic material into a major non-target vessel.
- After selective catheterization has been achieved, it is essential to test if the position of the tip of the catheter will remain in position. For "solid materials" like embolization coils, this is usually done by advancing the guidewire that will be used for coil deployment to the tip of the catheter.
- Liquid materials, e.g., PVA are assessed by initially using a test injection of contrast of a similar volume and rate to that anticipated for the embolic material.

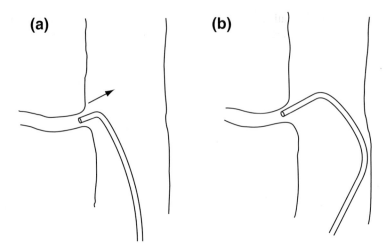

Fig. 1.2 (**a**) Vertebral catheter at vessel origin; the catheter is easily backed out as it does not reach the contralateral aortic wall. (**b**) Cobra catheter at the same site; the catheter curve is supported by the contralateral aortic wall and achieves a more stable position

- If the catheter backs out during the test, then more stable positions can be achieved by modifying the shape of the delivery catheter, e.g., exchanging a vertebral catheter for a cobra catheter as the wider cobra shape is better supported by the aortic wall (Fig. 1.2); when this is not possible consider using a co-axial system either guidecatheter/sheath around a standard catheter or a microcatheter through a standard catheter. Sometimes it is necessary to use a tri-axial system comprising guide catheter, standard catheter, and microcatheter.

Single End Hole Catheters

Regardless of the shape of catheter used, it is essential to use an end hole-only catheter during embolization procedures.

- Catheters with side holes can result in non-target embolization via the side holes if used with particulate or liquid materials.
- Side hole catheters are equally hazardous with coil embolization as the end of the coil may get caught in the side hole trapping the coil within the catheter either before extrusion or as the coil tail exits the catheter lumen.
- Either way it is a sure fire way to make a controlled procedure more difficult, time consuming, and hazardous.

Avoiding Wedged Catheter Positions

Finally, in the search to achieve the perfect catheter position, it is possible to impact or wedge the catheter into the vessel.

- In this position, the catheter occupies the entire lumen and no blood can get past.
- Flow-directed embolization is then very hazardous, as pressure can build up in the distal vascular bed leading to the following:
  - rupture the target vessel
  - non-target embolization by back-pressure reflux of embolic agent when the catheter is removed or by opening collateral channels
- If the target vessel is so small that a conventional catheter is wedging, then the simplest solution is to use a microcatheter.

Microcatheters

Microcatheters have extended the range of embolization into small and tortuous vascular beds and permit targeted embolization in even the most challenging circulations.

- In general, it is far better to accept using a microcatheter early than provoke vasospasm or catheter wedging by persisting with a conventional catheter in a difficult circulation.
- A large range of microcatheter designs are available; generic microcatheters are small caliber, usually less then 3F, unshaped catheters.
- Microcatheters are generally straight and therefore not steerable. They are usually used in conjunction with steerable 0.014–0.018 wires to allow selective catheterization of the distal circulation.
- Microcatheters have to be delivered within a conventional catheter to a branch in the proximal circulation. It is best to use a Tuohy Borst adapter to allow circulation of saline between the conventional "guiding catheter" and the microcatheter, as this both helps prevent thrombus formation and provides lubrication to allow the microcatheter to slide easily within the conventional catheter lumen.

Delivery of Embolic Materials

Embolization requires careful control of the materials used and this is usually achieved by direct visualization of the delivery under continuous fluoroscopy. Some embolic agents are already opaque, e.g., coils, but most other materials are not opaque in themselves. Particulate embolic materials such as gelfoam, PVA, and microspheres are all suspended in contrast to allow controlled delivery.

Sclerosant agents pose a different problem; dilution with contrast will reduce their effectiveness and there are several approaches to permit safe embolization.

- *Mixing with a contrast agent.* Opacification with tantalum powder, which is very radioopaque, is sometimes used.
- *Performing test injections with contrast.* Test injections can be used to see the distribution of a known volume and rate of injection. The same volume of

unopacified sclerosant is then injected at the same rate. Remember that the injection rate and volume may change during the procedure due to vasospasm and occlusion. Repeat test injections should be performed frequently.

- *Reducing the flow*. Venous outflow can be occluded with a simple tourniquet in the periphery. Occlusion balloons can be used in less accessible sites. This combination can permit safe delivery of sclerosant without diluting effectiveness.

Preserving Vessels

If there is a macroscopic vessel lesion such as a pseudoaneursym in a vital vessel, then preservation of the vessel may be possible. The technique used will depend on the size of the vessel and the tortuousity of the access vessel.

- A stent graft offers the simplest solution to exclude the lesion from the circulation and preserve flow. Currently stent grafts are limited to fairly large vessels, certainly greater than 4 mm, and struggle to get round more than one or two gentle curves.
- The alternative approach is to very gently fill up the space of the psuedoaneurym with either coils or specialized liquid embolic agents such as Onyx. The vessel lumen can be preserved by either balloon modeling during coil placement or initially placing a stent across the neck of the pseudoaneurysm which helps constrain the coils. This is certainly a far more complex technique; however, this technique is being used very successfully for intra-cerebral aneurysms, and undoubtedly the interventional neuroradiologists have the greatest experience and the best equipment for this type of situation.

Non-target Embolization

- Non-target embolization may be unavoidable, but should be minimized by careful planning and execution.
- Occasionally it is not possible to limit non-target embolization simply by using selective catheterization. This typically occurs when there are multiple small vessels arising proximally that are too small and often too many to individually catheterize (Fig. 1.3).
- It is very rarely possible to exclude these vessels with a stent graft.
- It can still be possible to achieve target-only delivery of embolic material by intentionally occluding the circulation distal to the lesion, which will direct blood flow and the embolic agent into the target circulation.
- Depending on vessel size and collateral circulation, this occlusion can either be temporary via balloon occlusion, which is often more difficult and requires further vascular access, or by using gelfoam plug occlusion which will recanalize in time.

Fig. 1.3 The small vessels at the vessel origin cannot be individually catheterized; temporary occlusion at *point A* will permit delivery into the tumor circulation while minimizing collateral damage

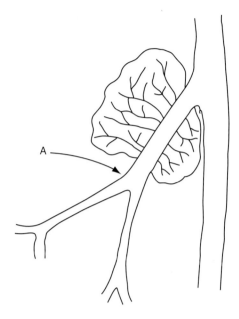

A

The chapters which follow will expand on these principles; they are not complicated and if kept in mind will keep you and your patient safe.

Keypoints

Embolization creates some of the greatest technical and intellectual challenges for the angiographer.

Careful adherence to the core principles will ensure simpler, safer, and effective treatments.

Planning is the key to success and requires a thorough knowledge of the condition and the treatment options. Use all the available information from clinicians, diagnostic tests, imaging, and operative notes.

Use high-quality imaging at key points in the procedure, e.g., injecting particles.

Preserve as much tissue and many collaterals as possible by taking care and paying attention to scrupulous technique.

Chapter 2
Coils, Occluders, and Plugs

David Tuite and Kevin O'Regan

Introduction

Coils, plugs, and vascular occluders are permanent mechanical embolic agents. This chapter considers the following:

- Mechanism of action
- Physical properties
- Deployment
- Associated complications and strategies for minimizing these

The ideal vascular occlusion device should have the following attributes:

- Simple deployment mechanisms
- Require a low profile delivery system
- Allow precise placement before final deployment
- Resist migration after deployment
- Have a low rate of recanalization
- Should not cause significant vessel damage or inflammatory response
- Have sufficient expansile force to securely attach to the vessel wall in high pressure and high volume flow studies
- Cost competitive

The choice of embolic material depends on the clinical scenario and the desired end-point of the procedure.

Mechanism of Action

There are three mechanisms by which these devices occlude vessels:

- Intimal injury
- Promotion of thrombus formation
- Mechanical occlusion

Transcatheter Embolization and Therapy,
Techniques in Interventional Radiology, DOI 10.1007/978-1-84800-897-7_2,
© Springer-Verlag London Limited 2010

The first two of these are the most important and are closely interrelated. Although it is important to create a tightly packed nest of coils, physical occlusion of the vessel by the coils themselves will not occur without thrombosis occurring. *Hence coils may be ineffective if clotting is deranged.* Embolization coils can be utilized outside of the vascular system in certain circumstances; however, in these circumstances they work by a different mechanism (Fig. 2.1).

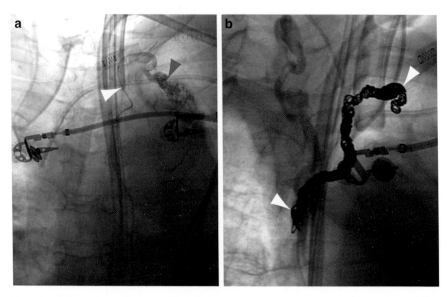

Fig. 2.1 (**a**) Microcatheter access into the thoracic duct demonstrates source of chyle leak post-thoracic surgery. (**b**) Coil embolization was successful in treating this. Two points are noteworthy. First embolization in this setting takes approximately 1 week to work as no thrombus can form. The coils cause an inflammatory reaction in the thoracic duct which leads to fibrosis of the duct. Second, coils can be used outside of the vascular system

Intimal Injury and Thrombus Formation Are Interrelated

A properly deployed device damages the endothelial surface causing

- Platelet adhesion (platelet glycoprotein 1b binding with von Willebrand factor in the subendothelial matrix) and activation (PDGF, TGF-β, and thromboxane-A_2).
- Exposure of tissue factor to the blood stream and the initiation of the coagulation cascade resulting in the formation of a fibrin-rich thrombus.
- Thrombin is generated in large amounts at the site of injury. Arterial wall-associated thrombin activity remains elevated for at least 48 h and returns to baseline after 1 week.

A tightly packed nest of coils

- Has a large thrombogenic surface area.
- This surface area is further increased by the addition of fibers.

Physical Properties of Embolization Coils and Plugs

Materials

- Manufactured from metals; platinum, tungsten, gold, tantalum, and stainless steel.
- They are all radiopaque (platinum coils are more opaque than stainless steel coils).
- Coil conspicuity can be further increased by the use of various radiopaque fillers such as tantalum, tungsten, barium sulfate, bismuth oxide, or bismuth carbonate.
- Nitinol (nickel/titanium alloy) is used in some of the newer plug devices.
- Stainless steel coils maintain greater radial force than platinum coils.
- Some coils have very little radial force These coils come in long lengths and can be packed very tightly, e.g., liquid–metal coils (Berenstein Liquid Coil, Target Therapeutics, Fremont, CA, USA), Nestor coils (Cook UK Ltd, Letchworth, UK). The diameter of these coils is nominal, since the coil will instead simply fill any space into which it is injected.
- Nestor coils will extrude from the catheter as a straight wire; they must engage something within the lumen of the vessels to start forming curves and causing occlusion of the vessel. For this reason, it is often advantageous to place a standard coil as a "backstop" against which the Nestor can start to reform its shape and cause occlusion.

Novel Materials

Examples of these include the following:

- Bioabsorbable polymeric GDC coils (Boston Scientific, MA, USA) which aim to obtain a more rapid and controlled wound healing at the site of aneurysmal repair.
- Hydrophilic hydrogel-coated platinum coils (Microvention, CA, USA) in which a hydrogel polymer expands from 0.014 to 0.027 inch in the presence of blood.
- Silk suture has been used as an embolic material, typically for intracranial aneurysms or high-flow AVMs. Silk suture is highly thrombogenic but has the disadvantage of being radiolucent. Up to 24% of patients have a transient fever after the intravascular administration of silk. This is usually maximal at days 5–8 post-embolization and is not associated with infection.

Material Issues

Nickel allergy. Nickel allergy has been documented as a complication of nitinol device placement. This device syndrome results in local irritation and mild leukocytosis which is maximal 2–3 days post-procedure. It is rare and can be treated with systemic prednisolone. In the setting of embolization, these symptoms are obscured.

MRI compatibility. Modern stainless steel coils are MRI safe but may generate artifact.

Thrombogenicity

- Coils vary in their thrombogenicity. Untreated tungsten microcoils have superior clot-promoting activity compared to untreated stainless steel or platinum microcoils.
- Various strategies have been employed to further improve thrombogenicity:
  - *Coatings:* thrombin, gelatine, and polyurethane.
  - *Fibers* (Fig. 2.2): typically individual fibers or bundles of 5–100 fibers are used. Suitable fibers include synthetic materials Dacron, polyesters, polyamides, and natural fibers such as silk and cotton.

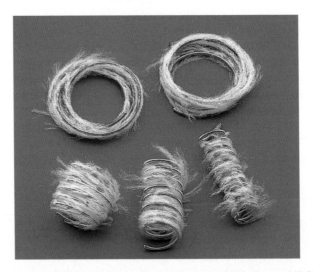

Fig. 2.2 An array of Nestor coils (Cook Medical Incorporated, Bloomington, NJ, USA) showing the typical helical design with fibers (Image courtesy of Cook Medical Inc.)

  - The fibers are looped in a generally serpentine manner along the coil. The fibrous loops are affixed to (or looped through) the coil at spaced intervals along the coil.

   o Adding filaments to the exterior of the coil also increases the friction of the
     fibrous coil against the catheter lumen. The ideal balance of these two
     factors is difficult to achieve.
 • Use non-heparinized saline while performing coil embolization or you will
   inhibit thrombus formation.

Coils Shapes and Sizes

Coils have a predetermined shape that they adopt after release from the deployment
device. This predetermined shape can be achieved by either crimping the coil at
various intervals or heat-treating the coil on a mandril during the manufacturing
process. For this reason, an alloy of platinum with a small amount of tungsten is
often used as tungsten reduces the ductility of the resultant coil.

   Coils come in a variety of shapes which are intended for slightly different
indications.

   Helical coils: these are the most commonly used and designed for deployment
within non-aneurysmal long vessels (Fig. 2.2).

   Spiral coils: such as the tornado coil (Cook). The spiral design maximizes coil
exposure to cross-section of the lumen for greater disruption of blood flow. In
addition they are more suited for embolization of tapered vessels.

   More complex shapes are used for more complex aneurysmal vessels (Fig. 2.3).
The most complex shapes are typically used in intracranial berry aneurysms.

   Straight coils are also available for the embolization of small vessels such as
those in the colonic mesentery. These are often injected out the end of a catheter
rather than pushed out with a wire or coil-pusher.

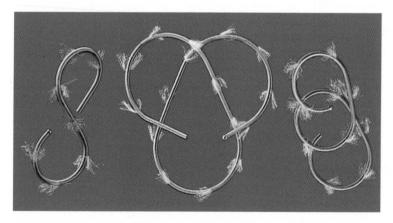

Fig. 2.3 More complex-shaped microcoils for use in the embolization of aneurysms. The cor-
rugated surface of the coil is designed to injure the endothelium (Image courtesy of Cook
Medical Inc.)

Coil Size

Sizes are described by three parameters:

Coil diameter. This is the diameter of the outstretched coil (equivalent to the guidewire size) that you are using, e.g., 0.014–0.038-inch diameter. This will determine with which catheters and pushers the coil can be used. The coil diameter

- Must match delivery system. An oversized coil will not fit in the catheter. An undersized coil will try to reform in your catheter and may block it.
- Must match the coil pusher size to the coil and both must be compatible with the delivery system. An undersized coil pusher will jam alongside the coil in the catheter.

Terminology

- o Coils for use in a 0.035- or 0.038-inch delivery system are referred to as standard coils.
- o Coils used in a 0.014- or 0.018-inch delivery system are referred to as microcoils.

Unconstrained coil length. This is the length of the individual coil when held out straight. Length varies considerably depending on the type of coil being used, but in general it increases with increasing coil diameter.

Reformed coil diameter. This is the diameter of the coil when it reforms to its predetermined shape.

- This must be larger than the target vessel.
- The coil should not adopt its predetermined shape. If it does, then it is undersized.
- Undersized coils
  - o Are at risk of migration and non-target embolization
  - o Fail to injure the vessel wall and thus not induce thrombosis
- Oversized coils will act like a guidewire and pass further distally into the vessel.

Coil size is typically given as a series of those three numbers. A 35-4-8 coil will pass through a 0.035-inch inner lumen catheter, will measure 4 cm in length, and have an 8-mm coil diameter.

Coil Deployment

Five steps are taken to ensure appropriate embolization with coils:

1. *Establishing Stable Catheter Position*

   - The target vessel is catheterized in the conventional manner.

- Once the intended deployment position is reached, catheter stability is checked by passing the coil pusher through to the end of the catheter. If the catheter position moves, then it is too unstable to deploy a coil.
- Additional stability can be obtained by using
  - Co-axial catheter systems
  - A more stable catheter shape, e.g., reverse curve catheter
- When the coil pusher is approximately 15 cm from the catheter tip, the position of the back end of the pusher should be marked on the table. During coil deployment, it is not necessary to use fluoroscopy until this point is reached. This significantly reduces radiation dose.

2. *Introducing the coil*

- The coil comes preloaded in a cartridge when opened from the packaging.
- The cartridge is firmly engaged in the deployment catheter hub and held in position.
- Some microcoil cartridges are screwed onto the delivery catheter hub and come with a small stiff wire to push the coil from the cartridge.
- The back (stiff) end of the coil pusher is used to push the coil out of the cartridge and into the catheter for a distance of approximately 30 cm.
- At this point, the coil pusher is turned around and inserted front end first.
- The cartridge is snapped or kinked prior to being discarded so that there is no confusion as to which cartridges have been used and which still contain coils.

Coil pushers

- For standard catheters, a straight guidewire can be used as a coil pusher. A wire with a long taper may decrease the risk of catheter dislodgement.
- For microcatheters, a special coil pusher is needed as microcatheter guidewires will not work.
- Microcoil pushers have a soft flexible tip with a stiff shaft.
- Remember to use the pusher to establish catheter stability before deploying a coil

3. *Extruding the Coil*

- Good fluoroscopy is essential at this point.
- The coil is extruded by advancing the pusher, as the coil deploys the catheter will tend to migrate backward.

- It is essential to have control of any guide catheter, delivery catheter, and also the coil pusher at this stage. Gentle forward pressure on the delivery catheter is helpful to stabilize the delivery system.
- If the coil is correctly sized, then it will begin to form loops. The number of loops is approximately the coil length divided by the coil diameter multiplied by π (length/[diameter × π]).
- A correctly sized coil will form an irregular shape as it is constrained by the vessel wall.
- Once the first coil is deployed further coils can be placed to build up a tightly packed nest of coils.
- As the nest becomes bigger it may be necessary to allow the catheter to migrate backward to allow coils to be extruded.
- Variant techniques

  ○ If the catheter system is in a strong stable position, then some coils may be hydrostatically injected into position. Once the coil is loaded into the catheter, a 1-ml Luer-lock syringe filled with saline is forcefully injected pushing the coil into position.
  ○ Other methods include introducing multiple coils into the catheter before pushing them into position with the coil pusher. This method is used when it is obvious that multiple coils will be needed for a large target vessel.
  ○ Liquid–metal coils (Berenstein Liquid Coil, Target Therapeutics, Fremont, CA, USA) are long, soft coils which are delivered by a slow saline infusion. This slow stream is sufficient to drive the coil to the catheter tip with minimal friction between coil and catheter. This makes it particularly useful for long tortuous vessels. They come in sizes up to 30 cm and this long length makes embolization of large vessel quicker and more efficient.
  ○ Interlocking detachable coils greater than 10 cm are available, but friction between coil and microcatheter may limit their use. These coils come in two sizes and can be used in both conventional microcatheters and flow-directed microcatheters. They allow a very dense coil pack to be created. The main benefit of detachable coils is that they can be placed into the vessel to be embolized, and detached only if the operator deems placement to be appropriate.

4. *Anchoring Techniques*

- *Coaxial technique.* This is the standard technique used for the placement of embolization coils and is detailed above.
- *Scaffold technique.* This is the use of a large coil initially to create a scaffold into which smaller coils can be placed to build up the coil nest. The initial coil should ideally have a high radial force so as to secure the scaffold position. As such a stainless steel coil is a good choice. The subsequent coils such as soft, fibered platinum coils are a suitable choice here.
- *Anchor technique.* The initial coil is initially deployed in a small side branch of the target vessel. As the coil is deployed, the catheter is withdrawn into the larger

target vessel. This helps to secure the first coil in position in the target vessel. The subsequent coils are deployed as normal (Fig. 2.4).

- *Stent-supported embolization technique.* This technique is best used for wide-necked aneurysms, fusiform aneurysms and pseudoaneurysms, where unsupported coil deployment is not possible. In this technique, a stent is placed across the aneurysm. A microcatheter is then passed through the interstices of the stent and embolization can now proceed without fear of coil migration or malposition (Fig. 2.5).

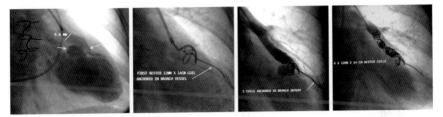

Fig. 2.4 Anchor technique. A large left pulmonary arteriovenous malformation (both arterial and venous components *arrowed*) is shown in the first panel. A Nestor coil is initially anchored in a side branch and then fully deployed in the arterial limb of the malformation. A second coil is placed in a similar position to stabilize the coil nest before a further six coils are added to achieve embolization

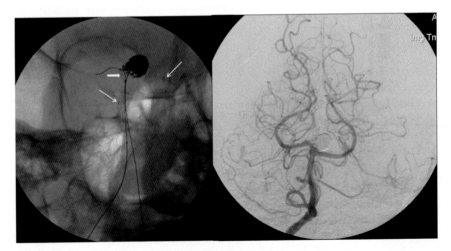

Fig. 2.5 Stent-supported embolization technique in the treatment of basilar tip aneurysm. The posterior cerebral circulation has been accessed via each of the vertebral arteries. A stent has been placed extending from the basilar artery into the left posterior cerebral artery (*small arrows* denote the stent ends). A balloon has been inflated at the origin of the right posterior cerebral artery (*large arrow*). A microcatheter has been passed through the stent into the basilar tip aneurysm and coils have been used to embolize the aneurysm. Completion angiography shows successful exclusion of the aneurysm

- Why not use a covered stent? Covered stents are much stiffer than uncovered stents and it may not be possible to position the stent graft. Also stent grafts will cover small perforators, which in intracranial intervention may prove catastrophic.

5. *Endpoint Of Deployment*

- Coils are added until the nest looks sufficient to occlude the vessel or the coils reach a vessel intended to be spared.
- Post-embolization angiography is performed. The catheter should be withdrawn slightly to avoid dislodging newly formed thrombus so that the real flow dynamics are observed.
- Brisk flow through the coils indicates the need for further embolization.
- If slow flow is noted, wait a few minutes to allow thrombus to form and check again.
- If necessary, continue adding to the nest until occlusion is obtained. If there is not much room for additional coils, or if the patient is coagulopathic, consider using some gelfoam.

Additional Techniques

Most coils are deployed as described above. In certain circumstances additional control is desirable, for which several devices and techniques exist including the following.

Detachable Coils

- These come in all shapes, sizes, and materials.
- The coil is attached to the delivery wire allowing it to be positioned and withdrawn if necessary prior to deployment.
- There are several systems for detaching the coil
  - Mechanical: via a microscrew or via the core mandril (Fig. 2.6).
  - Electrolytic and heat mechanisms: Guglielmi detachable coils are platinum coils soldered to a stainless steel delivery wire. Once the coil has been placed into the target vessel and the position confirmed, a 1-mA current is applied to the delivery wire. The coil then detaches by electrolysis and the wire can be removed. Heat mechanisms work by burning a filament that attaches the coil to the delivery wire.

Amplatzer vascular plug (AVP) (AGA Medical)

- The AVP is a self-expanding nitinol wire mesh (Fig. 2.7). The second-generation AVP has two waists within it making it a tri-lobed structure.

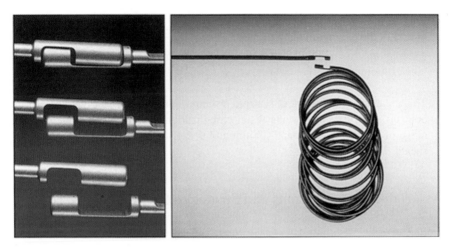

Fig. 2.6 Simple mechanical detachable coil system. This is the Interlock system from Boston Scientific Corporation. More complex systems are available where detachment of the delivery wire from the coil is achieved by either heat or electrolysis (Image courtesy of Boston Scientific Corporation)

- The AVP plug comes in sizes ranging from 4 to 16 mm in 2-mm increments (AVP II ranges from 4 to 22 mm). Plugs should be oversized by 30–50% (e.g., an 8-mm vessel should be embolized with a 10- or 12-mm AVP).
- A 5Fr guide catheter is needed for 4–8 mm devices, 6Fr for 10–12 mm devices, and 8Fr for 14–16 mm plugs.
- The AVP is deployed through a guide catheter attached to the end of a 135-cm long nitinol wire by a microscrew.

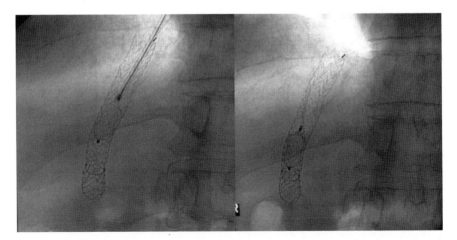

Fig. 2.7 Amplatzer vascular plug (AVP). A single AVP is used to occlude a TIPS in a patient with intractable encephalopathy post TIPS creation. In the first panel, the plug has been uncovered from the delivery sheath; however, it remains attached to the delivery wire. It is repositioned prior to complete deployment

- The AVP is released by anticlockwise rotation of the delivery wire, which unscrews the plug from the wire.

    Amplatz vascular obstruction device (Amplatz spider) (Cook Medical Inc., Bloomington, IN, USA)

- This creates a stainless steel scaffold system onto which a nest of coils can be built up. The device prevents distal embolization of coils. It is available in a range of sizes between 9 and 20 mm and is delivered through a 5Fr introducer sheath.

Associated Complications and Strategies for Minimizing These

Unable to obtain selective catheter position: The use of guide catheters, hydrophilic wires, and microcatheters can all be employed at this stage. Guide catheters provide support; hydrophilic wires and microcatheters improve the chances of accessing a difficult vessel. Often the use of different microwires can prove helpful. If optimal position cannot be obtained, then consideration can be given to more proximal embolization; however, this will increase the potential for collateral tissue damage.

Unable to obtain stable catheter position: Initially a guiding catheter should be used. Ensure that the shape of the catheter and guide catheter is optimized. If this does not work, then an approach from a different access point should be considered, i.e., brachial approach vs femoral approach.

Misplaced coil: Misplaced coils occur as a result of oversized coils, undersized coils, or unstable catheter position. They can be removed using a snare but this can cause additional problems and may even dislodge the coil nest! If the coil is not likely to cause a problem, then leave it alone.

Catheter is pushed back during deployment: Gentle forward pressure is necessary as is the support from your base catheter. It may be necessary to enlist assistance from a second operator to stabilize the catheter system during coil deployment.

Coil occludes the catheter: This is a result of coil–catheter mismatch, when there is a kink or tight bend in the catheter or when the inner lumen of the catheter has been damaged by particulate matter or coils.

- First determine the site of obstruction with fluoroscopy.
- Attempt disimpacting the coil using a saline flush.
- If there is a kink in the delivery catheter, provide gentle forward pressure on the pusher wire while the deployment catheter is withdrawn slightly. The back (stiff) end of the pusher wire can also be tried.
- If the coil is impacted in the catheter outside of the patient, then the catheter can be cut distal to the coil, a wire passed, and the catheter replaced.
- If the coil is impacted in the catheter within the patient, then the catheter must be removed and position re-established with a new catheter.

Other Problems

Coagulopathic patients. Thrombus formation is essential for coil embolization to be successful. In the coagulopathic patient this will not occur.

- One strategy for dealing with this is to deploy a nest of coils, then gelfoam pledgets, and then pack with coils again, thus creating a gelfoam sandwich. The coils prevent the gelfoam from embolizing distally and the gelfoam provides mechanical occlusion of the vessel.
- Remember to use non-heparinized saline for flushing.

Keypoints

- Plan, plan, and plan again.
- Obtain good angiographic images that detail the anatomy and pathology.
- Choose site of embolization.
- Ensure stable catheter position.
- Select appropriate coils and appropriate deployment method.
- Check completion angiogram.

Suggested Further Reading

Kessel D, Robertson I. Interventional Radiology: A survival Guide. 2nd edition, Elsevier, Amsterdam 2005 ISBN 0-4431-0044-6.

Berenstein A, Lasjaunias P, Ter Brugge KG. Surgical Neuroangiography: Clinical and Endovascular Treatment Aspects in Adults vol. 2, Springer-Verlag Berlin and Heidelberg GmbH & Co. K; 2Rev Ed. 2004 ISBN-10: 3540416684.

Schmutz F, McAuliffe W, Anderson DM, Elliott JP, Eskridge JM, Winn HR. Embolization of cerebral arteriovenous malformations with silk: histopathologic changes and hemorrhagic complications. AJNR Am J Neuroradiol. 1997 Aug;18(7):1233–7.

Osuga K, Mikami K, Higashihara H, Maeda N, Tsuboyama T, Kuwabara M, Onishi H, Hori M, Kim T, Tomoda K, Murakami T, Nakamura H. Principles and techniques of transcatheter embolotherapy for peripheral vascular lesions. Radiat Med. 2006 May;24(4):309–14. Review.

Chapter 3
Permanent Particulate Agents

Audrey Fohlen and Jean-Pierre Pelage

Introduction

Embolization materials can be classified according to their physical and biological characteristics. They are chosen according to the following:

- Characteristics of the target vessels: size, flow, and type of vessel (artery or vein).
- Permanent particulate agents are not resorbed and are intended to provide durable occlusion (Fig. 3.1).
- The level of arterial occlusion obtained with particulate agents varies from proximal to distal according to the chosen agent.
- Recanalization can occur due to expulsion, distal migration, fragmentation of the embolization material, and formation of a new vessel lumen.
- Occlusion can be purely mechanical or may be a conjunction of different mechanisms with vessel wall destruction by inflammation or sclerosis.

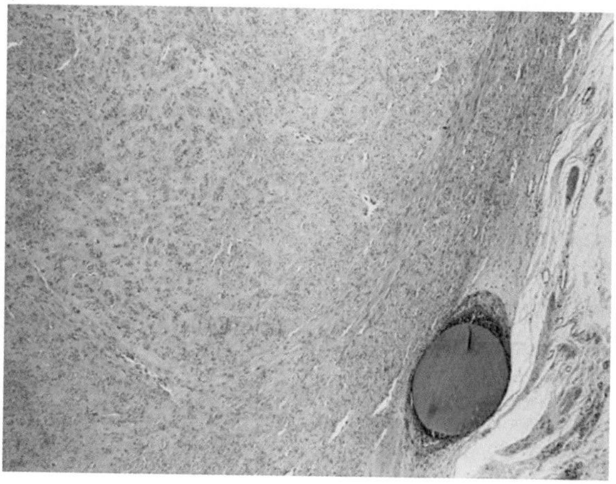

Fig. 3.1 500–700 μm Tris-acryl microspheres Embosphere (Biosphere Medical, Louvres, France) located in the perifibroid arterial plexus in a patient treated with pre-myomectomy embolization

Transcatheter Embolization and Therapy,
Techniques in Interventional Radiology, DOI 10.1007/978-1-84800-897-7_3,
© Springer-Verlag London Limited 2010

This chapter outlines the different permanent particulate embolization agents available, their characteristics, and how to choose and use them.

Not all particles are equal; they differ in physical and biological properties.

Particle Physical Properties

- *Size*: all particles come in a range of sizes. The diameter of vessel that will be occluded depends on this and other properties (including compressibility and elastic recovery).
- *Uniformity*: some particles are very uniform in size (calibrated). Others are variable and described according to mean particle size (Fig. 3.2).
- *Compressibility*: some particles (mainly microspheres) compress during deployment which makes delivery of large sizes through microcatheters easy but may block vessels smaller than the nominal particle diameter if the elastic recovery is slow.
- *Aggregation*: some particles tend to clump which will affect the level of embolization (Fig. 3.3).
- *Visibility*:
  - Most particles are suspended in 50% contrast to allow visualization during injection (Fig. 3.2).
  - Some particles are intended to be visible on computed tomography (CT) or magnetic resonance (MR) follow-up.

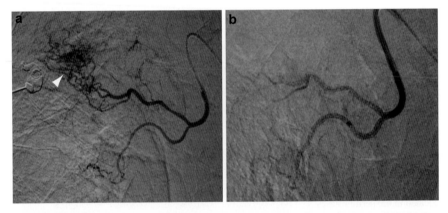

Fig. 3.2 Bronchial artery embolization for hemoptysis. (**a**) Superselective catheterization of the bronchial artery shows abnormal lung vascularity. (**b**) Targeted devascularization is obtained using 700–900 μm tris-acryl microspheres seen as uniform filling defects in the arterial lumen

Fig. 3.3 Conventional
polyvinyl alcohol particles
are of irregular shape

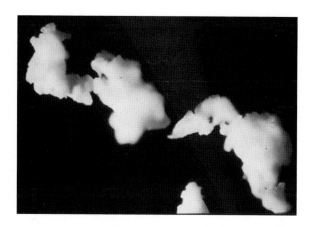

Mechanism of Action

- Simple mechanical occlusion
- Active agents: drug eluting, radioactive

Commonly Used Agents

Polyvinyl Alcohol Particles (PVA)

PVA is an inert plastic which has been used as an embolic agent for 20 years and has a long-track record of safety and efficacy in embolization procedures.

Non-spherical Polyvinyl Alcohol Particles

- Non-spherical PVA particles do not completely occlude the lumen of the occluded arteries. Occlusion is completed by thrombus formation within the interstices of the particles.
- Non-spherical PVA particles cause moderate perivascular inflammatory change.
- Recanalization can occur after several months or years due to the following:
  - Distal migration, fragmentation or extravascular migration of PVA particles
  - Resorption of thrombus
  - Calcification of PVA particles has been reported but is of uncertain significance
- The irregular shape of the material is associated with a larger granulometric range of the particles than advertised (Fig. 3.3). Some of the particles are smaller than the advertised size. Small fragments of PVA may cause non-target embolization of normal tissue (e.g., the ovaries during uterine artery embolization).
- Aggregation of PVA particles can lead to obstruction of the delivery catheter and potentially to uncontrolled level of arterial occlusion. With non-spherical particles, clumping of the embolic material may result in a false angiographic end-point at the conclusion of the embolization.

PVA Microspheres

- PVA spheres have been recently introduced (Contour SE, Boston Scientific, Nattick, MA, USA and Bead Block, Biocompatibles, Farnham, UK).
- PVA microspheres are easily visible because of their white (Contour SE) or blue (Bead Block) coloration (Figs. 3.4 and 3.5).

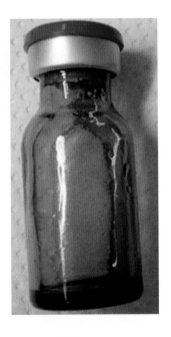

Fig. 3.4 Polyvinyl alcohol microspheres Contour SE (Boston Scientific, Nattick, MA, USA)

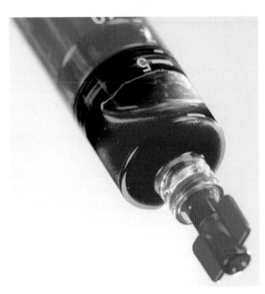

Fig. 3.5 Acrylamido polyvinyl alcohol microspheres Bead Block (Biocompatibles, Farnham, UK)

- The following size ranges are currently available: 100–300, 500–700, 700–900, and 900–1200 μm.
- Even large PVA microspheres are easy to inject through microcatheters and tend to travel more distally than the irregular PVA particles or tris-acryl microspheres of theoretical same diameter.

Tris-Acryl Microspheres

- Tris-acryl microspheres are made from precisely calibrated microporous cross-linked acrylic beads embedded with gelatin (Embosphere, Biosphere Medical, Roissy, France).
- The following size ranges are currently available: 40–120, 100–300, 500–700, 700–900, and 900–1200 μm. The diameter of occluded arteries correlates well with the microsphere size.
- The spheres are compressible, which allow easy passage through a microcatheter with a luminal diameter smaller than that of the microspheres.
- Angiographically, apparent clumping may occur with microspheres. The embolic material redistributes depending on the infusion rate and the concentration.
- In the long-term, there is no chronic inflammatory reaction and no degradation of the polymer (Fig. 3.1).

Hydrogel–Polyzene F Microspheres

- Calibrated microspheres consisting of a hydrogel core of polymethylmethacrylate with a thin coating that may reduce inflammation for better biocompatibility (Embozene, Celonova, Newnan, GA, USA).
- The following sizes are currently available: 40, 100, 250, 400, 500, 700, 900, and 1100 μm.
- As opposed to the other types of microspheres, a tight size distribution exists; this means that each vial or syringe contains microspheres that are consistently the same size.
- Particles are color-coded by particle size (Fig. 3.6). This is useful to avoid inappropriate mixing, contamination of saline and contrast syringes, and confirmation that optimal suspension is reached before embolization.

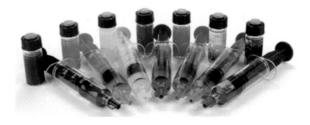

Fig. 3.6 Hydrogel–polyzene F microspheres Embozene (Celonova, Newnan, GA, USA)

Novel Agents

Bio-active Particles

These embolic agents combine vascular occlusion with other local effects such as drug delivery or irradiation. The embolic property causes particles to lodge in a specific location, they then act a as platform to deliver high-intensity therapy in a selected location.

Drug-Eluting Microspheres

The theoretical advantages of drug-loaded particles are numerous, including a higher local drug concentration and a lower total dose of drug compared to a systemic administration and the potential to use drugs that are potentially toxic using the systemic route. Several such agents are under investigation including the following.

- *Anti-tumor drugs*: doxorubicin and irinotecan-loaded microspheres are being currently investigated in pre-clinical evaluations and clinical studies.
- *Analgesic agents*: ibuprofen-loaded microspheres (Biocompatibles, Farnham, UK) are being assessed to evaluate the clinical effects on post-embolization pain following UAE.

  Other possibilities include

- Agents that enhance or prolong the duration of arterial occlusion: vasoactive drug, such as prothrombotic agents and anti-angiogenic factors.
- Agents that prevent local tumor regrowth such as hormones, growth factor inhibitors, or anti-mitotic agents.

Two Types of Drug-Eluting Microspheres are Available

- Those that behave "like sponges" able to osmotically absorb large amounts of drug in solution (Hepasphere/Quadrasphere, Biosphere Medical, Roissy, France). These can be considered as a ready-to-load platform for any type of water-soluble drugs, but elution of the agent can occur before and during injection.
- Those produced from polymers able to adsorb a given drug which reaches high concentration inside the biomaterial (DC Beads, Biocompatibles, Farnham, UK) (Fig. 3.7). Drug release is more controlled and allows long-term delivery, but only selected drugs can be successfully loaded and released.

Fig. 3.7 Doxorubicin-eluting microspheres DC-Beads (Biocompatibles, Farnham, UK)

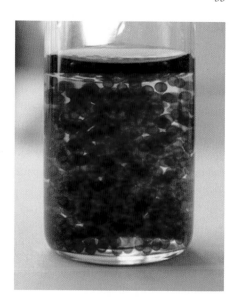

Several Factors May Influence the Ability to Deliver Drugs in Practice

- The diffusion area is composed of the vessel wall and the perivascular space, which comprises veins, lymphatic ducts, and interstitial tissue.
- Within a few hours, a foreign body reaction develops around the microsphere.
- This inflammatory response may modify the drug release by creating a barrier that reduces the diffusion of the drug or by eliminating the drug in the process.

For these reasons the drug release is very promising strategy, but its efficiency needs to be demonstrated experimentally first in animals and second in patients. In animals, the following has to be proven:

- The systemic level of the drug is null or much lower than after a systemic administration.
- The microsphere can release the loaded drug in significant amounts
- There are proven signs of the biological action of the drug
- No adverse local or general event or side effect occurs
- Finally the primary effect of the microspheres is not changed by the loaded drug.

Therefore, it remains to be proven in large cohort of patients that chemotherapy-loaded microspheres are safe and effective in terms of symptoms or prevention of tumor recurrence.

Radioactive Microspheres

Radioembolization consists of intra-arterial delivery of carrier spheres onto which radioactive particles are attached. There are two types of currently available radioactive microspheres that can be used in the treatment of primary and metastatic liver diseases. They both contain Yttrium-90 (^{90}Y) as the active element but differ in the type of carrier particle. Average activity per sphere is known allowing the delivered dose to be calculated. ^{90}Y is predominantly a beta-particle emitter with an average tissue penetration of 10 mm. ^{90}Y becomes inactive approximately 10 days after radioembolization. The indications, patient selection, preparation, and technique are identical for both preparations.

- ^{90}Y glass microspheres (TheraSphere, MDS Nordion, Canada) are glass spheres with a diameter of 25 ± 10 μm impregnated with ^{90}Y. Theraspheres embolize at the arteriole level.
- ^{90}Y resin-based microspheres (SIR-spheres, Sirtex Medical, Australia) with a diameter of 29–35 μm.
- SIR-spheres have a much lower specific activity per bead, meaning that many more beads must be injected to achieve the same radiation dose when compared to TheraSpheres. This leads to a much greater "embolic effect" when using SIR-spheres as compared to TheraSpheres.

Considerations Relating to ^{90}Y Microspheres

Radioactive microspheres have been used to treat liver tumors and metastases. Experience has been limited because of very restrictive conditions of use, strict patient selection, and costs. As in the case for transarterial chemoembolization, radioembolization takes advantage of the preferential hepatic arterial supply of hepatocellular carcinoma (HCC) or vascular metastases to deliver targeted therapy to the tumor, relatively sparing the normal liver parenchyma, that is mostly supported by the portal venous system.

- The total dose to be delivered depends on the tumor burden and the liver volume based on imaging evaluation (CT or MRI).
- A total dose of 120–150 Gy is considered to be optimal.
- The degree of shunting between the hepatic artery and hepatic vein needs to be precisely assessed by performing a perfusion study of the liver with ^{99}T-m macroaggregated albumin (MAA) particles. The MAA particles are injected through a catheter located in the arterial branch that will be used for radioembolization. The patient is then taken to the nuclear medicine department and planar images of the liver and lungs are obtained [14, 15]. Normal lungs can tolerate a total dose of 30 Gy. If the calculated liver dose is 120 Gy, the shunt fraction should then be less than 25%.

- All extrahepatic arteries originating from the hepatic artery such as gastroduo-denal, right gastric or falciform branches should be embolized prior to yttrium therapy.
- At the time of radioembolization, a very specific technique of use with an infusion set-up apparatus is used.
- Intra-arterial radioembolization has been recently promoted in patients with HCC or colorectal metastases who do not respond to TACE or systemic chemotherapy.

Detectable Microspheres

None of the agents above are radio-opaque; hence they are not detectable by flu-oroscopy, CT or MR scan, and operators cannot localize them during and after embolization. Delivery is normally guided by mixing with a contrast agent; the alternative is to use particles prepared to be radio-opaque and MRI detectable for embolization. Potential advantages of detectable agents are as follows:

- Detection of non-target embolization.
- Control of the homogeneity of distribution of the particles.
- Evaluation of the intra- or extratumoral location of the microspheres.
- Follow-up of the migration of the microspheres during time. The information regarding the distribution of the particles obtained at the time of emboliza-tion may have a significant impact on clinical practice with optimization of embolization protocols.

To obtain a radio-opaque microsphere, it is necessary to add a specific component that often changes radically the mechanical properties of the microspheres (com-pressibility and injectability); no such product is currently available. In vitro and in vivo pre-clinical results with MRI-detectable microspheres are encouraging and it has been possible to detect microspheres in different organs such as the kidneys, the uterus, and the liver.

Using Permanent Particulate Agents

All the particulate agents can be effective but there are some practical considerations to bear in mind. Four phases should be considered.

- Selection of the agent
- Preparation
- Delivery
- Post-injection

Choice of Particle Size for Embolization

PVA spheres typically occlude at a more distal level than tris-acryl spheres probably because of different compressibility properties. In clinical practice, the interventional radiologist should consider choosing larger particles when PVA microspheres are used instead of tris-acryl spheres (Table 3.1).

In practice, smaller particles are used to occlude more distal vessels and to induce tissue ischemia and necrosis..

Indicative size tris-acryl particles are uterine fibroid embolization (UFE) >500 μm, bronchial artery embolization (BAE) 500–700 μm, liver embolization 100–300 μm or 300–500 μm. As a general rule, larger particles are used in the presence of AV-shunting to avoid pulmonary embolization.

Table 3.1 Recommended particle size for uterine fibroid embolization

Agent	Recommended particle size for UFE (μm)
Non-spherical PVA particles	300–500 or 500–700
PVA microspheres	700–900
Tris-acryl microspheres	>500
Hydrogel–polyzene F microspheres	900

Preparation of the Agent

During delivery, the agent will normally be mixed with conventional contrast. This acts to suspend the particles, to carry them to the target, and to allow flow to be visualized during injection. The strength and volume of contrast used depend on personal preference and patient factors such as the size of tumor and renal function. As general rules

- Each vial of PVA particles is mixed in 20–30 mL of a 50% iodinated contrast medium and 50% of saline solution.
- Two syringes and a three-way tap are used to suspend the agent evenly. Typically use a 20-ml syringe as a reservoir and a 2–5-ml syringe to inject the mixture.
- Prior to each injection, the mixture is agitated to maintain homogeneous particle suspension. Failure to do this will result in all the PVA floating on the surface of the contrast.
- The quantity of embolic agent used for a typical case varies considerably depending on the clinical indication and angiographic end-point selected.

Injection of the Agent

- The delivery catheter
  - o Must be chosen to allow injection of the chosen agent.
  - o Should be positioned such that injection only opacifies tissue to be embolized.
  - o Should not be wedged. Particles should be able to be carried by flow, and a wedged catheter can result in abnormal pressure in the vessel that can open up shunts or lead to extravasation.
- Particles must be injected
  - o Under high-quality fluoroscopic control.
  - o In small aliquots.
  - o At a rate determined not to cause reflux on a test injection. Note that this will change during the embolization.
  - o Until a predetermined endpoint is reached. This is normally near stasis of flow. In practical terms, the contrast should be seen not to wash out for several seconds.

Following Injection

- o The catheter remains full of the embolic agent! If you have injected to stasis, any further injection or flushing of the catheter will lead to reflux and non-target embolization.
- o If stasis has been reached, then the catheter *must* be removed before it is flushed.
- o Even following thorough flushing, some particles may remain in the catheter or hub; this will interfere with subsequent passage of guidewires and embolization coils. If in doubt change the catheter.

Keypoints

- Many permanent embolic agents are available but they are not identical in their performance.
- Calibrated agents offer some potential advantages.
- Active agents may increase the therapeutic potential particularly in terms of pain control and effectiveness of cancer therapy.
- Agents that can be seen on X-ray and MRI imaging may simplify delivery and improve follow-up.

Recommended Reading

1. Siskin GP, Englander M, Stainken BF, et al. Embolic agent used for uterine fibroid embolization. Am J Roentgenol 2000; 175: 767–73.
2. Castaneda-Zuniga WR, Sanchez R, Amplatz K. Experimental observations on short and long-term effects of arterial occlusion with Ivalon. Radiology 1978; 126: 783–5.
3. Segni RD, Young AT, Qian Z, Castaneda-Zuniga WR. Embolotherapy: agents, equipment and techniques. In: Castaneda-Zuniga WR, Tadavarthy SM, Qian Z, Ferral H, Maynar M (eds) Interventional Radiology. Williams and Wilkins, Baltimore, 1997, pp 29–103
4. Repa I, Moradian GP, Dehrer LP, et al. Mortalities associated with use of a commercial suspension of polyvinyl alcohol. Radiology 1989; 170: 395–9.
5. Laurent A, Wassef M, Saint Maurice JP, et al. Arterial distribution of calibrated tris-acryl gelatin and polyvinyl alcohol microspheres in a sheep kidney model. Invest Radiol 2006; 41: 8–14.
6. Kroencke TJ, Scheurig C, Lampmann LE, et al. Acrylamido polyvinyl alcohol microspheres for uterine artery embolization: 12-month clinical and MR imaging results. J Vasc Interv Radiol 2008; 19: 47–57.
7. Bendszus M, Klein R, Burger R, Warmuth-Metz M, Hofmann E, Solymosi L. Efficacy of trisacryl gelatin microspheres and polyvinyl alcohol particles in the preoperative embolization of meningiomas. Am J Neuroradiol 2000; 21: 255–61.
8. Pelage JP, Laurent A, Wassef M, et al. Acute effects of uterine artery embolization in the sheep: comparison between polyvinyl alcohol particles and calibrated microspheres. Radiology 2002; 224:436–45.
9. Stampfl S, Stampfl U, Bellemann N, et al. Biocompatibility and recanalization characteristics of hydrogel microspheres with polyzene-F as polymer coating. Cardiovasc Intervent Radiol 2008; 31: 799–806.
10. Varela M, Real MI, Burrel M, et al. Chemoembolization of hepatocellular carcinoma with drug eluting beads: efficacy and doxorubicin pharmacokinetics. J Hepatol 2007; 46: 474–81.
11. Taylor RR, Tang Y, Gonzalez MV, Stratford PW, Lewis AL. Irinotecan drug eluting beads for use in chemoembolization: in vitro and in vivo evaluation of drug release properties. Eur J Pharm Sci 2007; 30: 7–14.
12. Wassef M, Pelage JP, Velzenberger E, et al. Anti-inflammatory effect of ibuprofen-loaded embolization beads in sheep uterus. J Biomed Mater Res B Appl Biomater 2008; 86: 63–73.
13. Grosso M, Vignali C, Quaretti P, et al. Transarterial chemoembolization for hepatocellular carcinoma with drug-eluting microspheres: preliminary results from an Italian multicentre study. Cardiovasc Intervent Radiol 2008; 31: 1141–9.
14. Geschwind JF, Salem R, Carr BI, et al.Yttrium-90 microspheres for the treatment of hepatocellular carcinoma. Gastroenterology 2004;127: S194–205
15. Sato KT, Lewandowski RJ, Mulcahy MF, et al. Unresectable chemorefractory liver metastases: radioembolization with 90Y microspheres—safety, efficacy, and survival. Radiology 2008; 247: 507–15.
16. Namur J, Chapot R, Pelage JP, et al. MR imaging detection of superparamagnetic iron oxide loaded tris-acryl embolization microspheres. J Vasc Interv Radiol 2007; 18: 1287–95.

Chapter 4
Temporary Embolic Agents

Mark Brinckman

Sometimes it is unnecessary or undesirable to permanently occlude a blood vessel. In these circumstances, using an agent which causes temporary vascular occlusion is preferable. On other occasions, the risk of a procedure may be reduced by using agents which cause only temporary vascular blockade. It must be recognized that although some of the agents described as "temporary" may be resorbed, their effects on the vascular endothelium may be irreversible.

Circumstances in which temporary agents may be indicated

- *Pre-operative embolization:* e.g., embolization of a renal tumor immediately before resection. In these circumstances, there is no advantage in permanent obliteration of the tumor circulation and any non-target embolization is less likely to be harmful.
- *High-flow priapism:* in this circumstance, the desirability of restoring blood flow is obvious.
- *Trauma:* it is usually only necessary to arrest bleeding until a stable clot forms and the vessel can heal. Remember that speed is of the essence here.
- *Upper gastrointestinal tract haemorrhage*

Temporary Agents

Autologous Blood Clot

Physical Description and Properties
- Clotted blood: this can be macerated or injected intact
- Readily available, sterile, non-immunogenic, cost-effective
- Can be used alone, modified by thrombin, or combined with other agents for a more permanent effect

Transcatheter Embolization and Therapy,
Techniques in Interventional Radiology, DOI 10.1007/978-1-84800-897-7_4,
© Springer-Verlag London Limited 2010

Mode of Action

- Mechanical obstruction of target vessel.

How to Prepare and Use It

- If you anticipate using autologous clot, instruct the ward staff to draw 10–15 cc of the patient's own blood into a sterile container, e.g., a clean syringe/vacutainer with no additives. Ensure that the specimen is correctly labeled.
- Obtain the specimen at the beginning of the procedure, before giving any heparin or using heparinized saline.
- Allow the blood to clot. 15–90 min may be required for adequate clot formation, depending on the status of patient's endogenous clotting factors. In patients with severe coagulopathy, sufficient clotting may not occur.
- Heating with steam for 1 min or adding clotting factors such as thrombin may be used to augment the clot formation process.
- 1–2 cc of clot is usually sufficient to achieve desired hemostasis. Higher amounts may be required, but this should be determined by angiographic evaluation in order to balance hemostasis versus end-organ ischemic injury.
  - Example: 5–10 ml of autogenous clot will most likely result in hemostasis following renal trauma; however, it may also result in a much higher amount of long-term renal parenchyma loss or complete loss of renal function in the target kidney. A smaller amount may very well achieve hemostasis of the segmental arterial bleed, while preserving a large portion of the kidney.
- Autologous clot can be administered through standard catheter systems that allow for super selection of the intended vessel. Due to the size and viscosity of clot, using autologous clot with a microcatheter system may be difficult. A 1-ml syringe is essential.
- A balloon catheter system may be employed in those instances where there may be a higher chance of reflux and unintended (non-target) embolization, e.g., during embolization of the gastroduodenal artery to prevent reflux into the hepatic artery.

When and When Not to Use It

- Autologous clot is an ideal agent in those situations where hemostasis in a target vessel is desired on the order of hours to days, and especially when early recanalization may be beneficial to save as much of the involved end organ as possible, e.g., renal trauma.
- Autologous clot has been successfully used in many wide ranging applications as follows:
  - Acute gastrointestinal bleeding—Rosch et al. pioneered the use of autologous clot embolization for this means
  - Pelvic trauma. Embolization following fractures of the pubic rami that have resulted in uncontrollable bleeding from the obturator artery

o Renal trauma
o Post-traumatic priapism
o Biopsy-track embolization to prevent pneumothoraces following CT-guided lung biopsy

Detecting and Preventing Problems

- Clot not forming in a timely fashion:
  o Consider the coagulation status of the patient.
  o Has the patient's endogenous clotting ability been hampered by multiple transfusions, liver dysfunction, or hypothermia?
- Non-target embolization:
  o Consider the use of a balloon catheter delivery system to prevent reflux.
- Early rebleeding:
  o Consider a different agent.
  o Consider modified autologous clot.
  o Thrombin/clot, clot/Gelfoam combinations.
  o Evaluate with angiography whether another bleeding vessel may now be involved with the change in hemodynamics following previous embolization.

Gelatin Sponge

Commercially sold as Gelfoam (Upjohn, Kalamazoo, MI, USA) or Surgifoam (Ethicon, Sommerville, NJ, USA)

Gelatin sponge is a commonly used agent and can be used in three different forms:

- Slurry–medium sized vessel agent
- Pledgets–larger vessel, proximal occlusion agent
- Powder–arteriolar/capillary, distal agent

Each form causes mechanical vascular occlusion but of different sized vessels.

Gelfoam is made from purified porcine skin gelatin, and so is contraindicated in patients with allergy to porcine collagen products.

Slurry

Physical Description and Properties

- "Slurry" is prepared by mixing gelatin sponge and contrast together.
- Consistency can be fine-tuned for specific uses by adjusting the amount of fluid added.
- Slurry provides an excellent middle consistency agent (between powder and pledgets) that can easily be delivered through a microcatheter.

- The injected slurry is intended to form a cast of the embolized vessel just beyond the delivery catheter tip.

Mode of Action

- As with other gelatin sponge agents, embolization is largely by mechanical occlusion. Thrombus induction and inflammation of vessel wall are secondary contributors.
- Off-label use, but is standard technique in many circumstances.
- Recanalization will begin as early as 2 days and may take up to several weeks.

How to Prepare and Use It (Figure 4.1)

- Gelatin sponge cubes (approximately 1 mm in size) are placed in one 10-ml syringe.

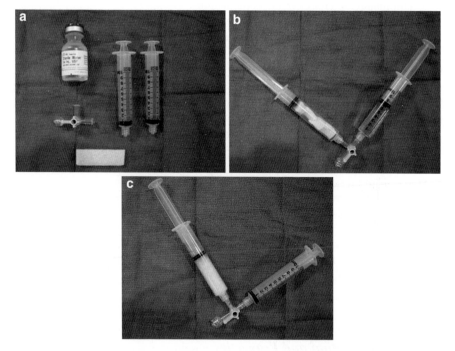

Fig. 4.1 Gelfoam slurry. **a)** The materials required to make a Gelfoam slurry. Contrast is often used in lieu of water or saline to increase visibility of the injectate. **b)** The Gelfoam is torn into several pieces and back-loaded into one of the syringes. Contrast (5–10 cc) is drawn into the second syringe, and the two syringes are connected to a three-way stopcock. **c)** Using a to-and-fro motion, the Gelfoam and contrast are mixed together until a consistent slurry is formed. Air will invariably be trapped in the Gelfoam slurry

- A second 10-ml syringe is filled with 5–10 cc of contrast.
- Two catheters are connected via a three-way stopcock.
- Back and forth agitation through the stopcock results in a slurry (consistency of pudding) that can then be loaded into one of the syringes and injected into standard catheter and microcatheter systems.
- Delivery with a smaller syringe (e.g., 1–5 cc) may be helpful, especially if a microcatheter system is being used.
- If a longer time period of occlusion before recanalization is desired, ε-aminocaproic acid (a plasmin inhibitor) can be added to the slurry mixture. This has been demonstrated to extend the typical recanalization times for Gelfoam and probably renders this a permanent agent.

When and When Not to Use It

- Slurry is a good embolization agent for medium-sized vessels.
- The level of embolization is relatively proximal; hence necrosis is uncommon except in end arteries.
- Useful for gaining temporary occlusion of highly selected second order vessels, e.g., highly selective embolization of the supraduodenal artery supplied by the gastroduodenal artery in the treatment of a bleeding peptic ulcer.
- Slurry can be combined with pledgets, torpedoes, coils, etc, to accomplish hemostasis in a wide range of applications.
- Trauma
- Pre-operative embolization
- Gastrointestinal hemorrhage
- Postpartum hemorrhage

Detecting Problems

- Use carefully collimated high-quality fluoroscopy to detect reflux during delivery.
- Stop embolization before short of complete hemostasis to avoid reflux and non-target embolization.
- Remember that the catheter remains full of embolic material so
  o Flush with saline under fluoroscopic control until no contrast is seen.
  o If there is reflux either aspirate until freely flowing blood is obtained or remove the catheter before flushing.

Tip should be pointed up during injection to avoid aggregation at the back of the catheter.

Powder

Physical Description and Properties

- Made from purified pork skin.
- Powder made by milling gelatin sponge.
- Jar of powder (1 g) mixed with contrast solution to obtain desired consistency.
- Powder particles measure 40–60 μm. Due to particle clumping/aggregation, 100–500 μm vessel (arteriolar or capillary level) occlusion results.

Mode of Action

- Off-label use as an intravascular product, but accepted standard of care.
- Exact mode of action is not completely understood, but thought to be largely mechanical. Thrombus induction and inflammation of the vessel wall are also thought to contribute.
- Size allows for high level of distal occlusion and hemostatsis at the capillary and/or arteriolar level.
- As a temporary agent, recanalization may begin as soon a few days, but often requires 2–4 weeks.
- Unknown what percentage of embolized vessels actually recanalize.
- Capillary level occlusion makes necrosis more likely.

How to Prepare and Use It

- Powder mixed with contrast to allow for ease of delivery and visualization through standard microcatheter systems.
- Once mixed, the tip of syringe should be pointed upward during delivery to prevent aggregation in the back part of the syringe.
- Special care should be taken to ensure delivery to correct location, given the high order of occlusion, poor visualization of agent during embolization, and irretrievable nature of the agent.
- Delivery should be stopped prior to any angiographic evidence of significant reflux, as inadvertent reflux can result in significant morbidity.

When and When Not to Use It

- Use intended mainly for situations where complete target ischemia desired.
- Useful as a high-order embolization agent in pre-operative embolization of tumors or organs.

- Not a good agent for GI bleeding, because of the real risk of non-target bowel necrosis. Rarely, situations can arise where a major coagulopathy or uremia may make proximal control of bleeding unsuccessful, necessitating more distal, high-order embolization in massive GI hemorrhage, etc.
- Should NOT be used in individuals with high arteriovenous fistula potential.

Detecting Problems

- Of all the three gelatin agents, powder results in the most distal level of embolization, beyond most collateral vessels and therefore may result in more severe ischemia.
- As with all gelatin sponge products, an idiopathic, temporary rise in temperature can sometimes be seen (as high as 39° C) and may persist as long as 1–2 days. This post-embolization fever will often resolve spontaneously with blood cultures and WBC count remaining unremarkable.

Pledgets

Physical Description and Properties

- Purified pork skin, packaged into sterile sheets.
- Sizes can be tailored. Typical sizes for Gelfoam cubes range in size from 0.5 to 2.0 mm. Typical pledget sizes are $1 \times 2 \times 5$ mm rectangles. Torpedos can be formed for tailored proximal occlusion, but typically are 3–4 mm in size.

Mode of Action

- Off-label use, but considered standard of care.
- Mechanical, temporary occlusion that can be tailored to occlude medium and larger sized vessels or tissue tracts.
- Inflammation of vessel wall and superimposed thrombosis are also likely contributors.
- As with all gelatin sponge products, recanalization can occur in a matter of days and take as long as 4–6 weeks.

How to Prepare and Use It

- Cubes, pledgets, and torpedoes are cut from the gelatin sponge and may be soaked in contrast to improve fluoroscopic visibility. Remove the plunger from the tube of the syringe, load the cube, pledget, or torpedo as desired. Replace the plunger.
- Deliver with contrast to facilitate transfer through the catheter and visibility.

- Delivery syringe sizes of 1–3 ml are typical with a Luerlock tip that keeps the syringe from dislodging from the catheter during injection.
- Following syringe preparation, the tip should be kept up to keep the agent in the leading part of the delivery and prevent aggregation if suspended cubes are used.
- If a slightly longer lasting occlusion is desired, then the contrast/saline/Gelfoam mixture can be mixed with ϵ-aminocaproic acid.
- Agent should be delivered until antegrade flow ceases. Further injection risks reflux and/or non-target embolization.
- Larger pledgets and torpedoes can be delivered and placed with lodging in the natural taper of the vessel and therefore must be appropriately sized.
- Smaller cube/contrast solutions are often best delivered in a pulsatile fashion.
- When large vessel occlusion is beyond the upper limit of tailored torpedo capability alone (e.g., transected vessel from trauma), a coil may be used as a scaffold or backstop on which Gelfoam can be packed ("coil-Gelfoam sandwich").

When and When Not to Use It

- As with all temporary agents, other agents should be considered if long-term occlusion is required.
- Widely used in gastrointestinal bleeding, early post-partum hemorrhage, and trauma, particularly pelvic trauma.
- Good agent for use to occlude percutaneous biopsy tracks.

Detecting Problems

- Reflux or non-target embolization can generally be precluded with direct angiographic visualization during delivery.
- If reflux or non-target embolization does occur, then suction embolectomy can be considered.
- Gelfoam embolization may result in a temporary, idiopathic fever. This should only last 1–2 days and culture/white count are usually unremarkable.
- Detection of air in the biopsy track following Gelfoam placement is usually airtrapped in the pledgets and not of significant concern.

Microfibrillar Collagen

Commercially sold as Avitene.

Physical Description and Properties

- Derived from bovine hide collagen.
- Dry, thinly shredded flakes packaged in 1–5 g containers.
- Fiber size: 5×70–200 μm.

Mode of Action

- Avitene is a potent thrombogenic agent that causes occlusion by mechanical means, but unlike gelatin sponge, has been demonstrated to cause a granulomatous arteritis.
- The granulomatous reaction is followed by fibrosis as the inflammation subsides at 3 months.
- Recanalization begins in roughly a week and may take up to 8 weeks.

How to Prepare and Use It

- Roughly 0.5 g of microfibrillar collagen is mixed with 10 ml of contrast to form a semi-liquid suspension (applesauce consistency).
- 0.1–1.0 ml can be injected through a microcatheter or catheter delivery system followed by ~5 ml; a saline bolus chaser to flush the catheter, advance embolus, and prevent catheter occlusion.

When and When Not to Use It

- Avitene is suitable for tumor embolization, where a high order of occlusion for hemostasis during surgery is desired.
- Not suitable for GI embolization, for reasons similar to Gelfoam powder. The distal third- or fourth-order vessel occlusion increases risks for inadvertent gastrointestinal ischemia.

Detecting Problems

- Catheter occlusion—the potent thrombogenic nature and consistency of the suspension may lend itself to occlusion. This can be avoided by a saline bolus and exchanging the delivery catheter using a guide catheter or sheath system.
- Reflux/non-target embolization –
  - o Stop short of complete embolization of target and/or if any reflux is noted.
  - o Consider a balloon occlusion catheter delivery system to prevent significant reflux.
  - o Consider other agents if the risk of ischemia beyond collateralization outweighs any benefit of using microfibrillar collagen (e.g., GI embolization).

Keypoints

1. Temporary embolization agents are most beneficial when a vessel can safely be sacrificed but permanent occlusion is not necessary (e.g., trauma).
2. Temporary agents may result in permanent vascular damage even though they are resorbed.
3. All temporary agents are non-radioopaque, and as such should be mixed with contrast material for injection.
4. When used correctly and in the right clinical circumstances, temporary agents are easy, quick, and cheap to use.

Chapter 5
Liquid Embolic Agents

Kimi Kondo

It is easy to understand how particles, coils, and other solid agents can lead to vascular occlusion. Liquid embolic agents can also be very effective at occluding vessels and act by a variety of mechanisms.

- Sclerosant agents: e.g., absolute alcohol, sodium tetradecyl sulphate (STD)
- Glues: *N*-butyl cyanoacrylate (NBCA)
- Elastic polymers: ethylene vinyl alcohol/dimethyl sulfoxide (Onyx®)
- Iodized poppy seed oil droplets: lipiodol

Liquid agents pose particular challenges and are perhaps the hardest embolic agents to use. They can be very unforgiving as there is little to no control once they start to flow away from the delivery catheter.

Sclerosing Agents

- They include the following:

    - Detergent agents
    - Hyperosmolar agents
    - Chemical irritants

- Sclerosants act by damaging endothelial cells.
- Many chemicals can achieve this; to realize how effective this can be, one only has to think about the obliteration of veins in an intravenous drug abuser or patient receiving chemotherapy.
- When using sclerosants, the intention is to destroy the endothelium to expose subendothelial tissues which in turn will lead to irreversible vascular fibrosis.
- The sclerosant effect will depend on the following:

    - The strength of the agent
    - The time it is in contact with the endothelium

- The volume and rate of injection will influence outcome and also the propensity to damage adjacent non-target vessels.

Transcatheter Embolization and Therapy,
Techniques in Interventional Radiology, DOI 10.1007/978-1-84800-897-7_5,
© Springer-Verlag London Limited 2010

Absolute Alcohol (Dehyrated Alcohol)

Physical Description and Properties

- C_2H_5OH—anhydrous ethanol
- Clear colorless liquid
- Completely miscible with water and organic solvents

Mode of Action

- Causes vasospasm
- Causes cell death by dehydration, denaturing proteins, and precipitation of protoplasm.
- Cytotoxic—damages any tissue it contacts.
- Injection into a vessel denudes the endothelium, which leads to thrombosis and eventual fibrosis.
- Toxic effect can extend beyond the blood vessels into the perivascular spaces.
- When injected in close proximity to nerve tissues, it can produce neuritis and nerve degeneration (neurolysis).

How to Prepare and Use Alcohol

- Usually supplied in glass ampoules (1 and 5 ml); can draw up into a syringe. A filter needle should be used to filter any glass shards from the ampoule.
- Can be diluted and opacified with contrast up to 1:1 ratio.
- Normally administered by direct intralesional injection.
- Can be used with
  - Balloon occlusion catheter to prevent reflux and non-target embolization
  - Tourniquet to prolong dwell time

Dosage and Side Effects

- Use with caution at high doses (0.5–1 ml/kg body weight) as alcohol is absorbed systemically.
- Alcohol intoxication.
- Hemolysis.
- Systemic and pulmonary hypertension.
- Hyperthermia.

When to Use Absolute Alcohol

- Embolization:
  - Renal cell carcinoma
  - Aldosterone-producing adrenal adenomas
  - Vascular malformations

Absolute alcohol can also be used for the following:

- Nerve blocks (e.g., celiac plexus block, trigeminal nerve block).
- Sclerosis of hepatic or renal cysts, seromas.
- Percutaneous ethanol injection (PEI):
  - Hepatocellular carcinoma (HCC)
  - Recurrent cervical lymph node disease for thyroid cancer
  - Cystic thyroid nodules
  - Parathyroid adenomas

When Not to Use It

- When optimal catheter or needle placement is not possible.
- High risk of non-target embolization.

Sodium Tetradecyl Sulfate

- Brand names: Sotradecol (Angiodynamics, Queesnbury, NY, USA), FibroVein (STD Limited, Hereford, UK), Trombovar (Aventis Pharma, Le Trait, France), Thromboject (Omega, Montreal, QC, Canada).

Physical Description and Properties

- Anionic surfactant; detergent.

Mode of Action

- Intravascular injection causes intimal inflammation and superimposed thrombus formation.
- Dissolution of endothelial cell membrane.
- Subsequent formation of fibrous tissue results in partial or complete vessel obliteration that may or may not be permanent.

- Foam preparation also displaces blood in the vessel that enhances sclerosing power.
- May have effect up to 20 cm from injection site.

How to Prepare and Use It

- Commercially available in concentrations between 0.2% (2 mg/ml) and 3% (30 mg/ml) depending on manufacturer.
  - o Maximum single treatment should not exceed 300 mg (10 ml of 3% solution) (American manufacturer recommendations), 120 mg (British manufacturer recommendations).
- Dissolves rubber stoppers; therefore, use latex-free syringes.
- Foam: one part sclerosant: four parts air mixed through 20 passages in two syringes (2–10 ml) connected by three-way stopcock (Tessari method).
- Injected directly into vessel.

When to Use

- Varicose veins and telangectasias: concentrations between 0.1% and 3.0% used depending on the size of the vein to be treated; foam.
- Varicoceles and pelvic congestion syndrome: 2–3% concentration; foam.
- Peripheral venous vascular malformations: 2–3% concentration; foam.

When Not to Use It

- Previous hypersensitivity reaction to the drug
- Acute infection
- Asthma
- Large superficial veins with wide-open communication to deeper veins

N-Butyl Cyanoacrylate

Brand name: TRUFILL n-Butyl Cyanoacrylate (n-BCA) Liquid Embolic System (Cordis Neurovascular, Inc., Miami Lakes, FL, USA).

Physical Description and Properties

- Free-flowing clear liquid adhesive similar to "superglue."

Mode of Action

- Polymerizes into a solid material upon contact with any ionic media such as contrast, body fluids or tissues.
- Adheres to most body tissues.

How to Prepare and Use It

- Do not use with any device containing polycarbonate, as it will cause polycarbonate to deteriorate. Use polyethylene or polypropylene syringes.
- Use a sterile 25–50 cc glass beaker or equivalent as a mixing container to prepare the mixture.
- Radiopacification of n-BCA accomplished by adding lipiodol and if necessary tantalum powder.
- Addition of lipiodol and/or tantalum powder extends the polymerization time of n-BCA.
- Mix lipiodol and tantalum powder in the glass beaker by aspirating in and out of a syringe until the mixture is homogenous.
- Add desired amount of n-BCA and mix by aspirating in and out with a syringe.
- Compare the mixture fluoroscopically to a similar syringe of contrast to determine adequate radiopacity.
- Flush catheter and rinse outside of the catheter hub with 5% dextrose.
- Aspirate n-BCA/lipiodol mixture into syringe using a 21- or 23-gauged needle and verify that the mixture is well suspended and free of air bubbles.
- After injection under fluoroscopy, immediately aspirate with injection syringe and rapidly withdraw the catheter.
- Discard used catheter; do not flush the catheter or perform check angiography after use, in case residual glue remains in the lumen or hub and causes non-target embolization.

When to Use

- FDA approved for embolization of cerebral arteriovenous malformations (AVMs) when presurgical embolization is desired.
- Embolization:
  - Vascular malformations
  - Thoracic duct ablation for postoperative chylothorax
  - Trauma
  - Upper gastrointestinal bleeding

When Not to Use It

- Previous history of reactions to cyanoacrylates.
- When vasospasm stops blood flow.
- When optimal catheter placement is not possible.

Ethylene Vinyl Alcohol/Dimethyl Sulfoxide (Onyx®)

- Brand name: Onyx Liquid Embolic System (Micro Therapeutics, Inc., Irvine, CA, USA).

Physical Description and Properties

- Non-adhesive elastic polymer.
- Non-thrombogenic.
- Comprised of EVOH (ethylene vinyl alcohol) copolymer dissolved in DMSO (dimethyl sulfoxide) and suspended micronized tantalum powder.
- Two product formulations
  o Onyx 18 (6% EVOH) and Onyx 34 (8% EVOH).
  o Onyx 18 is less viscous than Onyx 34 and will embolize more distally.

Mode of Action

- DMSO solvent dissipates into the blood causing the EVOH copolymer and suspended tantalum to precipitate in situ into a spongy, coherent embolus.
- The polymeric embolus solidifies from the outside to the inside, while traveling distally.
- Final solidification occurs within 5 min.
- Unlike n-BCA, Onyx causes a mechanical occlusion without significant tissue adherence.

How to Prepare and Use It

- Use DMSO compatible delivery microcatheter (Marathon, Rebar, or Ultraflow HPC catheters [Microtherapeutics]) and syringes.
- Shake Onyx at least 20 mins on an Onyx mixer (at a setting of 8) and mix until ready to inject.
- Flush contrast from microcatheter with 10 cc NS.
- Fill microcatheter deadspace volume with DMSO.

- Hold catheter hub in a vertical position and overfill and wash the luer hub with DMSC to create a meniscus of DMSO.
- Attach Onyx syringe to microcatheter, meniscus to meniscus and then quickly point the syringe vertically.
- Inject Onyx at a steady, slow rate of 0.16 ml/min (0.25 ml/90 sec). Do not exceed 0.3 ml/min. Once Onyx passes through the catheter hub, the syringe may be held in a more comfortable position.
- Do not allow more than 1 cm of Onyx to reflux back over the catheter tip.
- Upon completion of injection, wait a few seconds, slightly aspirate syringe, and gently pull the catheter to separate it from the Onyx cast.
- Do not interrupt Onyx injection for longer than 2 min prior to re-injection.
- Stop injection if increased resistance is observed.

When to Use

- FDA approved for presurgical embolization of cerebral arteriovenous malformations.
- Visceral and cerebral arteries aneurysms.

When Not to Use It

- When optimal catheter placement is not possible.
- When vasospasm stops blood flow.
- History of reaction or hypersensitivity to DMSO.
- Premature infants (<1,500 g) or individuals with significant liver and kidney function impairment.

Note

- DMSO has a characteristic aroma not unlike a patient with ketoacidosis. Warn the patient that it is normal for them to smell of this until all DMSO has been excreted from the body.

Lipiodol

- Brand name: Ethiodol (Savage Laboratories, Melville, NY, USA).

Physical Description and Properties

- Sterile, injectable, low-viscosity radio-opaque diagnostic agent.
- Contains 37% iodine (475 mg/ml) organically combined with ethyl esters of the fatty acids of poppy seed oil.
- Straw to amber colored oily fluid.

Fate of Injected Lipiodol

Lymphatic Injection

- Following intralymphatic administration, lipiodol enters the bloodstream and is transported to the liver, lungs, spleen, and adipose tissue.
- In the lungs, the lipid droplets are dispersed in the pulmonary alveoli. Disappearance of droplets in the lungs or other tissues occurs slowly.
- During metabolism, iodine is released, which is excreted through the urinary system.

Hepatic Arterial Injection

- When injected into the hepatic artery, lipiodol is selectively retained by hepato-cellular carcinoma (HCC) and other lipiodol-avid tumors.
- Selective uptake of lipiodol is thought to be due to a siphoning effect created by the increased blood flow in a hypervascular tumor.
- The lipidol droplets divide into smaller globules as they travel in the blood vessels and lodge in the liver parenchyma.
- Lipiodol is normally cleared through the hepatic lymphatics; Kupffer cells might also contribute to the clearance of lipiodol from hepatic lobules. HCC does not contain hepatic lymphatic tissue and thus is still stained with lipiodol even after clearance from background liver tissue.

How to Prepare and Use It

- Can be injected as a single agent but often mixed (through two syringes with a three-way stopcock) with other agents such as chemotherapy to form an emulsion in ratios ranging from 1:1 to 1:4.
- Lipiodol can be prepared with I^{131} a beta particle emitter and used to deliver radiotherapy.

When to Use

- Chemoembolization.
- Diagnostic arteriogram for HCC.
- In combination with n-BCA to delay n-BCA polymerization.
- In combination with absolute alcohol to opacify alcohol delivery.

When Not to Use It

- History of reaction or hypersensitivity to iodine or lipiodol.
- Do not use for bronchography.
- Due to risk of lipiodol bypassing the liver via arteriovenous fistulae and lodging in the pulmonary vasculature, lipiodol should be used with care in patients with impaired lung function.

Keypoints

Liquid embolic agents are a valuable addition to the armamentarium of the vascular radiologist.

They have widely differing modes of action.

They provide a different set of considerations and challenges from conventional embolic agents.

Before using liquid agents, ensure that you have a thorough understanding of the mechanism of action, use, and complications associated with the agent.

Suggested Reading

Weiss RA, Feied CF, Weiss MA. *Sclerosing Solutions*. In: Vein Diagnosis and Treatment: A Comprehensive Approach. New York, NY: McGraw-Hill; 2001:119–130.

Society of Interventional Radiology (SIR) 33rd Annual Scientific Meeting Workshop book. Chapters: Glue: Neuro and Beyond; Regional Cancer Therapy; Arterial Embolotherapy. 2008.

Pollak JS and White RI Jr. The Use of Cyanoacrylate Adhesives in Peripheral Embolization. J Vasc Interv Radiol 2001; 12:907–13.

Ray CE Jr. and Bauer JR. Embolization Agents. In Mauro MA, Murphy KP, Thomson KR, et al. (eds). Image-Guided Interventions. Vol. 1, Philadelphia, Saunders, Elsevier, 2008, 131–9.

Chapter 6
Miscellaneous Embolic Agents: Laser and Radiofrequency

David West

Embolization, the deliberate therapeutic occlusion of vessels, is normally undertaken using mechanical occlusion devices like coils, plugs, particles, or liquids such as glues. An alternative approach is sclerosant therapy; this can be accomplished using liquid agents such as alcohol or sodium tetradecyl sulphate or by temperature change. Thermal ablation is most commonly used in the treatment of varicose veins (see Chapter 45).

Sclerosis can be achieved by the following:

- Heating
  - Laser
  - Radiofrequency (RF)
- Cooling
  - Cryotherapy

This chapter will consider laser and RF, as cryotherapy is not in common usage for vascular occlusion.

The effects of heating tissues with laser or RF are dependent on the local temperature achieved (Table 6.1).

Table 6.1 Effect of Heating Tissues to different Temperature

Temperature (°C)	Effect
45	Vasodilation
60	Denaturation of proteins
80	Contraction of collagen
100	Steam production, dehydration
>100	Carbonization

Remember the following when depositing heat energy:

- Tissue heating will depend on the rate of deposition of energy.
- Heating is effective over a limited radius. Thermal therapy is most effective and controlled, if the target tissue is in direct apposition with the heating agent.

- Conduction of the local tissues (e.g., fast-flowing blood will act as a coolant).
- Surrounding tissues may be affected unless protected.

When using laser or RF, the principle is to introduce the probe or fiber to the target site and then to pull back at a controlled rate while depositing energy in the tissues. This rate will depend on the following:

- The desired energy deposition
- The power of the device
- The diameter of the target vessel
- Factors affecting local heat conduction

Laser

LASER is an acronym for Light Amplification by the Stimulated Emission of Radiation. The absorption of laser light energy heats tissues, and different tissues absorb different wavelengths of light. Blood absorbs best around 810–1064 nm, and water in the cells of the vein wall absorbs best around 1320 nm. Most of the lasers used for permanent occlusion of blood vessels are diode lasers operating at a wavelength between 810 and 980 nm. Nd/YAG lasers, operating at 1064 and 1320 nm, can also be used. Diode lasers are very compact and relatively cheap and, being solid state, robust.

About Lasers

Lasers produce light with certain characteristic properties.

- Monochromatic (i.e., one specific wavelength/color).
- Highly coherent (i.e., all the photons are moving in phase with one another).
- Highly directional (i.e., almost all photons are traveling in a parallel beam).
- They can be highly focused and all the energy within the light beam can be targeted on a very small area of tissue, resulting in localized heating.

Laser light is delivered to the target via simple bare-tipped optical fibers. The diameter of the fiber influences flexibility, durability, and energy deposition. Normally these are 600 μm (0.6 m) diameter (which are quite robust), but 400 μm and even 200 μm fibers are quite capable of delivering the necessary energy.

- The fibers are introduced through vascular sheaths or catheters of sufficient luminal diameter (usually 4–6Fr) (Fig. 6.1). The fiber has to protrude out of the end of the catheter by a minimum of 2 cm to avoid burning the plastic sheath.
- Most manufacturers produce kits comprising the laser fiber, the introducer sheath, needle, and guidewire. They tend to modify their lasers to prevent the use of other manufacturer's fibers. To reduce costs and limit supply problems, look for laser

Fig. 6.1 Laser fiber in position in calibrated sheath

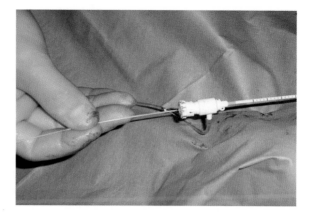

manufacturers that allow use of generic fibers. Also check the numerical aperture of the laser. The two common numerical apertures are 0.22 and 0.37 (NA). Either works well but 0.37 NA lasers can only be used with 0.37 NA fibers, whereas 0.22 NA machines can use either 0.22 or 0.37 NA fibers.

Laser Power (Fig. 6.2)

- The power output required to induce vessel wall death and permanent occlusion is 8–30 watts.
- The power and the length of time the power is applied for (determined by the pull back rates) are adjusted to deliver a certain number of joules of energy deposition per centimeter of vessel treated.
- The greatest shrinkage and fewest perforations occur using a power of 8–12 watts and a slow pull-back rate.

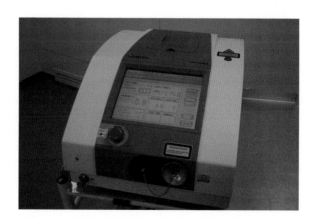

Fig. 6.2 Typical diode laser for EVLA with settings indicating a power of 12.0 watts, 1.0 s pulse, and 1.0 s pulse interval

Using Lasers

- When treating veins, the aim is to maximize damage to the vein wall while minimizing thrombosis within the vessel lumen and damage to adjacent tissues.
- To achieve this, the vessel should be emptied and ideally compressed against the laser fiber. This is easily achieved by injecting large quantities of saline into the fascial envelope surrounding the vessel.
- Addition of adrenaline to this solution further helps contract the vessel, and addition of anesthetic to the solution ("tumescent anaesthesia") prevents pain.
- The vessel diameter influences the energy deposition required to occlude it, contributes to the likelihood of collateral damage and vessel perforation. Typical doses to cause permanent occlusion are shown below:

Vein diameter (mm)	Pulsed	Continuous
3	15 J/cm 15 W	50 J/cm
5	50 J/cm at 15 W	100 J/cm 150 J/cm

- Higher doses will damage the full thickness of a vessel wall (e.g., in continuous mode a 5 mm diameter vein needs minimum 100 J/cm to permanently damage intima and 150 J/cm to permanently damage the media and adventitia).
- In practice, most operators tend to err on the side of effectiveness rather than minimal energy deposition. Whether pulsed or continuous, a minimum energy deposition of 80 J/cm is used.
- Perforations will occur in many patients leading to bruising, but other collateral damage is very rare at these levels and permanent vessel occlusion is virtually guaranteed.

Safety

The types of laser used for vessel occlusion are high-powered and potentially dangerous class 4 lasers. As such, any establishment using them must be registered. In the UK, this registration is with the Healthcare Commission. Certain legal obligations are also in force. You must have a qualified laser protection advisor, an in-house laser protection supervisor, designation of laser controlled areas, an operating manual specifying exactly how the laser will be used for different treatments, a register of users, register of every time the laser is used, and any local rules and regulations are followed. Regular risk assessments must be undertaken. Although daunting to start with, these requirements are actually quite simple and cheap to comply with and essential to avoid harm to staff or patients.

The dangers specific to the use of lasers for vessel occlusion are as follows:

- Permanent eye damage. Safety spectacles are essential for anyone in the room. These spectacles must protect against the specific wavelength of laser light being used.
- Collateral damage to other tissues (e.g., adjacent nerves, skin). Restrict energy delivered and apply copious tumescent anesthesia which acts as a heat sink and minimizes this risk.
- Fire. It is possible to set combustible materials alight by a stray laser beam. Skin cleaning solutions must be non-flammable.

Radiofrequency (Fig. 6.3)

Mode of action: this is akin to diathermy. Radiofrequency (RF) uses high-frequency alternating electric current passed through an electrode inserted into the vessel and positioned against the vessel wall. The electrical current passes through the vein wall and back into a second electrode on the instrument. The current causes heating of the tissue which has the same effect on the tissue as described under laser above. Like laser, the probe is inserted through a vascular sheath and the vessel wall is brought into contact with the probe by perivascular fluid injection.

The probe can be used like a guidewire and advanced directly to the target site. If this fails, conventional catheter and wire techniques are used to place a sheath at the target and the RF probe is inserted through this.

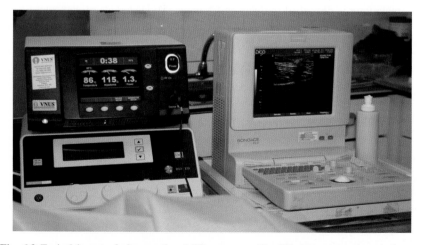

Fig. 6.3 Typical layout of ultrasound and RF generator. The RF generator settings indicate a temperature of 86° C, impedance of 115 Ω, and power of 1.3 watts

Monitoring Treatment

- As the tissue is heated, it dehydrates and the resistance to flow of electricity (impedance) increases.
- Sensors in the probe can also measure temperature within the tissue.
- The treatment is controlled by measurement of either impedance, temperature or a mixture of both.

Comparison of laser and radiofrequency for varicose veins		
	Laser	Radiofrequency
Capital cost	High	Low
Consumables cost	Low	High
Regulations of use	Tight	None specific
Vessel occlusion effectiveness	Almost 100%	Almost 100%
Serious complications	Very rare	More common (e.g., burns, deep venous thrombosis, nerve injury)
Minor side effects (bruising, discomfort)	Moderate	Very mild
Recanalization	Very rare	Very rare
Speed of procedure	10–30 min per leg	10–30 min per leg

Applications of Temperature-Induced Vessel Occlusion

By far and away the commonest application is in the treatment of varicose veins (the technique is described in detail in Chapter 45). Due to its effectiveness, ease of use, low cost, and permanence of heat-induced vessel occlusion, heat-induced vessel occlusion is likely to have an increasing role in the following:

- Fallopian tube occlusion for female sterilization
- Permanent ureteric occlusion to seal fistulae
- Certain arterial situations
- Hemorrhoids
- Gastric varices

Keypoints

- Laser and RF ablation are relatively new techniques that are likely to have an increasing role in endovascular therapy as well as tumor ablation.

- These techniques will be useful in cases where permanent occlusion is desirable; so like coils they should not be used when repeat vascular access is likely to be necessary.
- The limitations of these techniques will be due to difficulty accessing some of the target vessels with a sheath of sufficient size to allow the RF probe or laser fiber to be positioned. At present these will typically be 4–6 F for laser fibers, and 7F for RF probes.

Chapter 7
Future Embolic Therapies

Rajan Gupta and Louis Lucas

This chapter will consider potential future developments for embolotherapy. These could take the form of the following:

- Novel agents: these are covered in the other chapters in this section and include permanent embolic agents, particulate agents, and liquids. It is clear that there will be developments in all these areas which will

  o Improve the safety and efficacy of temporary and permanent vascular occlusion.
  o Increase the ability to deliver drugs to a target site as "magic bullets."

- Novel technologies: these might not be limited to embolization with the objective of vascular occlusion but rather to deliver therapeutic vectors which will modify or even cure disease processes. These are some of the most exciting potential avenues for interventional therapy. Examples include the following:

  o Gene therapy
  o Nanotechnology
  o Cellular infusion

Gene Therapy

The first clinical trials using gene therapy were in 1988 and evaluated the use of gene transfer to treat severe combined immunodeficiency (SCID). The fact that it is not widely practiced indicates that the obvious theoretical advantages may be difficult to achieve in practice. Gene therapy holds significant promise but many hurdles must be overcome before its widespread use in clinical practice hence this remains a highly theoretical and experimental field. Technical issues are not the only problem; there are significant emotive ethical issues which need to be overcome before gene therapy can become accepted.

Transcatheter Embolization and Therapy,
Techniques in Interventional Radiology, DOI 10.1007/978-1-84800-897-7_7,
© Springer-Verlag London Limited 2010

Mode of Action

Gene therapy involves either the modulation of existing genes or the transfer of foreign genetic material into patient's cells and tissues. The net result is modified protein expression (the gene product) with the purpose of treating disease. An obvious barrier to success is the limited effectiveness for multigene disorders!

Challenges lie ahead in terms of controlling the expression of any modified or induced genes in particular:

- *Sustained production of the gene product,* e.g., "cures" for systemic diseases such as cystic fibrosis. For this to occur, genes need to be integrated into viable long-term cell populations and expressed through subsequent generations of cells.
- *Limiting expression of the gene product.* Concern regarding the risk of tumorgenesis, uncontrolled gene expression is after all a cause of proliferation of cancer cells, e.g., use of vascular endothelial growth factor (VEGF) to promote neovascularization in patients with peripheral ischemia can lead to development of angiomas rather than useful collaterals.
- *Cell survival.* Populations of injected cells might ultimately be able to replace organ transplant for certain conditions. Unfortunately foreign cells are immunogenic and likely to be rejected unless the patient is treated with immunosuppressants.
  - o This has been the case in attempts to cure diabetes mellitus using islet-cell therapy and liver-cell therapy to treat acute liver failure.
  - o Use of modified cells derived form the patient in a manner akin to autologous marrow transplant would avoid this.

Mechanisms of Gene Transfer/Modulation

Two principal methods exist.

1. Transfer of foreign genetic material in order to replace deficient or faulty genes via

   - Genetically altered cells.
   - Viral and plasmid vectors. Viruses were first used because they have adapted the unique ability to insert their own genetic material into host DNA for replication.

2. Modulation of expression of existing genes using

   - Growth factors.
   - Nanotechnology.

Potential Roles for Interventional Radiology

- Direct injection of vectors into tumor or tissues.
- Selective intra-arterial or intravenous injection of altered cells or vectors

  o Early experiments in treating familial hypercholesterolemia consisted of harvesting a patient's liver tissue, genetically altering the cells outside the body, and infusing them back into the portal vein. Unfortunately, this trial was limited by negligible clinical effect.

- Use of embolic agents to enhance the potency of the gene therapy

  o Lipiodol administered with vectors has been shown to improve efficiency of cancer selective gene transfer in both rabbit and rat models.
  o This effect is thought to be related to prolonged dwell time of the vector in the neoplastic tissue.
  o Injection of adenoviral human hepatocyte growth factor soaked in gelatin sponge particles has also been shown to improve gene transfer. Prolonged dwell time and time-dependent decrease in Kupffer cell activity are thought to be possible mechanisms of action by gelatin sponge administration.

- Use of embolization to induce cell replication enhancing gene therapy

  o Gene therapy may be enhanced in replicating tissues. Several studies have shown that partial portal vein embolization induces hepatocyte replication in the nonembolized tissue (Chapter 41). In theory, genetic transfer may be increased in the nonembolized tissue demonstrating higher cell turnover.

- Use of stents/coils as platforms to deliver or act as vectors

  o Several investigations have shown that vectors can be attached to stents or coils.
  o Nanopatterning could be used to modify the surface of the implant into a biologically active material capable of modifying cellular behavior. For example the surface could be engineered to resemble a drug or cell receptor or gene product.
  o Many potential applications have been proposed, including inhibition of intimal hyperplasia could prevent in-stent restenosis, and promotion of intimal hyperplasia or enhanced matrix metalloproteinase inhibitors could promote stabilization of coiled aneurysms.

- Use of gene therapy for vascular embolization

  o In vivo mice models have induced selective tumor specific blood vessel coagulation resulting in massive tumor necrosis. Therefore, gene therapy could be used as a mechanism of vascular embolization.

Nanotechnology

Nanotechnology is an emerging highly multidisciplinary field based upon the construction of particles, devices or surfaces on the atomic or molecular level (generally <500 nm, often smaller). For reference, a RBC diameter is 6000–8000 nm. Nanopatterning has already been described above.

Nanoparticles

- It is important to emphasize that nanoparticles and nanocapsules are not generally intended as embolic agents because they are too small to cause vessel occlusion. Rather, they are engineered to make drugs more available and/or selective for tumors, while at the same time decreasing systemic toxicity.
- Nanoparticles can be administered either intra-arterially or directly into a tumor to maximize delivery to target tissues.
- It should be noted that the field of nanotechnology has markedly advanced the development and manufacturing of embolic materials, particularly in regards to the manufacturing of novel spherical and drug-eluting embolic devices.
- In the future, paramagnetic nanoparticles may be used for magnetic drug targeting and tumor imaging. Also, nanoparticles may be used as an adjunct in the targeted thermal ablation of tumors.

Keypoints

Gene therapy and nanotechnology are likely to evolve in parallel with developments in embolic agents and have the potential to radically alter the types of therapy provided by interventional radiology.

This will require interventional radiologists (IRs) to have a thorough understanding of the disease processes which they are involved in treating.

The natural inventiveness of IRs will lend itself to expanding the range of techniques and treatments in ways that will not occur to clinicians or scientists.

Recommended Readings/References

Abrahams, JM et al. Endovascular microcoil gene delivery using immobilized anti-adenovirus antibody for vector tethering. Stroke 2002;33: 1376–1382.

Brigger I, Dubernet C, Couvreur P. Nanoparticles in cancer therapy and diagnosis. Adv Drug Deliv Rev 2002; 54: 631–651.

Damascelli, B et al. Feasibility and efficacy of percutaneous transcatheter intraarterial chemotherapy with paclitaxel in albumin nanoparticles for advanced squamous-cell carcinoma of the oral cavity, oropharynx, and hypopharynx. J Vasc Interv Radiol 2007; 18: 1395–1403.

Gwinn, MR Nanoparticles: Health effects – pros and cons. Environ Health Perspect 2006; 114(12): 1818–1825.

Moghimi SM et al. Nanomedicine: Current status and future prospects. FASEB J 2005; 19: 311–330.

Park et al. Vascular administration of adenoviral vector soaked in absorbable gelatin sponge particles (GSP) prolongs the transgene expression in hepatocytes. Cancer Gene Therapy 2005; 12: 116–121.

Service RF. Nanotechnology takes aim at cancer. Science 2005; 310: 1132–1134.

Shiba H. et al. Efficient and cancer-selective gene transfer to hepatocellular carcinoma in a rat using adenovirus vector with iodized oil esters. Cancer Gene Therapy 2001 Oct; 8(10): 713–718.

Sinha R. Nanotechnology in cancer therapeutics: Bioconjugated nanoparticles for drug delivery. Mol Cancer Therapy 2006; 5(8): 1909–1917.

Wickline S, Neubauer, A. Applications of nanotechnology to atherosclerosis, thrombosis, and vascular biology. Arterioscler Thromb Vasc Biol 2006; 26: 435–441.

Chapter 8
Vascular Access, for Embolization: Techniques and Equipment

Nick Chalmers

A successful embolization procedure depends as much on achieving satisfactory catheterization of the required vessels as on delivering an appropriate embolic material. Successful catheterization depends on making the right decisions and on manual dexterity.

Decisions regarding equipment principally concern the types of catheter/s and guidewires required. The choice will be affected by many factors.

Catheter Choice

Several factors need to be considered in order to select the correct catheters for a particular case. These include the following:

- *The anatomy of the target vessel:* this requires careful pre-procedural preparation and review of all available imaging to determine the following:

  - Exactly which vessels are to be catheterized?
  - Factors likely to lead to difficulty during catheterization – angulation, tortuosity, stenosis, aneurismal dilatation, calcification?
  - The shapes of catheters that are likely to succeed (Fig. 8.1); this is discussed later.
  - Other factors such the length, torque control, and trackability of the catheter.
  - The optimal approach for the procedure.
  - In the absence of any pre-procedural imaging, selection of access route and equipment is a "best guess" based on previous experience.

- *The need for diagnostic angiography:* this will probably require a catheter with end and sideholes. These catheters may be non-selective such as a pigtail catheter or a selective shaped catheter. *Embolization should be performed using an endhole-only catheter.* Catheters with sideholes should not be used for embolization, particularly with coils: one end of the coil may emerge through a sidehole and the other through the endhole, making deployment impossible and requiring removal of the catheter.

Transcatheter Embolization and Therapy,
Techniques in Interventional Radiology, DOI 10.1007/978-1-84800-897-7_8,
© Springer-Verlag London Limited 2010

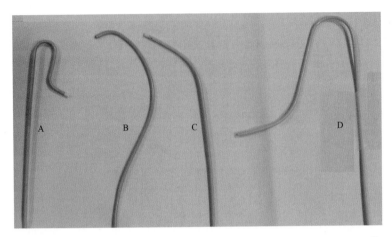

Fig. 8.1 Selective catheter shapes. This range of commonly used selective catheters will permit the great majority of selective catheterizations: (**a**) Sos or USL, (**b**) Cobra, (**c**) multipurpose or hockey-stick, (**d**) Sidewinder or Simmons 3

- *The type of embolic agent to be used:* the catheter must be compatible with the embolic agent in terms of lumen diameter, length, and material.

  - The catheter lumen must accommodate appropriate coil diameter and particle size.
  - The catheter must be chemically compatible with the agent; this is most important with liquid agents. For instance, lipiodol is used as an embolic agent in liver tumor chemoembolization and can be used to opacify cyanoacrylate glue. Lipiodol is made from poppy seed oil and has unpredictable effects on some catheter hubs, taps, and syringes, which can become very brittle and may fragment during the procedure, necessitating exchange of the catheter (Fig. 8.2). Onyx is suspended in DMSO which can also lead to catheter failure.

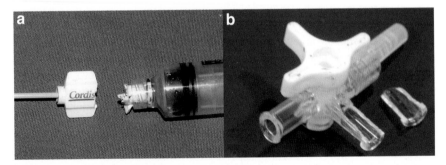

Fig. 8.2 Lipiodol effect on catheter hubs and taps. Fragmentation of the luer-lock hubs of a catheter (**a**) and a three-way tap (**b**) due to contact with Lipiodol

- Take care when using coils after other embolic agents, as any residual material in the lumen of the catheter may cause the coils to lodge in the catheter.

- *The need for a co-axial catheter system.* Make sure that

  - The chosen catheter/microcatheter will fit through your guiding catheter.
  - The chosen catheter/microcatheter is long enough to reach the target through the guiding catheter. This is a common source of frustration.
  - Guidewires and coil pushers are long enough to reach the target and also to allow catheter exchanges.

- *The need for adjunctive measures:*

  - Procedures such as balloon occlusion will influence access and sheath size.

In practice, it is useful to have a mental list of the available options so that if "Plan A" fails, one can move on to "Plan B" and so on.

Catheter Properties

A range of catheters with different properties is required. Remember, every operator has their individual preference and there is usually more than one way of working. It is important that you experiment with different approaches and become comfortable with at least one.

Catheter Shapes and Technical Tips

The shape of the catheter (Fig. 8.1) is initially often a "best guess" based on anatomy and operator's experience.

Reverse Curve Catheters

The celiac axis and superior mesenteric artery (SMA) often have a markedly downward course with sharp angulation at their origin. To negotiate this from the femoral artery requires a reverse curve catheter such as a sidewinder, a SosOmni or a visceral curve.

Technical note: Forming a sidewinder catheter: The sidewinder catheter requires a specific technique to reform its hook shape.

a. Advance the catheter over a guidewire up to the distal part of the aortic arch.
b. Pull back the guidewire into the shaft.
c. Simultaneously rotate and push the catheter from the groin until the tip doubles back on the shaft.
d. Pull back the catheter carefully under fluoroscopic control.

Care must be taken to prevent selection of an arch branch during this maneuver.

Remember that it may be simpler and safer to approach from the arm than to struggle to form a sidewinder catheter in a diseased aortic arch.

Double-curve catheters: less caudally angulated vessels such as the renal arteries require a less angulated catheter, such as a cobra or renal double-curve shape. These catheters do not have to be "formed" into shape.

Single-curve catheters: these are the simplest shapes to use and have a single bend; they are excellent for engaging forward-facing vessels and are typified by the multipurpose and Berenstein shapes.

Scenarios

It is impossible to cover every eventuality; however, some of the commonest encountered during embolization are included below. Remember that selective catheterization of youthful, elastic arteries is generally much easier than older, rigid, and calcified vessels. Vessels in younger patients are, however, more prone to spasm. A sharply angulated vessel will present little challenge when the arteries are healthy, but may prove very difficult or even impossible to catheterize when the arteries are diseased (especially if there is significant dilatation or stenosis).

Crossing the Aortic Bifurcation

The optimal catheter for crossing the aortic bifurcation will depend on the shape of the bifurcation and the elasticity of the arteries. In young women undergoing uterine artery embolization (UAE), the cobra or Roberts catheter is usually appropriate. Most operators will start from a right femoral approach and first catheterize the left uterine artery. In elderly patients or in patients who have undergone an aorto-bi-iliac/bifermoral bypass operation, a reverse curve catheter such as the SosOmni may be necessary.

Catheterizing the ipsilateral internal iliac artery: during UAE the cobra catheter can usually be used to select the ipsilateral internal iliac either in the normal fashion or by forming a "Waltman Loop." A Roberts catheter may also be used without forming a loop. In other scenarios, the contralateral approach is usually simpler.

Technical Note: Waltman Loop Technique

- With the catheter tip in the left internal iliac, advance the stiff end of a guidewire into the catheter as far as the aortic bifurcation.
- With the combination of a slight twist and a gentle push, the cobra catheter will form a loop in the aorta.

- Further pushing will advance the catheter tip into the lower abdominal aorta. The catheter can then be pulled back and steered into the right internal iliac artery.

Catheterizing the celiac axis and SMA using the sidewinder catheter: pull the catheter back until the tip engages the vessel origin. If you engage non-target aortic side branches, push the catheter back in to disengage and make small rotational adjustments before pulling back again.

Selective catheterization of a celiac artery branch requires further manipulation.

- Continued traction on the hub will pull the tip of the sidewinder further into one of the celiac branches, usually the splenic.
- In order to then catheterize the common hepatic artery
  - Either pull the catheter back at the groin until the curve of the catheter is lost, and so that the tip of the catheter is pulled back into the main celiac trunk. Repeated small injections of contrast will enable this to be done with precision. Remember that pulling back shortens the loop of the catheter and can lead to instability. The common hepatic artery can then be selected with a steerable guidewire (see below) and the catheter advanced into the hepatic artery by pushing it forward over the wire.
  - Or push the catheter back until the tip is in the celiac trunk, then use a wire to select the hepatic artery. The catheter is then pulled down along with the wire until the tip enters the hepatic artery.

Catheter Characteristics

Different stages in a procedure may require catheters with different mechanical properties. For example, accessing a visceral vessel, particularly in the presence of diseased or tortuous arteries, may require a catheter with a high degree of stiffness and torque control. However, advancing a catheter into a second- or third-order branch for selective embolization may require a catheter with different properties: flexibility, trackability, lubricity.

The handling properties of catheters vary considerably according to the following:

- *Diameter*: the French gauge of the catheter is its outer circumference in millimeters (or approximately the diameter in millimeters multiplied by three).
- *Construction*: material, braiding, shape, and coating.

In general, larger gauge catheters have greater stiffness, pushability, and torque control, whereas smaller gauge catheters will track over a guidewire into more tortuous anatomy. A 4 or 5Fr catheter is usually an appropriate first choice for selective catheterization of first- and second-order branches of the aorta.

Hydrophilic catheters are covered with the same coating as hydrophilic guidewires. This coating decreases friction between the outer catheter and the vessel wall, making selection of tortuous vessels easier. The trade-off (other than increased cost) is that hydrophilic catheters generally provide somewhat less torque than standard catheters.

Never hesitate to exchange catheters if you are having difficulty catheterizing a vessel or maneuvering within it. This will likely decrease the risk of catheter-induced complications such as spasm or dissection.

Microcatheters

These are very low-profile catheters that pass through standard catheters with an inner lumen diameter of 0.035 or 0.038″ (just under 1 mm or 3Fr). Many microcatheters are available with different wires and coatings. Figure 8.3 demonstrates the use of the Terumo Progreat microcatheter. This braided hydrophilic catheter has an outer diameter of 2.7Fr (0.9 mm) and an inner lumen diameter of 0.65 mm. It is supplied with a hydrophilic guidewire. Both the tip of the guidewire and the tip of the catheter can be shaped by the operator to conform to specific requirements.

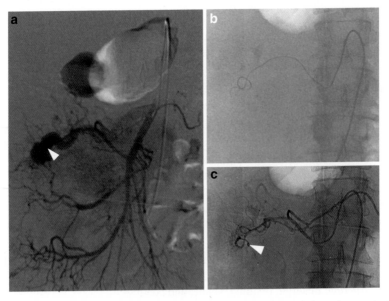

Fig. 8.3 Microcatheter in use. The microcatheter can be advanced through very tortuous anatomy. (**a**) An iatrogenic arterio-portal fistula is seen arising from a distal branch of the middle colic artery (*white arrowhead*). A sidewinder catheter has engaged the origin of the middle colic artery. (**b**) The microcatheter and guidewire combination has been advanced through tortuous anatomy to the fistula (*white arrowhead*) and (**c**) microcoils have been deployed to occlude it (*white arrowhead*)

Advantages of Microcatheters

1. *Unfavorable vascular anatomy*
   Selective catheterization of even second-order visceral branches may prove impossible with standard catheters in the presence of arterial disease, particularly in the elderly. However, if a stable catheter position can be achieved in the first-order branch, a microcatheter can be used to achieve a more selective position.
2. *Super selective catheterization*
   Microcatheters can be advanced into small distal vessels, sometimes through remarkably tortuous anatomy (Fig. 8.3). This enables very focused embolization.
3. *Maintaining antegrade flow during embolization*
   Uterine fibroid embolization can be accomplished in most cases using standard 4/5Fr catheters. Many operators favor a microcatheter to avoid wedging the catheter. This causes stasis within the uterine artery due to the small caliber of the vessel or due to concomitant spasm. This makes it impossible to judge the endpoint of embolization. On the other hand, due to their smaller size, embolic materials introduced through a microcatheter will not induce stasis so readily.
4. *Permitting multiple catheter exchanges without loss of access*
   Certain embolic agents (for example Onyx) cause catheter occlusion. If repeated injections are required, a new catheter must be used. The use of microcatheters enables exchange of the blocked catheter without losing the selective position achieved with the standard catheter.

Disadvantages of Microcatheters

1. *Reduced range and size of embolic agents*
   Standard embolization coils are designed for catheters with a 0.035″ lumen. Microcatheters therefore require microcoils; these have a lower volume for a given coil length and diameter and exert less radial force than conventional coils. Some particulate embolic material tends to clump, for example PVA particles (as opposed to microspheres) and gelatin sponge. This can block the microcatheter.
2. *Reduced contrast medium flow rates*
   Microcatheters can achieve flow rates of only about 3 ml/s at best using an injection pump. Hand injection of contrast requires high pressure, which usually entails using a 1-ml syringe. This limits the quality of diagnostic angiograms performed through a microcatheter.
3. *Cost*
   The use of microcatheters adds significantly to the cost of an embolization procedure.
4. *Vessel wall perforation*
   Microcatheter wires can quite easily produce vessel wall perforation. They should not be advanced against resistance.

Using Microcatheters

- The use of microcatheters requires stable catheterization of at least the first-order branch vessel with a standard catheter. Microcatheters cannot be used from the aorta directly.
- Microcatheters can be advanced using the guidewire and catheter in combination.
- There comes a point where it is possible to advance the guidewire, but the catheter fails to track over it.
- In this situation it is possible to get the catheter tip to advance further by a combination of pushing the catheter to compress it along its length and then pulling back on the wire. As the wire retracts, the catheter tip slides forward.
- The wire can then be advanced again and the procedure repeated stepwise. However, performing this procedure multiple times may lead to vessel spasm.

Occlusion Balloons

Some situations require occlusion of arterial inflow during embolization. Occlusion balloons are soft latex balloons with very different properties from the more familiar angioplasty balloons. Occlusion balloons may require a larger sheath size. They require only a small volume of dilute contrast material for inflation. There is very little resistance to inflation, so it is easy to over-inflate or burst them.

Uses of Occlusion Balloons in Embolization

1. To occlude arterial inflow in the renal artery prior to alcohol ablation of a kidney.
2. Prophylactically, prior to Caesarian section in high-risk cases (placenta accreta or percreta), occlusion balloons can be deployed uninflated in both internal iliac arteries. Following delivery, if there is major hemorrhage, the balloons can be inflated to control hemorrhage. The same catheters can be used to deliver embolic material such as gelatin sponge.

Vascular Sheaths and Guiding Catheters

These are used to facilitate vascular access, catheter exchange, and catheter stability.

- A vascular sheath with a hemostatic valve is useful for any selective catheterization procedure to facilitate catheter exchanges. A standard length (10 cm) short sheath is routine.
- *Sheath diameter*: the sizing of sheaths refers to the size of the lumen; thus, a 5Fr sheath will accommodate a 5Fr catheter. Choose a sheath with a lumen able to accommodate the largest catheter size anticipated; 5Fr is adequate for most applications. Rarely, a larger sheath will be required in particular circumstances

(see below). However, it makes sense to use the minimum sheath size in order to minimize the size of the arterial puncture.

- *Long sheaths*: although these are not usually required, they provide additional support for the catheter and may allow angiography around the catheter (e.g., contralateral internal iliac embolization may be facilitated by a long sheath (30–45 cm in length and 6Fr in size) positioned over the aortic bifurcation). This will provide some stability for the selective 5Fr catheter as well as having room around the catheter for injection of contrast medium for control angiograms during the procedure.
- *Shaped sheaths*: these are long sheaths with tips formed into a shape. The commonest is a single smooth curve "multipurpose" shape. The shape is used to help guide the catheter toward its target.
- *Guiding catheters*: these perform the same function as long sheaths and come in a variety of shapes akin to selective catheters.

  - The French size of a guide catheter refers to its outer diameter, not to the lumen. Thus a 5F catheter cannot pass through a 5F guiding catheter as it is of the same diameter.
  - The lumen diameter of a guiding catheter is usually given in inches and millimeters.
  - Many guiding catheters have to be introduced through a sheath!
  - Many guiding catheters do not come with any hemostatic valve. To use them, you need either a detachable valve or a Tuohy–Borst adapter.
  - Some guiding catheters come with an integral dilator and hemostatic valve and effectively function as a long sheath.

Do not forget that these are co-axial systems, and when using guiding catheters and long sheaths make sure that your working catheter is long enough to reach its target with the sheath in position.

Guidewires

A vast range of guidewires exists from non-steerable workhorses such as a standard 0.035″ 3 mm J-wire to exotic 0.010″ wires for use with microcatheters. Almost all wires needed for embolization are chosen for one of the following properties:

- Steerability
- Support
- Catheter exchange
- Microcatheterization
- Deploying embolization coils

Initial vascular access is typically obtained using a standard safety-J tip Teflon-coated steel guidewire.

A range of additional wires is required for selective catheterization and for catheter exchanges.

Steerable Hydrophilic Wires

The most useful wire for selective catheterization is the hydrophilic-coated nitinol wire exemplified by the Terumo Glidewire. When the wire is wet, the low friction coating enables it to be advanced into small branch vessels. The combination of slipperiness and springiness means that it has a propensity to end up on the floor. The most popular wire has an angled tip which is steered by rotating the wire. As it is extremely slippery, this is simplified by using a pin vise to grip the wire. Hydrophilic wires must be handled with care and steered rather than pushed in order to avoid causing arterial dissection or perforation. However, their properties have revolutionized selective catheterization; so practice will pay off.

Support Wires

These wires have stiffer shafts that are useful for maintaining position when introducing guide catheters and long sheaths. Remember that the stiffness is for supporting catheters and not for forcing across lesions. Support wires have floppy tips of variable lengths that protect the target vessel.

Exchange Wires

It is often necessary to exchange catheters during embolization procedures. This requires a longer wire. Remember that the properties that make hydrophilic wires so useful make it difficult to use them for catheter exchange. Once the target vessel has been catheterized, consider exchanging for a standard wire before swapping catheters.

Some operators favor the Cook Bentson wire for selective catheterization. It is of standard Teflon-coated steel construction but has a 6 cm atraumatic floppy tip with a stiffer shaft for pushability. The disadvantage of the Bentson wire is that it cannot be steered.

Keypoints

There is a large range of equipment that can help with embolization procedures.

Plan the approach and ensure that you have appropriate

- Catheters: shapes, lengths, handling properties, and diameters.
- Guidewires: selective, steerable, hydrophilic and supportive.
- Embolic material to use with the catheters.

Make sure you achieve a stable catheter position before embolizing.

Chapter 9
Pre-procedure Imaging: When, Why, and How?

James Jackson

Introduction

Most of the chapters in Section 2 will outline imaging related to a specific clinical scenario. This chapter and the subsequent chapter on "Trauma Imaging" (Chapter 10) will focus on the philosophy behind the imaging strategies. The clinical scenarios chosen to illustrate this are some of the less common indications for embolization and those in which contemporary imaging is of particular benefit and likely to change clinical practice.

Pre-procedure Imaging: When?

Pre-embolization imaging should be performed whenever it is likely to provide information that will simplify the procedure, improve its outcome, and reduce complications.

Pre-procedure Imaging: Why?

There are several common indications for embolization, including the treatment of primary and secondary liver tumors and uterine fibroid disease, where the major role of pre-procedural cross-sectional imaging by CT and/or MR is to demonstrate the extent of the disease; these applications will not be discussed further.

In other circumstances, the target vessel will be obvious, e.g., the source of hemorrhage following a renal or liver biopsy and there will be less benefit from pre-procedure imaging. It follows then that the major benefit will be in patients in whom

- There is uncertainty regarding the target for embolotherapy.
- There is uncertainty regarding the vascular anatomy.
- The embolization procedure is likely to be complex.

Transcatheter Embolization and Therapy,
Techniques in Interventional Radiology, DOI 10.1007/978-1-84800-897-7_9,
© Springer-Verlag London Limited 2010

This is the case in several scenarios including gastrointestinal bleeding, trauma, and hemoptysis. The answer to "why?" is also to make patient care simpler and safer by the following:

- Demonstrating the cause of the clinical problem
- Demonstrating the target vascular anatomy
- Deciding whether endovascular therapy is indicated
- Anticipating the approach, equipment, and techniques which will be required for effective treatment

Pre-procedure Imaging: How?

Having decided that imaging is desirable, the focus shifts to how to image the patient. A full description of contemporary imaging techniques is beyond the scope of this book, but important points relating to the particular clinical scenarios presented below will be discussed.

- It is important for interventional radiologists to recognize that they will increasingly be required to
  - o Advise on the most suitable imaging, be familiar with local protocols, and be involved with the introduction of new imaging algorithms.
  - o Interpret the resultant studies.

In essence, the interventional radiologist will need to have high-level diagnostic skills coupled with clinical acumen and the ability to triage patients to treatment of the highest priority problem.

Less than a decade ago, the only pre-embolization imaging in the acute situation would be a diagnostic angiogram. Improvements in the availability, speed, and quality of non-invasive imaging modalities have transformed the situation. Multidetector computed tomography (MDCT) has had a dramatic effect on transcatheter embolization practice. With MDCT, data can be acquired during arterial and/or venous phases of contrast medium enhancement and images can almost instantly be reconstructed in any plane. These reformats greatly simplify interpretation of the images and will also give an overview of the arterial anatomy; this is invaluable in planning the optimal approach and best technique for successful treatment. Remember when making image reformats that their quality is dependent on using the source data from the scan rather than the reduced dataset which is available following reconstruction as thick slices.

In contemporary practice, it is essential to be familiar with the use of the computer console to perform the common image reconstructions and to make measurements from them.

Imaging Technique

Clearly the most suitable imaging modality will vary depending upon the pathology requiring embolization, and examinations will often have to be specifically tailored to the patient but a little time spent planning how to obtain the most appropriate and best quality images will often save considerable time during the subsequent interventional procedure.

Contrast Enhancement

Intravascular contrast medium will be necessary in the majority of pre-embolization imaging examinations but important exceptions include the assessment of venous and lymphatic malformations by magnetic resonance imaging (Chapters 17 and 46) and the diagnosis and pre-embolization planning of pulmonary arterio-venous malformations (Chapter 15). An initial unenhanced study is advisable in certain instances including the imaging of patients with acute gastrointestinal hemorrhage (vide infra). Positive oral contrast should be avoided as this may mimic or obscure a source of bleeding.

Clinical Scenarios

Thoracic Embolization

Hemoptysis

Pre-procedure Imaging: When?

While pre-procedural imaging should not delay a patient with ongoing hemorrhage from undergoing bronchial artery embolization, the majority of individuals will stabilize after an initial bleed and MDCT should then be performed.

Pre-procedure Imaging: Why?

Demonstrating the target vascular anatomy

- *Bronchial artery anatomy.* This is highly variable and may be difficult to assess accurately on a catheter thoracic aortogram at the time of embolization because of respiratory movement.
    - ○ Hypertrophied bronchial arteries are usually well visualized on axial, coronal, and sagittal reformatted images on a good-quality CT scan.
    - ○ Conventional and anomalous bronchial artery origins can be documented.
- *Non-bronchial systemic artery supply.* Hypertrophied "non-bronchial" systemic arteries providing a transpleural supply to areas of abnormal lung are a common finding in patients with severe hemoptysis due to chronic inflammatory pulmonary disease. Even when they are hypertrophied, these vessels are easily overlooked on CT unless specifically assessed.

- o The vessels most commonly recruited include the intercostal, internal mammary, costocervical, thoracic branches of the axillary and inferior phrenic arteries.
- *Pulmonary arterial abnormality.* Pulmonary artery pseudoaneurysmal disease occurs in approximately 10% of this group of patients.
  - o Pulmonary artery pseudoaneurysms may be small and very difficult to visualize on CT especially as they are often in very diseased and disorganized lung.
  - o Larger pulmonary artery pseudoaneurysms often fill very sluggishly and may be much more difficult to see on pulmonary arteriography, particularly if later images are degraded by motion artifact, a common problem in this group of patients (Fig. 9.1).
- *Side and site of hemorrhage.* Although it may be useful to know the side and site of hemorrhage, this is not essential before bronchial artery embolization as it is usual to occlude all hypertrophied bronchial and non-bronchial systemic arteries at the time of the procedure.

Anticipating the approach, equipment, and techniques which will be required for effective treatment

- Recognition of a hypertrophied bronchial artery arising from, for example, the undersurface of the aortic arch can save a great deal of time during the subsequent procedure (Fig. 9.2).
- The demonstration of hypertrophied non-bronchial systemic arteries will alert the angiographer that a variety of catheter shapes may be required (e.g., an internal mammary catheter).
- The knowledge that a pulmonary artery pseudoaneurysm is present on pre-procedural CT means that pulmonary artery catheterization will almost certainly be necessary, as embolization of co-existent hypertrophied bronchial arteries alone is rarely sufficient to prevent recurrent bleeding. Hence arterial and venous access will be required.

Pre-procedure Imaging: How?

The most common protocol would be to perform a volume acquisition study during the aortic phase of contrast medium enhancement, but ideally pulmonary arterial phase images should also be obtained for the reasons discussed above.

Pulmonary Arterio-venous Malformations (PAVMs)—Treatment of PAVM Is Covered in Chapter 15

Pre-procedure Imaging: When?

There are three main indications for imaging.

- To image the patient before embolotherapy
- To follow-up the patient after treatment
- To screen patients' relatives for PAVM

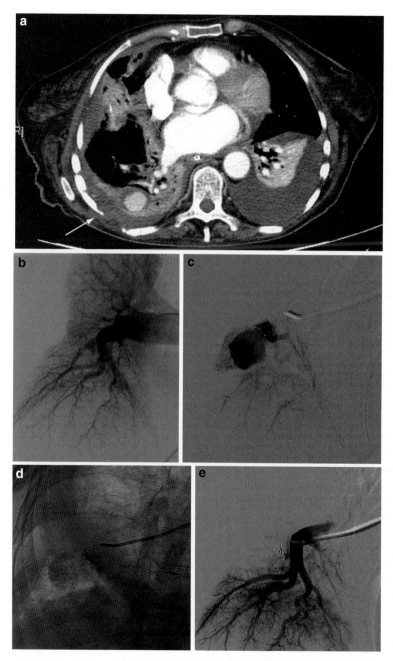

Fig. 9.1 Fifty-eight-year-old lady with massive hemoptysis following thoracoscopic drainage of right-sided empyema. (**a**) Contrast-enhanced MDCT demonstrates large pulmonary artery pseudoaneurysm in the right lower lobe (*arrow*). (**b**) Selective right pulmonary artery angiogram does not show the aneurysmal cavity. (**c**) Superselective arteriogram with the catheter tip in a subsegmental right lower lobe pulmonary artery branch demonstrates the pseudoaneurysmal cavity. (**d** and **e**) Control film and angiogram after coil embolization demonstrate successful occlusion of the pseudoaneurysm with preservation of normal adjacent pulmonary artery branches

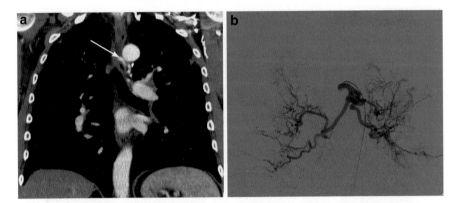

Fig. 9.2 Seventy-two-year-old man with pulmonary fibrosis and massive hemoptysis. (**a**) Coronal MDCT reformation shows hypertrophied bronchial artery (*arrow*) arising from the inferior aspect of the aortic arch. (**b**) Selective arteriogram of this hypertrophied anomalous combined right and left bronchial arteries trunks prior to embolization

Pre-procedure Imaging: Why?

Pre-procedural CT is extremely helpful to document the number and size of treatable lesions.

- *Number of feeding vessels.* There is often a dominant feeding artery to a PAVM but it is not uncommon to find additional small feeders, which may arise from a different segmental pulmonary artery branch, which will continue to perfuse the venous sac. These will gradually enlarge over time if missed and left untreated. A knowledge of the presence of multiple feeding arteries before intervention is very helpful so that this is avoided (Fig. 9.3).
- *Number of malformations.* CT is now the gold-standard imaging modality when it comes to the demonstration of treatable PAVMs. If there are no treatable malformations in one lung, then selective proximal pulmonary angiography of that side is unnecessary, thereby reducing radiation and contrast dose and procedural time.
  Deciding whether endovascular therapy is indicated
- *PAVM size.* Remember that it is the size of the feeding artery to a PAVM, rather than its venous sac, that is important when assessing these lesions and determining their suitability for treatment. It is generally recommended that all PAVMs with feeding arteries of 3 mm or greater in size are treated, as these are more likely to be a route for paradoxical embolization. Knowledge of the approximate diameter of the feeding arteries to each PAVM can be very helpful when determining the most appropriate embolic agent to use.
- *Exclusion of PAVM mimics.* Although PAVMs have characteristic features on CT with dilated feeding and draining vessels and an intervening venous sac, there are two uncommon lesions which may be a trap for the unwary and result in a referral for inappropriate angiography.

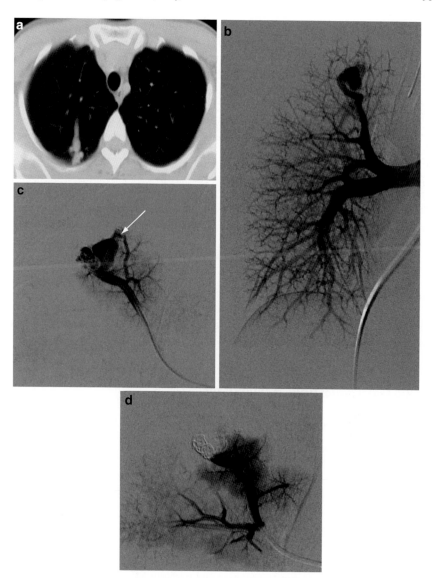

Fig. 9.3 Thirty-two-year-old lady with hereditary hemorrhagic telangiectasia and a single right upper lobe PAVM. (**a**) Single axial image from an unenhanced thoracic CT demonstrates a lobulated venous sac and a large outflow vein. Other images (not shown) suggested the presence of a dominant feeding artery with an adjacent smaller branch also supplying the venous sac. (**b**) Selective right pulmonary artery angiogram shows a single PAVM at the right lung apex with a dominant feeding artery. (**c**) Selective pulmonary angiogram after coil occlusion of the dominant feeding artery at the neck of the malformation shows persistent sac perfusion from an adjacent small vessel (*arrow*). (**d**) Selective pulmonary arteriogram after coil embolization of both feeding arteries confirms complete occlusion of the PAVM

o *Congenital pulmonary varix:* this is an intrapulmonary collateral vein bypassing a segment of atretic pulmonary vein. Close scrutiny of these vessels and
their communications will allow their correct diagnosis.
o *Congenital bronchial atresia:* the expanded branching bronchi distal to the
atretic segment will often contain fluid of high attenuation which may be
mistaken for vascular enhancement on a contrast-enhanced CT. The correct
diagnosis will usually be suggested by the fact that the branching bronchi do
not reach the lung hilum and that there is an area of surrounding hypertransra-
diancy due to air-trapping.

Pre-procedure Imaging: How?

Contrast enhancement is unnecessary. A volume acquisition during a single breath-
hold is all that is required and the study is best viewed on a workstation in axial,
coronal, and sagittal planes.

Abdominal Embolization

The two acute scenarios which require urgent assessment and intervention are acute
gastrointestinal tract hemorrhage and trauma.

Acute Gastrointestinal Hemorrhage

Pre-procedure Imaging: When?

Patients with recurrent episodes of acute gastrointestinal hemorrhage in whom
endoscopy has failed to determine the source are one of the most frustrating groups
in interventional radiology. By the time these patients have been admitted to hospital, bleeding has often stopped and visceral angiography is negative. MDCT has
become an invaluable tool in the management of these individuals and has become
the imaging procedure of first choice in many centers when endoscopy is negative
for the following reasons:

- *Time*: it is usually quicker to organize and perform MDCT than formal catheter
angiography.
- *Safety*: MDCT is less invasive and can be more easily repeated.
- *Sensitivity*: MDCT is almost certainly more sensitive than formal angiography at
determining the source and/or cause of hemorrhage because of the following:
  o Rapid access to imaging increases the likelihood of continuing bleeding at the
  time of study.
  o Reduction in respiratory artifact.
  o Demonstration of other significant pathology, for example, liver cirrhosis,
  varices, inflammatory or neoplastic bowel disease.

Pre-procedure Imaging: Why?

Demonstrating the target vascular anatomy

- Variants of normal visceral arterial anatomy are extremely common and should be looked for, as they may affect subsequent embolization.
  Anticipating the approach, equipment, and techniques which will be required for effective treatment
  - o The demonstration of the source of contrast medium extravasation helps considerably when performing embolization as this area can be targeted from the very beginning of the procedure.
  - o Close scrutiny of the vascular anatomy on axial, coronal, and sagittal reformatted images can be extremely useful to help plan the most appropriate route and catheter for subsequent catheter angiography and embolization (Fig. 9.4).
  - o For example, the demonstration of a pseudoaneurysm of the inferior pancreatico-duodenal artery originating from the first jejunal artery would suggest that a catheter with a "Cobra" configuration catheter might be the most suitable to start with, while an area of contrast medium extravasation within the distal transverse colon originating from an accessory middle colic artery might be best approached using a "Sidewinder"-shaped catheter.
  Deciding whether endovascular therapy is indicated
  - o MDCT allows appropriate referral for further therapy. In many cases this will be embolization, but occasionally a source of hemorrhage will suggest that an endoscopic or surgical approach is more appropriate (Fig. 9.5).
  - o In the absence of active extravasation, important underlying pathology may be identified but might be subtle. For example, a Meckel's diverticulum causing intermittent, short-lived episodes of acute hemorrhage may easily be missed unless specifically searched for with the help of multiplanar reformatted images (Fig. 9.6).
  - o Absence of a source of hemorrhage on MDCT makes it unlikely that catheter angiography performed immediately afterwards will be contributory.

Pre-procedure Imaging: How?

Timing. The best chance of "catching" active contrast medium extravasation is when there are clinical signs of ongoing hemorrhage, i.e., when the patient is hypotensive with a shock index (heart rate/systolic blood pressure) of >1. Clinicians involved with the patient's resuscitation should be aware of the importance of performing this study as soon as it is safe to do so. If the patient is "fit enough" to allow transfer to the radiology department for angiography and embolization, then they should undergo CT while the interventional suite is being prepared.

Technique. Volumetric acquisitions through the entire abdomen and pelvis should be performed without intravenous contrast medium and then during the arterial and portal venous phases of contrast medium enhancement. Oral contrast should not be used. Important points regarding image interpretation are as follows:

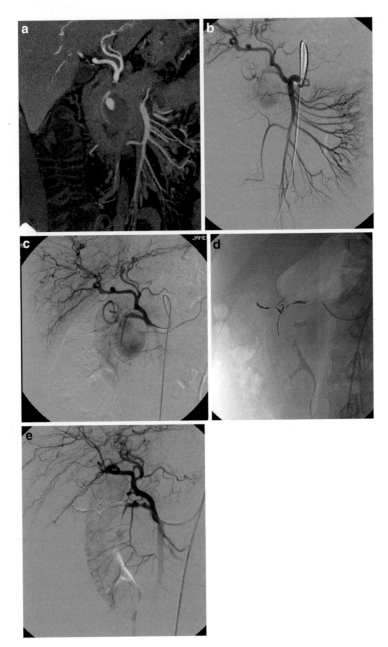

Fig. 9.4 Thirty-year-old man with several episodes of upper gastrointestinal hemorrhage during recovery from acute pancreatitis. (**a**) MDCT coronal reformatted image demonstrates a pseudoaneurysm arising from the gastroduodenal artery. Other images (not included) showed anomalous visceral arterial anatomy with the common hepatic artery arising from the proximal superior mesenteric artery. (**b**) Selective superior mesenteric artery angiogram confirms the anomalous anatomy and shows faint filling of the pseudoaneurysm cavity which has markedly increased in size

Fig. 9.5 Seventy-year-old man with massive bright red blood loss per rectum. Lower GI endoscopy before imaging showed copious blood but no source. (**a** and **b**) Axial and sagittal images obtained during the arterial phase of contrast medium enhancement show rapid contrast medium extravasation in the low rectum. A repeat endoscopy confirmed an actively bleeding rectal ulcer which was successfully treated

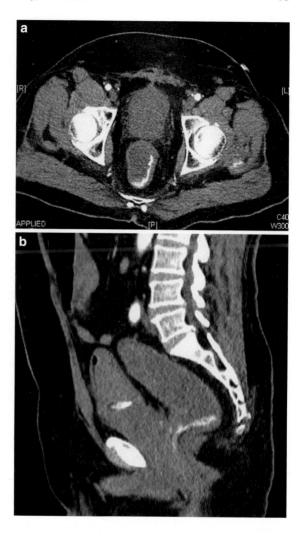

- Active contrast medium extravasation is most commonly seen on the arterial phase images but it can be subtle and may only be visualized during careful comparison of both the post-contrast and unenhanced studies (Fig. 9.7). Reformatted images often make the bleeding and the underlying cause much more obvious.

Fig. 9.4 (continued) since the MDCT. (**c**) A selective common hepatic artery angiogram shows the anatomy in greater detail. (**d** and **e**) Control film and angiogram after embolization confirm complete exclusion of the pseudoaneurysm from the circulation with coils in three separate branch vessels immediately beyond the pseudoaneurysm neck and within the distal gastroduodenal artery with preservation of the retroduodenal artery arising more proximally

Fig. 9.6 Twenty-eight-year-old
man with intermittent
episodes of acute lower GI
hemorrhage. MDCT
performed soon after
admission following further
bleed when patient
hemodynamically stable.
(**a** and **b**) Axial and coronal
images do not demonstrate
active contrast medium
extravasation but a
blind-ending fluid-filled
viscus is seen in the right
lower abdomen consistent
with a Meckel's diverticulum
confirmed at subsequent
surgery

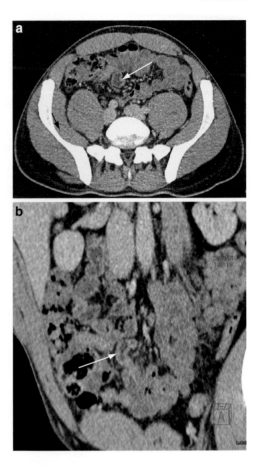

- The unenhanced study is also important so that high-attenuation material within the bowel lumen, such as vicariously excreted contrast medium following previous imaging, is not mistaken for active extravasation.
- Following surgery, think what anatomical changes will be present and also the likely source of bleeding.

Trauma (see also Chapter 10)

The advent of MDCT has been described as the greatest advance in trauma care that has occurred in the last 25 years. It has resulted in *diagnostic* angiography becoming almost obsolete, as most significant vascular injuries will be identified but, along with a trend toward non-surgical management, there has been an increase in the indications for embolization. The major indication for embolization following accidental or iatrogenic abdominal trauma is arterial bleeding from the liver, spleen, or kidneys. Severe bleeding following percutaneous biopsy of the liver or kidney is uncommon but, when it occurs, is generally easily controlled by

Fig. 9.7 Sixty-seven-year-old man with intermittent episodes of bright red bleeding per rectum. Pre- and post-contrast medium axial images demonstrate a subtle area of active contrast medium extravasation into a mid-transverse colon diverticulum (*arrow*) which would have been difficult to appreciate without the unenhanced study

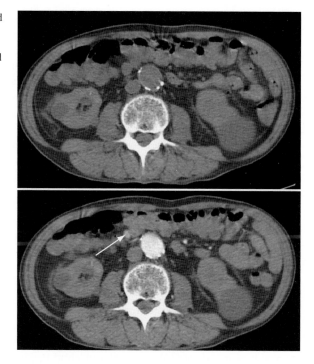

selective embolization. Pre-procedural imaging is rarely necessary, as the cause of sudden hemodynamic collapse within a few hours of biopsy is usually obvious; such patients should be transferred to the interventional suite for embolization as soon as possible after initial resuscitation. All other individuals with evidence of hemorrhage following accidental trauma or surgery should be assessed by MDCT before proceeding to embolization.

Pre-procedure Imaging: How?

Several algorithms are listed in the table in Chapter 10 (p. 108). The MDCT technique utilized needs to be tailored to the patient and will depend upon the nature of the trauma but, in the majority of cases, images obtained during the arterial phase of contrast medium enhancement are the most helpful.

Deciding whether endovascular therapy is indicated

Important points regarding image interpretation include the following:

- Active contrast medium extravasation within the liver and spleen is usually obvious and is an indication for urgent angiography and embolization.
- Pseudoaneurysms within the substance of the liver and spleen may be small but are usually easily visualized and are, once again, an indication for urgent angiography and embolization as they are at high risk of re-bleeding.

- Prophylactic splenic artery embolization is unnecessary in the absence of active contrast medium extravasation and pseudoaneurysm formation even in the presence of a high-grade splenic injury.
- A pseudoaneurysm involving the extrahepatic portion of the right hepatic artery is most commonly iatrogenic and is well recognized after laparoscopic cholecystectomy, particularly if there is a concomitant bile duct injury. It is at high risk of rupture causing extrahepatic hemorrhage or hemobilia, if it communicates with the biliary tree and should be treated by embolization. Such pseudoaneurysms may be small and difficult to visualize unless specifically looked for with the aid of multiplanar and 3D reconstructions.

True Aneurysms of the Visceral Arteries

True aneurysms of the visceral arteries are rare and are often an incidental finding on cross-sectional imaging. The splenic artery is the visceral vessel most commonly involved followed by extrahepatic and renal artery aneurysms.

Pre-procedure Imaging: When?

While the risk of hemorrhage from true visceral artery aneurysms is not known, it is recognized that their rupture is more common during pregnancy and in patients undergoing liver transplantation. Treatment of aneurysms of 2 cm in diameter or greater is recommended in women of child-bearing age who wish to become pregnant at some stage and in persons undergoing liver transplantation.

The indications for treatment outside these patient groups are not as clear-cut, but therapy is generally advised for aneurysms of greater than 2.5 cm in diameter, those who show a gradual increase in size on follow-up and those associated with symptoms due, for example, to peripheral embolic events.

Pre-procedure Imaging: Why?

If the decision has been made that treatment is necessary and that an endovascular approach is the most appropriate, pre-procedural imaging is essential in order to document completely the anatomy of the aneurysm, plan the best route of access, and ensure availability of all the equipment (sheaths, catheters, guidewires, and embolization agents) which is likely to be required to ensure a successful outcome.

Pre-procedure Imaging: How?

MDCT during the arterial phase of contrast medium enhancement should be performed through the area of interest, and multiplanar and 3D reconstructions should be viewed on a workstation. Important points regarding image interpretation include the following:

- Proximal parent vessel anatomy. Embolization is most commonly performed via a common femoral artery approach, but occasionally approach will be more favorable from the arm when the visceral artery requiring catheterization has an acutely angled origin from the aorta. Compression of the celiac axis origin by the median arcuate ligament of the hemidiaphragm is relatively common and its recognition on pre-procedural CT may indicate that an arm approach may be necessary. Look carefully for stenosis of the celiac axis and/or the superior mesenteric artery origins in the presence of pancreatico-duodenal artery aneurysmal disease.

- Vascular anatomy around the aneurysm neck.
  - Visceral arterial disease typically occurs at bifurcations (particularly common in splenic and renal arteries), and a complete understanding of the anatomy of such aneurysms before intervention is essential in order to determine the most suitable technique of embolization.

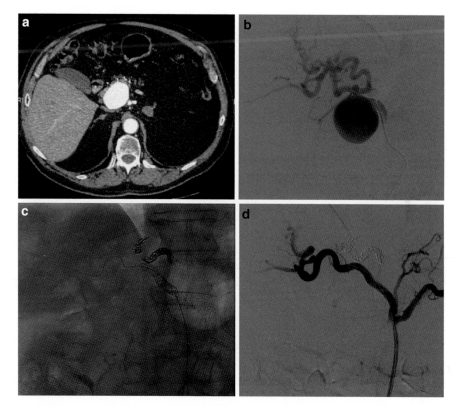

Fig. 9.8 Sixty-nine-year-old man with an incidental finding of a large hepatic artery aneurysm during investigation of renal pathology. (**a**) Axial image from arterial phase MDCT shows large aneurysm of common hepatic artery. Other images (not included) showed complex distal anatomy involving the bifurcation into the right and left hepatic arteries. (**b**) Selective common hepatic artery confirms extension of the aneurysm up to its bifurcation. (**c** and **d**) Control film and arteriogram after coil embolization of the left hepatic artery and the placement of covered stents from the proximal common hepatic artery into the right hepatic artery showing successful exclusion of the aneurysm

o The most common endovascular method of treating visceral arterial aneurysmal disease is by occlusion of the parent vessel on either side of the aneurysm's neck. Recognition of a complex branching anatomy before the procedure makes it more likely that the aneurysm will be completely excluded and that a vessel allowing continued sac perfusion is not missed.

o Pre-procedural CT might, however, suggest that the anatomy favors a different technique such as the embolization of the smaller of two distal arteries and then complete exclusion of the aneurysm by inserting a covered stent to maintain patency of the dominant branch vessel (Fig. 9.8).

o Alternatively, the CT may suggest that the use of a liquid polymer, injected into the aneurysm during protection of the main vessel lumen and distal branches by a balloon inflated across its neck, may provide a more successful method of treatment.

- Aneurysm neck size. This may be difficult to measure accurately on CT but it is usually possible to obtain some idea about the size of the defect in the parent vessel and determine how easy or difficult it is likely to "pack" the aneurysmal sac with embolic material without distal migration.

Keypoints

- *When*: Regardless of the indication for embolization, pre-procedure imaging is almost invariably helpful and should be performed whenever possible. It is especially helpful in the management of patients with acute gastrointestinal hemorrhage and abdominal trauma.
- *Why*: Accurate assessment of normal and variant anatomy and vascular pathology before intervention will often affect decisions regarding choice of approach and embolization technique resulting in a more targeted, shorter, safer, and successful procedure.
- *How*: Multidetector CT has had a dramatic effect on a wide range of embolization procedures because of its ability to produce exquisite multiplanar and 3D images. The technique must be tailored to the clinical issues to be resolved.

Suggested Further Reading

1. Remy-Jardin M, Bouaziz N, Dumont P, Brillet PY, Bruzzi J, Remy J. Bronchial and nonbronchial systemic arteries at multidetector row CT angiography: comparison with conventional angiography. Radiology 2004;233:741–9.

2. Khalil A, Parrot A, Nedelcu C, Fartoukh M, Marsault C, Carette MF. Severe haemoptysis of pulmonary arterial origin: signs and role of multidetector row CT angiography. Chest
   2008;133:212–9.
3. Jaeckle T, Stuber G, Hoffmann MH, Freund W, Schmitz BL, Aschoff AJ. Acute gastrointestinal
   bleeding: value of MDCT. Abdom Imaging. 2008;33:285–93.
4. Marmery H, Shanmuganathan K. Multidetector-row computed tomography imaging of splenic
   trauma. Semin Ultrasound CT MR. 2006;27:404–19.

Chapter 10
Imaging the Severely Injured Patient

Tony Nicholson

Introduction

This chapter focuses on the importance of imaging and intervention in the diagnosis and management of the severely injured patient. The conclusions are at variance with those currently recommended in the Advanced Trauma Life Support for Doctors Manual (ATLS) and are intended to be thought provoking and challenge the existing dogma.

Death from Trauma

Trauma is a major cause of death across all age groups. The primary determinant of survival and better quality of life for such trauma patients is the time from being injured to receiving definitive treatment by either surgery or intervention in a center with the appropriate specialist staff and equipment.

Trauma-related death has a trimodal distribution (Fig. 10.1).

- Many patients have unsurvivable injuries and die immediately at the scene of the accident.
- A second early mortality peak occurs within the first 24 h.
  - Death in both these groups results from predictable mechanisms, usually injury to the central nervous system and large vessels. Trauma victims who reach hospital alive are at risk of dying from internal hemorrhage during the 1 h after admission.
- The third mortality peak after days or weeks often results from poor hemorrhage control and management within the first 24 h. This eventually leads to multiorgan failure and subsequent death.

Transcatheter Embolization and Therapy,
Techniques in Interventional Radiology, DOI 10.1007/978-1-84800-897-7_10,
© Springer-Verlag London Limited 2010

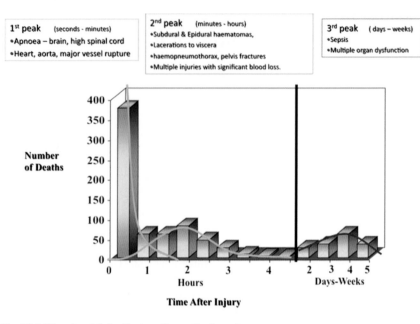

Fig. 10.1 The trimodal distribution of mortality in major trauma

Rationale for Early Imaging

- *Primary objective* is demonstration of
  - ○ Ongoing internal hemorrhage
  - ○ Other immediately life-threatening conditions
- *Secondary objective* is
  - ○ Recognition of all injuries present
  - ○ Ranking of injuries according to their clinical significance

Optimal Imaging

Whole-body multi-sliced CT scanning with contrast should become routine in all but the most unstable patient with multiple injuries. This will reveal the source of hemorrhage, demonstrate unsuspected injuries, speed up definitive care, and reduce additional unnecessary investigations.

This is at variance with the seventh edition of the Advanced Trauma Life Support for Doctors Manual (ATLS) which still recommends plain-film radiography in the severely injured patient, diagnostic peritoneal lavage as one method of determining whether a patient is actively bleeding, and states that MDCT should only be used when a patient is hemodynamically stable.

Evidence for this change in practice is emerging. One recent study by Weninger et al. evaluated 185 trauma patients managed conventionally as per ATLS protocols, and 185 managed by initial stabilization and early MDCT. Accurate diagnosis was significantly faster and emergency-room occupancy shorter in the group undergoing early MDCT. As a result, ITU stays and ventilation days were shorter and rates of organ failure significantly lower in the early MDCT group.

Specifics of Trauma Imaging

1. Conventional radiography

Following primary survey, imaging protocols at admission, which include frontal chest X-ray, AP pelvic, thoracolumbar and cervical spine series, are only applicable to patients who

- Are not severely injured
- Have Glasgow Coma scores of 15
- Normal pulse and blood pressure
- Can move all four limbs

Plain films add little information if a patient is going to have early CT scanning with appropriate protocols, early reconstructions, and early expert reporting.

2. Ultrasound

Focused assessment with sonography for trauma (FAST) is recommended by ATLS

- To identify the presence of free intraperitoneal, pleural, or pericardial fluid that is usually due to hemorrhage.
  However
- Fluid can easily be missed, particularly in the pelvis where volumes of up to 5 l can be missed.
- Thus, a FAST scan has low negative predictive value.
- Positive FAST scan indicates hemoperitoneum but does not identify the source of bleeding.

If a patient is going to have an MDCT scan, then the addition of pre-CT ultrasound and plain-film radiography simply introduces delay.

3. Contrast-enhanced multidetector computed tomography
   Scanning protocols (Appendix).

- Should include the head, neck, thorax, abdomen, and pelvis.
- Head scanning is performed without contrast and may require gantry angulation.

- Single arterial phase scans of neck, thorax, abdomen, and pelvis are performed following head scanning. The lower limbs are not routinely included unless there is continued bleeding or obvious ischemia.
- Bowel contrast is unnecessary. Many bowel injuries can be diagnosed by subtle changes in the bowel wall and gas pattern. Bowel injuries frequently only become apparent or clinically significant in the first 12 h. At that time, repeat scanning with oral contrast can be focused on intestinal complications.

Image Reconstruction

- Reconstructions should be performed routinely.
- During reconstruction, important head injuries, cervical spine injuries, and thoracolumbar spine injuries can be looked for and diagnosed.
- Reconstructions in coronal, sagittal, and oblique planes aid the diagnosis and classification of pelvic fractures.

What to Look For

Primary survey: remember that the purpose of this scan is to reveal those injuries that are immediately life threatening! In addition to the brain and spine, the following must be sought:

- *Active bleeding from*
  - Solid organs (Chapter 27 on solid organ trauma)
  - Fractures (Chapter 25 on pelvic trauma)
  - GI tract
  - Blood vessels (see Chapter 26 on extremity trauma)
- *Injuries likely to hemorrhage*
  - o Traumatic aortic injury including partial thickness tears
  - o Damaged arteries at any site; this includes vascular occlusions (see Chapter 26 on extremity trauma and Chapter 25 on pelvic trauma), which usually indicate significant arterial injury
  - o False aneurysm
- *Look particularly closely where there are injuries associated with increased risk of hemorrhage or important early morbidity*
  - o Injuries to solid organs. These can generally be managed conservatively if there is no active contrast extravasation and the patient is hemodynamically stable
  - o Fractured pancreas
  - o Bowel perforation or ischemia

Secondary Survey

- If the patient remains hamodynamically unstable, and no cause is noted from the primary survey, then repeat the primary survey and perform a delayed scan! The patient will still be on the CT table.
- Suspected bladder trauma can be investigated by CT cystography. This must not be performed until after active bleeding is excluded, as free contrast in the pelvis from a ruptured bladder may mask the site of bleeding during angiography and embolization.

4. Angiography
Indication for angiography

It should be accepted that angiography is no longer a diagnostic test and is simply a precursor to intervention. If intervention is not going to be performed, angiography has little value.

- CT should be used to determine whether angiography is required.
- Modern MDCT computer tomography is more sensitive than selective angiography in determining both active bleeding and its site.
- Angiography is unlikely to be of value following a CT scan that does not demonstrate active bleeding or injuries likely to bleed, ischemia requiring endovascular intervention, or more detail regarding the distal circulation.

What Next?

- In the unstable patient, stopping bleeding comes before fixing fractures or bowel surgery.
- The demonstration of arterial hemorrhage or a site of potential hemorrhage on CT should lead to angiography for embolization or stent grafting.
- Transfer to angiography must be rapid and efficient.
- Angiography rooms must be equipped for anesthesia and resuscitation.
- The angiography suite and staff should be prepared to receive the patient.
- Equipment including embolic agents should be immediately available.

Performing Angiography

- If CT has demonstrated the site of abnormality or extravasation, then aortography is usually not necessary. Go straight to the target site.
- In abdominal injuries, bowel paralytics are rarely necessary as the patient usually has an ileus.

- Because CT scanning is so sensitive to contrast extravasation, superselective angiography is often necessary and typically requires coaxial catheters.
- Embolization should be performed as quickly and as focally as possible, as described in other chapters in this book.

Considerations for Imaging Departments

- In an ideal world, "trauma centers" would have CT and angiography facilities located in resuscitation rooms.
- These should be designed so that the patient can be monitored from the operating consol so that the anesthetist is not limited in any way.
- Until this is achieved, patients will have to be transported. The dogma that patients cannot be safely transferred to angiography is no longer tenable.
- Surgeons, anesthetists, and sadly radiologists have to be made aware that intractable bleeding associated with solid organ or pelvic fractures and damage to other arterial structures are best treated by emergency arterial embolization or stent grafting.
- Full radiology information systems (RIS) and Picture Archiving and Communication Systems (PACS) should operate in the emergency environment.
- There should be no distinction made between diagnostic imaging and intervention.
- Interventional radiologists should be front-line members of trauma teams.
- There should be standardization of protocols for
  - Patient transfer to the CT scanner.
  - Scan acquisition: slice thickness, timing of contrast injection, site of contrast injection, viewing, reconstructing, archiving, and reporting.

Radiation Considerations

- MDCT has become vital in the management of the severely injured patient.
- In most patients, the benefit of CT scanning will outweigh any radiation risk, but it remains important to understand what that risk is.
- MDCT is associated with high radiation dose (mean effective dose in one study was 22.7 mSV) and the traumatized patients are by and large young.
- Doses in this range are estimated to result in approximately 190 additional cancer deaths per 100,000 individuals exposed.
- An audit of practice at one UK hospital suggested that the early CT scan in the severely injured patient resulted in fewer requests for delayed and post-operative CT scanning.

Keypoints

- In the severely injured patient, there is "speed and survival" or "delay and death."
- Properly organized and sited multidetector CT should be part of the secondary survey.
- When aortic or arterial vascular injuries are diagnosed, they should lead to angiography and definitive hemostasis.
- All other investigations in the hemodynamically unstable patient, including exploratory laparotomy, should be considered archaic and inappropriate.

Bibliography

1. Trauma-Who Cares December 2007.NCEPOD www.ncepod.org.uk
2. Advanced Trauma Life Support for Doctors 7th Edition, American College of Surgeons Committee on Trauma 2005.
3. Weninger P, Mauritz, W, Fridrich P, et al. Emergency Room Management of Patients with Blunt Major Trauma: Evaluation of the Multislice Computed Tomography Protocol Exemplified by an Urban Trauma Center. Journal of Trauma-Injury Infection & Critical Care 2007;62:584–91
4. Friese R, Malekzadeh S, Shafi S et al. Abdominal Ultrasound is an Unreliable Modality for the Detection of Hemoperitoneum in Patients With Pelvic Fracture. J Trauma 2007;63:97–102
5. Farahmand N, Sirlin CB, Brown MA, et al. Hypotensive Patients with Blunt Abdominal Trauma: Performance of Screening US. Radiology 2005;235: 436–443
6. Lee BC, Ormsby EL, McGahan JP, et al. The Utility of Sonography for the Triage of Blunt Abdominal Trauma Patients to Exploratory Laparotomy AJR 2007;188:415–421
7. Pryor J, Braslow B, Reilly P, et al. Journal of Trauma-Injury Infection & Critical Care 2005;59:102–4
8. Tien HC, Tremblay LN, Rizoli SB, et al. Radiation Exposure From Diagnostic Imaging in Severely Injured Trauma Patients. J Trauma 2007;62:151–6.
9. Sampson, M. Total body CT in trauma: is it justified. UKRC 2008
10. Ben-Menachem Y. Explatory and Interventional Angiography in Severe Trauma; Present and Future Procedure of Choice Radiographics 1996;16: 963–70
11. Roy-Choudhury SH, Gallacher DJ, Pilmer J, Rankin S, Fowler G, Steers J, Dourado R, Woodburn P, Adam A. Relative threshold of detection of active arterial bleeding: in vitro comparison of MDCT and digital subtraction angiography. AJR Am J Roentgenol. 2007 Nov;189(5):W238–46.

Appendix

Table 10.1 Exampleof a MDCT Trauma Protocol: In the severely injured polytrauma patient, a segmented scan of the head using the head protocol followed by the chest/abdomen/pelvis is required. If speed is mandatory, a single sweep with the arms by the side can be done, but diagnostic accuracy will be reduced by artifact

CT head	CT facial bones	Cervical spine	Chest abdomen and pelvis (will also image TL spine and pelvis)
• Arms down • Acquire 64 × 0.6 mm, no gantry angulation • Slice thickness/ reconstruction increment: 5/5 mm for brain (oblique) • 2/2 mm for bone (straight axial)	• Acquire 64 × 0.6 mm, no gantry angulation • Can be included with head CT by FOV • Slice thickness/reconstruction increment: • 2/2 mm and 0.75/0.5 mm (bone and soft tissue) • 2/2 mm coronal and sagittal bone and soft tissue • Reformats especially useful	• Acquire 64 × 0.6 mm • Slice thickness/ reconstruction increment • 2/2 mm and 0.75/0.5 mm (bone) • 2/2 mm (soft tissue) • Reformats: 2/2 mm coronal and sagittal bone	• Trauma team moves arms up • 100 ml IV contrast at 3 ml per second • Acquire at 1.2 mm at 50 s • Slice thickness/reconstruction increment: 1.5/1.2 mm 5/5 mm soft tissue 5/5 mm lung 1.5/1.2 mm bone Coronal lung 5/5 mm Coronal chest, abdomen and pelvis 5/5 mm • Delayed scanning useful for bleeding • MPRs and MP Reformats often useful Oral contrast unnecessary unless the patient is stable and specifically looking for bowel injury

Chapter 11
Safety in the Periprocedural Period

Stan Zipser

The possibility of adverse outcomes during or following embolization procedures is an unfortunate reality of the type of work that is performed in interventional radiology suites. Certain criteria may be followed, however, to help reduce the likelihood of such adverse outcomes. Some detrimental outcomes are due to technical factors, such as non-target embolization or ischemia caused by embolization procedures. Other harmful outcomes occur as a result of the medications and contrast agents used routinely during embolization procedures. This chapter focuses on the safe administration of medications routinely used for sedation and analgesia, as well as the intravascular administration of contrast media.

Introduction

- Many procedures can be performed without analgesia or sedation. The risks associated with such medication administrations must be taken into account with the benefits derived by their use.
- Adequate sedation and analgesia are typically necessary for patient satisfaction in anxious patients, and during any painful embolization procedure.
- Optimal patient care requires the following:
  - Anticipation that a procedure may require analgesia and sedation.
  - Awareness of factors that increase procedural risk.
  - Familiarity with analgesic and sedative drugs, and agents used for their reversal.
  - Organization of appropriate regimens for sedation and analgesia before, during, and after the procedure.
  - Appropriate patient monitoring during and after the procedure.
  - Alertness to and knowledge of potential complications.
- *It is a devastating outcome to perform a "successful procedure" technically only to have the patient suffer consequences from unsafe practices regarding the administration of sedation, analgesia, or contrast media!*

Transcatheter Embolization and Therapy,
Techniques in Interventional Radiology, DOI 10.1007/978-1-84800-897-7_11,
© Springer-Verlag London Limited 2010

Pre-procedural, Procedural, and Post-procedural Considerations

First and foremost, know your patient.

- The patient's history should be taken evaluating key factors (Table 11.1).
- A physical examination should also be performed, focusing on cardiopulmonary and airway status.

Table 11.1 Key factors in pre-sedation patient assessment

- Abnormalities of major organ systems
- Previous adverse experience with sedation and analgesia and general anesthesia
- Drug allergies
- Current medications
- Potential drug interactions
- Time and type of last oral intake
- History of tobacco, alcohol, or substance use

The American Society of Anesthesiologists Task Force on Sedation and Analgesia by Non-anesthesiologists has made recommendations that include the following:

Pre-procedure

- A patient's informed consent to administer sedation/analgesia should be obtained.
- Patients should be fasted before a procedure. Guidelines suggest clear liquids no later than 2 h and a light meal no later than 6 h before the procedure. In case of an emergency procedure, consider altering the target level of sedation/analgesia or consider pre-procedural endotracheal intubation to protect the airway against aspiration.

Procedural

- The practitioners responsible for the patient receiving sedation should understand the pharmacology of any drugs they use, their risks, and the role of reversal agents.
- A designated individual, other than the person performing the procedure, should monitor the patient at all times.
- At least one person capable of establishing a patent airway and positive pressure ventilation should be present.
- An ACLS-certified person should be readily available.
- Emergency equipment should be available.

- Patient's response to verbal commands and tactile stimulation should be monitored.
- The patient's oxygen saturation and blood pressure should be monitored in all patients, and oxygen administered if the pulse oximeter oxygen saturation falls below 96% (indicating arterial hypoxia).
- The blood pressure should be obtained before, during (at 5 min intervals), and after the procedure.
- Electrocardiographic activity should be monitored for patients in deep sedation.
- Medications should be given incrementally with sufficient time between doses to assess effects.

Post-procedural

- Patients should not be allowed to drive until the effects of sedatives have worn off.
- Patients should not be discharged from the post-procedure area until baseline vital signs are achieved.

Safe Sedation and Analgesia During the Procedure

- The guidelines given above should be adhered to as closely as possible.
- Most embolization procedures are performed under moderate (conscious) sedation with intravenous medication, with a nurse monitoring the patient.
- Moderate (conscious) sedation/analgesia is defined by the American Society of Anesthesiologists as "...a drug induced depression of consciousness during which patients respond purposefully to verbal commands, either alone or accompanied by light tactile stimulation. No interventions are required to maintain a patent airway, and spontaneous ventilation is adequate. Cardiovascular function is usually maintained."
- If a procedure requires deeper sedation than this, then anesthetist assistance should be requested. This is the case with very painful procedures, confused or agitated patients, and patients those who cannot keep still.
- In patients presenting with hemodynamic instability, it is wise to caution on the side of undersedation rather than oversedation. Although the procedure may be uncomfortable, the risk of administering medications with severe side effects may outweigh the benefits of temporary discomfort during the procedure.
- Certain patient populations (e.g., hemodynamically unstable, the very young or the very old) require increased attention during and following the procedure.

Staff

- Local protocols should be in place.
- According to the American Society of Anesthesiologists, as well as the Joint Commission for the Accreditation of Hospital Organizations, a person *other than*

the operator must be responsible for the administration of the sedation and analgesia medications, as well as for monitoring the patient following administration of the medications.

- At least one individual should be capable of establishing an airway.
- At least one individual should be advanced cardiac life support (ACLS) trained.
- If pediatric patients are being sedated, it is strongly encouraged to have at least one pediatric advanced life support (PALS) certified individual in the procedure room.
- Nurses should be appropriately trained in mixing and administering medications used in sedation and analgesia, as well as medications used in the treatment of complications such as hypotension, hypoxia, and dysrhythmias.

Equipment

It is vital to have all *appropriately sized* equipment readily available. This includes the following:

Routine Care Equipment

- Hemodynamic monitoring equipment
- Equipment for monitoring ventilation
  - Pulse oximetry and/or
  - Carbon dioxide monitor
- Oxygen supply, masks, and nasal cannulae

Emergency Equipment

- *Make sure you and your staff know where everything is and how to use it!*
- IV fluids
- Standard and pediatric size intubation trays
- External defibrillators
- Temporary pacemakers
- External pacing/defibrillation pads
- Pacing wires/catheters

Medications

- The ideal medications have a rapid onset of action, short half life, are reversible, and are effective in achieving their purpose.
- Since most medications used during embolization procedures have short half lives, they can be easily titrated to effect.

- If sedation and analgesia are being provided, then reversal agents should be readily available.
- Supportive medications, such as medications to treat hypertensive episodes (beta blockers, alpha blockers, calcium channel blockers) and hypotensive episodes (levophed, dopamine) should be readily available.
- Commonly used medications in moderate sedation and analgesia are presented in Table 11.2.

Table 11.2 Commonly used medications for sedation and analgesia

Drug	Dose (IV)	Onset	Duration	Comments
Hypnotics				
Midazolam (versed)	0.5–1 mg	1–3 min	45–60 min	Can cause respiratory depression especially in COPD patients
Lorazepam (ativan)	1 mg	5–10 min		
Diphenhydramine (benadryl)	25–50 mg	10–20 min	4–6 h	Also has anti-nausea effects
Analgesics				
Morphine sulphate	2–5 mg	5–10 min	4–6 h	
Fentanyl (sublimaze)	25–50 μg	2–5 min	45–90 min	Respiratory depression occurs at 5–15 min
Toradol	15–30 mg	5–10 min	6–8 h	Parenteral NSAID often used in UFE
Reversal agents				
Naloxone (narcan)	0.1–0.3 mg q30–60 s	2 min	30–45 min	Opioid reversal agent
Flumazenil (romazicon)	0.2 mg q1–2 min	1–2 min	10–30 min	Benzodiazepine reversal agent; 3 mg total dose
Anti-nausea				
Odansetron (zofran)	4 mg	30 min	4–6 h	32 mg daily dose limit; 8 mg in patients with severe hepatic cirrhosis

Complications

- Commonly encountered situations (e.g., hypotension) should be anticipated and algorithms created for sufficient treatment (Fig. 11.1).
- A spectrum of antibiotics, particularly those that treat gram-negative organisms (due to the potential for severe and rapid sepsis), should be available. These agents include third-generation cephalosporins, gentamycin, and levoquin.
- It may be helpful to have such algorithms for common problems posted in the procedure rooms.

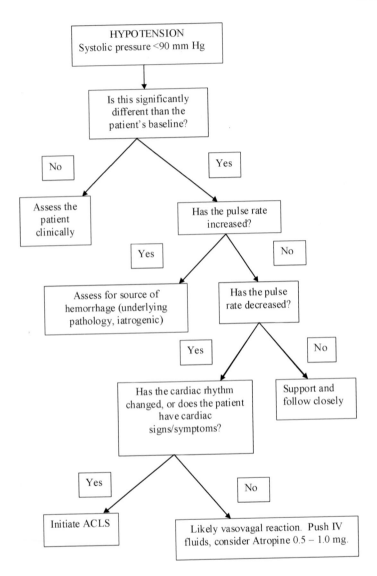

Fig. 11.1 Evaluation and treatment of hypotension

Anesthesiology Assistance During Sedation and the Use of General Anesthesia

Do Not Hesitate to Ask for Anesthesia Assistance!

Common indications for consultation with an anesthetist for monitored anesthesia care or general anesthesia during embolization procedures include the following:

- Hemodynamic instability, often due to trauma or from gastrointestinal or other bleeding source.

- Airway protection (intubation) during bronchial artery embolizations or any other procedure where there is potential respiratory compromise.
- Patient comorbidity causing possible loss of airway patency.
- Confused, agitated, or demented patient.
- Low pain threshold or inability to remain still, particularly in patients who are unable to be adequately controlled with moderate sedation.
- Neurointerventional procedures, such as AVM embolization.
- Embolization procedures in pediatric patients.
- Peripheral AVM embolization.

Safe Sedation and Analgesia Following the Procedure

- Post-procedural pain control is vital for both patient's safety and satisfaction.
- Post-procedural sedation is not typically needed unless pain management cannot be accomplished using standard analgesia regimens.
- If sedation and analgesia are used in combination in the post-procedural period, then it is vital to be aware of the increased likelihood of hemodynamic or ventilatory compromise.
- Analgesia is typically administered through the use of opiods.
  - o Different opiods have different strengths, onsets of action, and duration of action. Depending on these variables, medications can be tailored to fit the patient needs.
  - o It is important to evaluate the availability of nursing staff and/or medications if analgesia is ordered on an as-needed basis. If nurses will not be readily available, routine dosing of medications (e.g., morphine sulfate, 4 mg IV every 4 h) may result in a more predictable dose to the patient.
- *Patient-controlled analgesia (PCA) pumps* are frequently very helpful in the embolization patient population. Orders for these units are typically tailored for each patient. If opiods are used for a PCA pump, it is recommended to also write for as-needed orders for nausea that may result from the opioid administration. Typical PCA orders include a loading dose (a one-time dose the patient is given at the start of the PCA pump administration), basal rate (aliquot of medication given automatically, with the patient requesting it), a demand dose (the dose given each time the patient requests a dose), and a lockout period (the minimum amount of time between demand doses). Table 11.3 gives examples of typical PCA pump orders given following embolization procedures.

Table 11.3 Examples of patient-controlled analgesia orders administered in the post-procedural period

Medication	Loading dose	Basal rate	Demand dose	Lockout period
Fentanyl	10–50 μg	0–10 μg	5–20 μg	6–10 min
Hydrocodone	0.2–1.0 mg	0.2–0.4 mg	02.–0.4 mg	6–10 min
Morphine	0.2–1.0 mg	02.–0.4 mg	0.2–0.4 mg	6–10 min

Safe Administration of Contrast Media

Contrast-Induced Nephropathy

- Contrast-induced nephropathy (CIN) is often defined as an increase in serum creatinine by greater than 25%, or an absolute increase of >0.5 mg/dl, within 3 days of contrast administration.
- Most frequently, CIN is characterized by serum creatinine levels beginning to rise within 24 h, peaking within 96 h, and returning to normal within 7–10 days. However, temporary or permanent dialysis-dependent renal failure can result.
- There is a very low to no risk of CIN in patients with normal renal function. Risk increases as baseline renal function decreases—the worse the function, the greater the risk.
- The nephrotoxic effect of contrast is dose dependent: the higher the administered dose of contrast, the higher the risk of CIN.
- Risk factors for the development of CIN include the following:
  o Diabetes Mellituas
  o Dehydration
  o Concurrent use of furosemide with the contrast administration
  o Patients with multiple myeloma
  o Hypertension
  o Age > 70 years
  o Congestive heart failure
  o Hyperuricemia
  o Patients taking nephrotoxic medications (including NSAIDS)

Prevention of CIN

- Non-ionic agents have been shown to be less toxic than ionic agents, and therefore are generally favored over ionic agents.
- The use of low and iso-osmolar agents has been shown to decrease contrast-induced nephropathy and adverse contrast reactions.
- An IV fluid regimen of 0.9% saline (100 cc/h for 12 h before and after an angiographic procedure) has been shown to reduce the risk of CIN.
- The benefit of using pre- and periprocedural sodium bicarbonate IV drips and oral N-acetylcysteine is debatable. Due to the low likelihood of adverse reactions to both agents, many operators will use these agents even in the absence of firm data suggesting benefit.
- Patients with known renal dysfunction, or those who are at risk for CIN or who have significant comorbidities, should suspend metformin use for 48 h after the administration of iodinated contrast.
- Carbon dioxide gas is a non-toxic, low viscosity, highly soluble gas that acts as a negative contrast agent. It may be used in embolization procedures for patients with a contrast allergy or renal insufficiency.

Keypoints

Patient Safety and Comfort Are Paramount

- Published guidelines from the ASA and JCAHO regarding sedation and analgesia are readily available and should be followed.
- Sedation and analgesia may be necessary in the pre-, peri-, and post-procedural periods. The patient should have the opportunity to be treated for their pain/anxiety before and after the procedure, not just during the procedure.
- It is vital to remember what each drug class is used for! Most sedatives offer little or no analgesic effect. *If the procedure is going to hurt, solitary use of sedation will not be adequate!* In addition, there is a synergistic effect between benzodiazipenes and opiods, with each drug class accentuating the effect of the other. In the vast majority of instances, therefore, it is advantageous to use both medication classes together.
- Certain risk factors place patients at high risk for contrast-induced nephrotoxicity (CIN). Aggressive use of IV fluids is the only proven method to protect the kidneys from CIN. Certain risk factors are known, but the risk of NOT performing an embolization procedure should be weighed against the risk of administering contrast media.

Suggested Readings

1. Kelly AM, Dwamena B, Cronin P, Bernstein SJ, Carlos RC. Meta-analysis: effectiveness of drugs for preventing contrast-induced nephropathy. Annals of Int Med (2008):148(4):284–294
2. Morcos SK. Prevention of contrast media-induced nephrotoxicity after angiographic procedures. J Vasc Interv Radiol (2005);16:13–23
3. Rao QA, Newhouse JH. Risk of nephropathy after intravenous administration of contrast material: a critical literature analysis. Radiology (2006); 239:392–7
4. Shabanie A. Conscious sedation for interventional procedures: a practical guide. Tech Vasc Interv Rad (2006);9:84–8
5. Practice Guidelines for Sedation and Analgesia by Non-Anesthesiologists, Anesthesiology (2002);96:1004–17
6. Lee, SH, Hahn, ST, Park, SH. Intraarterial lidocaine administration for relief of pain resulting from transarterial chemoembolization of hepatocellular carcinoma: Its effectiveness and optimal timing of administration, Cardiovasc Intervent Radiol (2001);24:368–371
7. Keyoung, JA, Levy, EB, Roth, ER, et al. Intraarterial lidocaine for pain control after uterine artery embolization for leiomyomata, J Vasc Interv Radiol. 2001;12:1065–1073
8. Lang EV, Berbaum KS, Pauker SG, et al. Beneficial effects of hypnosis and adverse effects of empathic attention during percutaneous tumor treatment: when being nice does not suffice. J Vasc Interv Radiol (2008); 19:897–905

Chapter 12
Complications of Embolotherapy

Lakshmi Ratnam and Robert Morgan

Complications directly attributable to embolization essentially comprise the following:
- Consequences of non-target embolization
- Sepsis
- Infarction and/or necrosis of embolized tissue
- Extravasation of liquid agents
- Misplaced embolization coils

General complications of angiography related to access site and contrast nephrotoxicity will not be addressed in this chapter.

Prevention, Detection, and Recognition

Prevention: not all complications can be prevented but many can be anticipated and therefore avoided.

Pre-procedure

- *Planning*: review the diagnosis, options, and vascular approaches carefully.
- *Consent*: discuss the procedure and inform the patient of recognized risks.
- *Antibiotic prophylaxis*: this may be appropriate in solid organ embolization, especially if a large area of infarction is expected.
- *Anatomy*: thorough knowledge is the key to success and failure! Presence of anatomical variants may result in non-target embolization, if the operator is unaware of the pitfalls.

Transcatheter Embolization and Therapy,
Techniques in Interventional Radiology, DOI 10.1007/978-1-84800-897-7_12,
© Springer-Verlag London Limited 2010

Fig. 12.1 Angiogram of renal
metastasis in the femur. The
metastasis (*white
arrowheads*) is highly
vascular and early draining
veins (*black arrows*) are seen
indicating AV
shunting

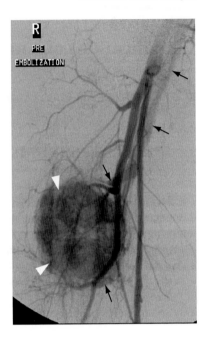

- *Collateral blood supply:* in the presence of tumor, neovascularization may be present (Fig. 12.1). In atherosclerotic patients, collateralization may be present as a result of arterial stenosis.
- *Arteriovenous shunting (AV):* in the presence of AV shunting (Fig. 12.1), the embolic material must be carefully chosen to avoid passage through the shunt, causing non-target embolization (e.g., stroke during embolization of pulmonary AVM).

During the Procedure

- *Choice of embolic agent:* this must be tailored to the clinical indication and anatomical site. Frequently, a final determination of the size of the embolic agent cannot be made until the final catheter position has been achieved and an angiogram showing the arterial territory supplying the lesion has been obtained.
- *Catheters*
  - o *Choice of catheters*
  - o *Size*: if you plan to use a co-axial catheter, then make sure that its diameter and length are compatible!
  - o *Lumen*: make sure that the embolic agent will pass through the catheter.
  - o *Type*: end-hole-only catheters are essential. Coils may partially extrude through a sidehole and block the catheter (Fig. 12.2). Particles and liquids will come out through the sideholes.

Fig. 12.2 Attempted coil deployment through a sidehole catheter (*black arrow*). The coil has partly extruded through the sidehole (*white arrowhead*) blocking the catheter. The catheter and coil are being removed through the femoral sheath

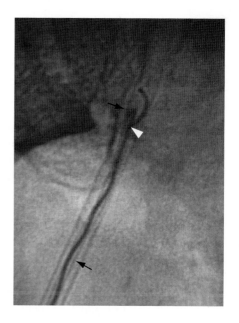

- *Catheter position:* ensure a stable catheter position before commencing embolization. Catheters can have a tendency to "jump back" if the position is not stable, which may result in non-target embolization.

  - *Avoid*: sharp angles and redundant loops of catheter. These predispose to loss of position as coils are introduced.
  - *Test stability*: check that insertion of the coil pusher wire does not displace the catheter. Only deliver coils with a flush technique, if the catheter remains in place during a forceful test injection of saline.
  - *Maintain and check* the catheter position during embolization.

- *Prevention of reflux*: this is a common cause of non-target embolization.

  - *Use good quality fluoroscopy* when injecting liquid and particulate agents. Look for flow toward the target. Slow or stop injection as flow slows.
  - *When flow slows*, flush the catheter with saline under fluoroscopic control to ensure that no embolic material remains in the catheter.
  - *If flow has stopped DO NOT FLUSH! Either* aspirate the catheter until free-flowing blood is obtained *or* remove the catheter and flush outside the patient.
  - *Consider occlusion balloons* to prevent reflux when embolizing with liquid agents.

- *Go with the flow*: if possible, try to embolize in the direction of blood flow:
  In principle, it is safer to embolize in free-flowing blood as flow will carry the embolic agent forward to the target.

- *Imaging*:
  - Consider use of road maps during embolization: subtraction techniques are very sensitive to contrast and help visualization of the embolic agent relative to normal anatomy.
- *Stopping*:
  - Embolize to a pre-determined endpoint.
  - Avoid over-embolization ("the enemy of good is better").
  - Resist the temptation to insert one more coil if the endpoint has been achieved. This last coil is frequently the one that migrates!

Detection and Recognition

During the Procedure

- *Tactile cues:* use caution when there is resistance to passage of coils or injection of particles or liquid. Consider that the delivery catheter may be blocking or kinked.
- *Visual cues*: use contrast and fluoroscopy especially when approaching the endpoint. Reduce the rate of embolization if flow is slowing or if there is intermittent reflux outside the vessel to be embolized. Coil/glue migration can be visualized with fluoroscopy.

Post-procedure

Clinical Assessment

- *Non-target embolization:* always assess and document the presence or absence of peripheral pulses at the beginning of arterial embolization procedures. Neurological status should be documented in neuroembolization procedures, and in cases where catheters or guidwires have been manipulated within the aortic arch.
- *Post-embolization syndrome (see Chapter 13):* this is usually benign and self-limiting. When it is not self-limiting, consider the possibility of sepsis and/or abscess formation.

Blood Tests

- White cell count and CRP to monitor for infection
- Blood cultures
- Urea and electrolytes

Imaging

- Plain films will demonstrate embolized coils (Fig. 12.3).
- Computed tomography (CT) or ultrasound for assessment of abscess formation.
- Magnetic resonance imaging (MRI) may not be an option if non-MRI compatible embolic agents have been used.
- Note: artifact from coils may limit the utility of CT and MRI.

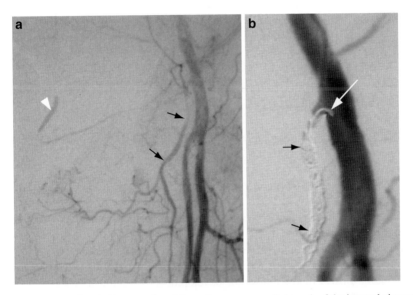

Fig. 12.3 (a) Bleeding (*white arrowhead*) from the corona mortis branch of the internal obturator artery (*black arrows*) following fracture of the pubic rami. (**b**) Following embolization, tightly packed coils in internal obturator artery (*black arrows*) the end of the last coil has trailed into the common femoral artery (*white arrow*). It was judged unlikely to lead to any problem and left where it was

Catheters Blocking

This is a common, important, and sometimes preventable problem. A blocked catheter may result in losing catheter position in a location accessed with great difficulty. Prevention is better than dealing with the consequences of a catheter that cannot be unblocked and has to be totally removed and exchanged for another.

- Ensure that the lumen of the delivery catheter is appropriate for the selected coils or other embolic agents (e.g., it is difficult to inject thick Gelfoam down a microcatheter, and it is impossible to pass a 0.038 "coil down a catheter with 0.035" lumen).

- Make sure coil introducers are held firmly in position in the catheter hub. Failure to do so will result in the coil being partly deployed in the hub. Maldeployed coils can usually be removed from the hub with a small pair of forceps.
- Remember that particles effectively narrow the catheter lumen.
- Frequently flush the catheter with saline. Use a 1-ml syringe to flush microcatheters.
- If a catheter does become blocked, then it may be safest to remove it. Forceful injection to clear may dislodge embolic material that has already been delivered and/or cause reflux into another vessel.

Non-target Embolization

It is important to recognize and record non-target embolization. The consequences will depend on the following:

- Vascular bed: some tissues are more vulnerable and a small amount of embolization can cause a major clinical problem (e.g., large intestine, kidney, nerve, and brain).
- Extent of the embolization: any tissue which is comprehensively embolized will be damaged.
- The risk of non-target embolization is reduced by the use of microcatheters in high-risk situations.
- In cases of coil migration, retrieval can be carried out if required.
  If non-target embolization is likely to have clinical sequelae, then the patient should be closely monitored for the development of complications.

Coil Retrieval

If the delivery catheter becomes displaced with a coil partially deployed, it may be possible to

- Push the catheter back into position and try again.
- Pull the catheter back into the introducer sheath with the coil in situ—apply suction with a large syringe as you do this. The coil will usually lodge in the tip of the sheath as the catheter is withdrawn. In this case, it can be snared close to the puncture site.

Completely deployed coils and other foreign bodies can be retrieved using a variety of commercially available devices.

- Loop snares, baskets, grasping forceps: these require a free segment of the coil to grasp.

- Hook-shaped catheters: these can be used to manipulate a coil into a position where it can be retrieved with a standard snare or basket.

Before attempting retrieval, consider pros and cons of leaving the coil where it is. Every case should be assessed on its own merits. A decision to retrieve a migrated coil is generally based on the following:

1. *The location of the coil.* The clinical situation is key here. A coil lodged in a solitary calf artery is more important than a similar coil in a branch gluteal vessel.
2. *The consequences of leaving it where it is.* If the patient is asymptomatic (Fig. 12.3) or the occlusion will not cause clinical sequelae, then the best course of action may be conservative (e.g., leaving the coil where it is)!
3. *The risks of attempting retrieval.* Removal might lead to further problems; complications of coil retrieval include

   - Disturbing the rest of the coil nest and exacerbating the problem.
   - Damaging other vessels: dissection, occlusion, spasm, rupture of the vessel caused by manipulation of the retrieval device.
   - Cardiac arrythmias if the coil has migrated to the heart.
   - Embedding or further distal embolization of the agent that you are trying to retrieve.

4. *Timing.* If retrieval is indicated, it is usually best to perform it immediately. Occasionally it is better to delay retrieval or chose an alternative option.
5. *Alternative options.* It may be safer to remove a coil surgically, especially if the embolization was performed pre-operatively.
6. *The patient's wishes.* The patient should always give informed consent.

Tissue Necrosis

Following successful embolization, significant tissue necrosis or intravascular thrombosis can result in the post-embolization syndrome. This must be distinguished from infection.

- Post-embolization syndrome is self-limiting (see Chapter 11).
- If symptoms persist or worsen, infection must be considered. In this case, blood cultures should be performed.

Consider imaging to assess for abscess formation. Note that gas formation can normally be seen following embolization of solid organs; in this instance, it is a benign entity unrelated to the presence of infection.

Necrosis due to extravasation of liquid agents will be considered elsewhere.

Keypoints

- Ensure that the indication for embolization is appropriate.
- Obtain fully informed consent.
- Careful planning of the procedure is essential.
- Review all available imaging before commencing procedure.
- Ensure all clinical information and imaging is up to date.
- Ensure adequate clinical back up is available should complications ensue.
- If necessary, discuss the case with an appropriate clinician/surgeon so that they are aware that their support may be required.

Chapter 13
Management of Post-embolization Syndrome

Sapna Puppala

Introduction

- Post-embolization syndrome (PES) is a common side effect of solid organ embolization.
- Clinical manifestations of PES are typically pain, fever, and sickness (nausea) sometimes described as a flu-like illness.
- It is important to differentiate PES from infection and tumor lysis syndrome, since these require different management.
- Occurrence and severity of PES cannot be predicted in any individual patient.
- Effective prevention and management of PES are crucial to fast patient recovery and improve patient satisfaction and quality of life.

Pathophysiology

- The etiology of PES is not fully established.
- Tissue hypoxia and cell death lead to release of tissue breakdown products, inflammatory mediators, and vasoactive substances from the tumor and adjacent normal tissues.
- Radiofrequency ablation of tumors leads to a syndrome similar to PES typically lasting 8–72 h and coinciding with the release of these bioactive substances.
- PES can continue up to 7–14 days post-procedure.

Clinical Features

The severity of symptoms can correlate with the volume of embolic agent and extent of target tissue embolization, but this does not predict whether PES will occur in any individual patient. The type of embolic agent does not correlate with the occurrence of PES but small particles and liquid agents are more likely to result in tissue necrosis. The key to success is to have flexible regimes to prevent and treat symptoms.

Transcatheter Embolization and Therapy,
Techniques in Interventional Radiology, DOI 10.1007/978-1-84800-897-7_13,
© Springer-Verlag London Limited 2010

- PES affects children and adults.
- Symptoms: varying degrees of pain, fever, nausea, malaise, arthralgia, and loss of appetite.

Pain

- Often characteristic pattern (e.g., uterine fibroid embolization (UAE)).
  - o 0–2 h: acute pain due to global uterine ischemia.
  - o 5–8 h: plateau phase.
  - o >8 h: rapid reduction due to resumption of blood flow to the myometrium.
- In 15–20% of patients after uterine fibroid embolization, this process can be more pronounced. The cause for this variation is not known.
- Uncontrolled pain or high fever indicates other complications such as infection and non-target embolization.
- Pain management must be flexible, responsive, and patient centred.

Fever

- Continuous or intermittent low-grade pyrexia <39°C (104 F) is typical.
- High or spiking fever suggests infection.

Nausea and Vomiting

- Sickness is common secondary to PES and the use of opiate analgesia.
- Can lead to dehydration and electrolyte imbalance.
- Require supportive therapy: antiemetics and IV fluids.

Diagnostic Evaluation

Laboratory

White Cells

- 20% of patients with PES have leukocytosis <24,000/microlitre in the first 24 h.
- A later rise in leukocytes must be viewed with caution and suggests infection.
- Neutropenia may occur a few days after chemoembolization.

U&E

- Dehydration, contrast media toxicity, and release of toxic mediators can lead to acute renal failure.

Imaging

Imaging is not usually necessary and should be reserved for cases in which it is necessary to exclude other pathology such as target organ infection and non-target embolization.

- Pulmonary embolism through arterio-venous shunts can mimic PES and is confirmed by ventilation/perfusion scan.
- For example, cystic artery embolization can lead to chemical cholecystitis (Fig. 13.1) which significantly exaggerates the symptoms of PES and is assessed by ultrasound and computed tomography (CT).

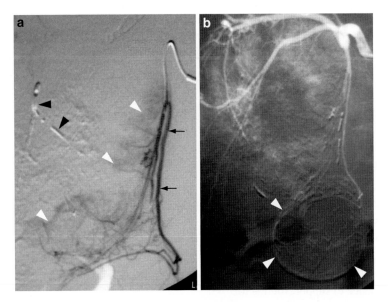

Fig. 13.1 Embolization of large hepatoma. (**a**) Collateral supply (*white arrowheads*) from a branch of the cystic artery (*black arrows*). Retained Lipiodol is seen in the main tumor (*black arrowheads*). (**b**) Following "selective" embolization of the branch artery, lipiodol is seen in the gallbladder. The patient developed chemical cholecystitis which was managed conservatively

Management of PES

Prevention

- Regimens involve pre-medication with analgesia, sedation, antiemetic therapy, and hydration.

Pre-procedural Care

1. *Informed consent*: patients should be fully informed of the risks of PES and its variable occurrence and severity. It is helpful to establish what the patient understands about PES and target explanation to any gaps in their knowledge.
2. *Hydration:* crucial in PES due to the risks of contrast nephropathy fluid loss from vomiting, loss of appetite, and secondary dehydration.
3. *Analgesia*: prophylactic analgesics are essential.

   - A combination of oral, IV, epidural, and/or patient-controlled analgesia can be used.
   - A local regime should be established with the pain control team and ward, and angiography staff should be familiar with the chosen protocol.
   - Our practice is to administer a non-steroidal analgesics either paracetamol (acetaminophen) 1 g IV or diclofenac 50 mg PR for procedures that are typically painful such as hepatic and renal tumor embolization. Acetaminophen helps control pain, reduces the inflammatory response, and provides an antipyretic action.
   - Patient-controlled analgesia (PCA) is set up and connected before the procedure.
   - Additional opiate analgesia is given from the start of the procedure according to patient requirement.

4. *Sedation*:

   - A small dose of intravenous benzodiazepine such as midazolam is given at the start of the procedure.
   - Additional doses are given as indicated.

5. *Antibiotics:* broad spectrum antibiotics may prevent infection but there is little evidence to support routine use.

Management of PES: Intraprocedural

Analgesia: PCA pump using morphine sulphate set at 1 mg/5 min lockout. This should be supplemented by additional opiate analgesia titrated to control pain. If a PCA pump is not used, then IV short-acting opiate and benzodiazepine protocols may be advantageous. *It is essential that someone other than the operator takes responsibility for pain control.*

Antiemetics: an IV antiemetic, e.g., Cyclizine 50 μg should be given. Ondansetron sodium is an alternative and administered as 16 mg per rectally or as 8 mg slow intravenous injection.

Management of PES—Post-procedure

Analgesia: should be continued until the patient is comfortable. PCA is discontinued when patient is able to tolerate oral analgesia. Use of an opiate combined with a NSAID is usually better than a single agent.

Antiemetics: should be continued as required using IV or IM routes until oral intake has resumed.

Hydration: is essential, intravenous fluids should be prescribed for sedated patients or those unable to manage oral fluids.

Reassurance: remind patients that PES is a normal and self-limiting side effect of embolotherapy.

Keypoints

- Post-embolization syndrome is an important and common side effect of embolization. It is a self-limiting phenomenon, and effective supportive measures for control of pain and nausea improve the overall outcome and also the quality of life after embolization. It is essential to have a clear local strategy for management pre-, peri- and post-procedure.
- Efforts should be focused on prevention of pain and sickness and supportive post-procedural care. It is essential not to discharge patients before symptoms have resolved sufficiently for them to be cared for at home. Further analgesics and antiemetics should be provided as necessary and the patient should be given clear verbal and written instructions regarding the normal evolution of PES.

Bibliography

1. Hemingway AP, Allison DJ. Complications of embolization: analysis of 410 procedures. Radiology 1988 Mar; 166(3):669–72.
2. Sohara N, Takagi H, Abe T, Hashimoto Y, Kojima A, Takahashi H, Nagamine T, Mori M. Nausea and vomiting induced by arterial chemo-embolization in patients with hepatocellular carcinoma and the antiemetic effect of ondansetron hydrochloride. Support Care Cancer 1999 Mar; 7(2):84–8
3. Romano M, Giojelli A, Tamburrini O, Salvatore M. Chomoembolization for hepatocellular carcinoma: effect of intrarterial lidocaine in peri and post procedural pain and hospitalization. Radio Med (Torino) 2003 Apr; 105(4):350–5
4. Bissler JJ, Racadio J, Donnelly LF, Johnson ND. Reduction of post embolization syndrome after ablation of renal angiomyolipoma. Am J Kidney Dis 2002 May; 39(5):966–71
5. Rauh S, Duhem C, Ries F, Dicato M. Complications and hospitalisation duration after chemoembolization for liver metastasis. Bull Soc Sci Med Grand Duche Luxemb 1999;(2):29–36
6. Sundset A, Haanaes OC, Enge I. Embolization of bronchial arteries in severe and recurrent haemoptysis. Tidsskr Nor Laegeforen 1992 Sep 30; 112(23):2958–62

7. Leung DA, Goin JE, sickles C, Raskay BJ, and Soulen MC. Determinants of post embolization syndrome after hepatic chemoembolization. Journal of vascular interventional radiology
   2001 Mar; 12(33):321–6
8. Marcio H M, Stanley P, Steel D A, Ortega JA. Feasibility and toxicity of chemoembolization
   for children with liver tumours. J clin oncol March 2000;18(6):1279–1284
9. Coldwell DM, Kennedy A, Vanecho D. Comparative side effects of yttrium-90 based intra-
   arterial brachytherapy. J Clin Oncol (July 15 Supplement) 2004;22(14S): 3760
10. Huo T-I, Wu J-C, Lee P-C, Chang F-Y, Lee S-D. Incidence and risk factors for acute renal fail-
    ure in patients with hepatocellular carcinoma undergoing transarterial chemoembolization: a
    prospective study. Liver Int June 2004;24(3):210–215(6)
11. Ganguli S, Faintuch S, Rabkin DJ, Lang EV. Post-Embolization Syndrome: Leukocytosis
    after Uterine Artery Embolization
12. Kimura F, Itoh H, Ambiru S et al. Long term results of initial and repeated partial
    splenic embolization for the treatment of chronic idiopathic thrombocytopenic purpura. AJR
    2002;179:1323–6.
13. Wah et al. Image guided percutaneous radiofrequency ablation and incidence of post ablation
    syndrome: prospective survey. Radiology 2005;237(3):1097.
14. Ganguli S, Faintuch S, Salazar GM, Rabkin DJ. Postembolization syndrome: changes in white
    blood cell counts immediately after uterine artery embolization. J Vasc Interv Radiol. 2008
    Mar;19(3):443–5.
15. The British National Formulary reference can easily be found by you
    http://bnf.org/bnf/bnf/current/104945.htm

Section II

Chapter 14
Peripheral Vascular Malformations

Peter Littler and Peter Rowlands

Background

- Peripheral vascular malformations are uncommon lesions and are thought to be due to a focal persistence of primitive vascular elements.
- Vascular malformations are not neoplastic. They are subdivided into high-flow and low-flow lesions. High-flow lesions are arterial; low-flow lesions are venous, capillary, or lymphatic.
- It is important that these lesions are evaluated and treated by a specialist with experience in embolotherapy working within a multidisciplinary team with access to anesthetic support and plastic surgery.
- The purpose of diagnostic evaluation is to assess suitability for treatment and to evaluate if the lesion is high flow (arteriovenous malformation) or low flow, as treatments are different for each group.

Low-Flow Lesions

Clinical Features

- Include venous, lymphatic (Chapter 46), and capillary malformations.
- Common sites of involvement include the limbs and head and neck.
- Patients with a venous or lymphatic malformation often present with swelling and/or pain.
- Other reasons for presentation include aesthetic appearance or hemorrhage.
- Pregnancy may exacerbate symptoms, particularly with lower limb lesions.

Transcatheter Embolization and Therapy,
Techniques in Interventional Radiology, DOI 10.1007/978-1-84800-897-7_14,
© Springer-Verlag London Limited 2010

Diagnostic Evaluation

Clinical Review

- A comprehensive history of the lesion is taken together with relevant past medical and drug history.
- The lesion is examined clinically for site, size, and appearance.
- Ultrasound (Fig. 14.1) should be considered to be a part of the clinical examination.

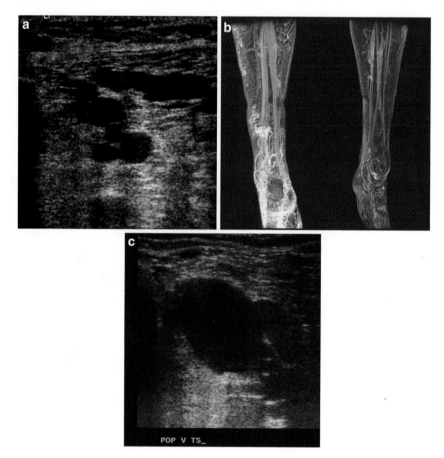

Fig. 14.1 (**a**) Ultrasound and (**b**) MRI demonstrating a venous malformation in a patient with Klippel–Trenaunay syndrome (Chapter 17). Note the right leg hypertrophy and large popliteal vein (**c**)

Laboratory

- It is important to check the platelet count in patients with very large vascular malformations as there can be a low platelet count secondary to sequestration.

- Clotting measurements and routine blood tests can be relevant if intervention is planned.

Imaging

- Ultrasound with greyscale and Doppler is a key step in evaluation of a peripheral vascular malformation (Fig. 14.1). Together with clinical examination, most lesions can be easily differentiated by ultrasound into high- and low-flow lesions. Limitations occur when evaluating deep lesions when the full extent of the lesion cannot be visualized.
- MRI of the lesion is routinely performed to assess morphology (Fig. 14.1) and any feeding and draining vessels (Fig. 14.2).

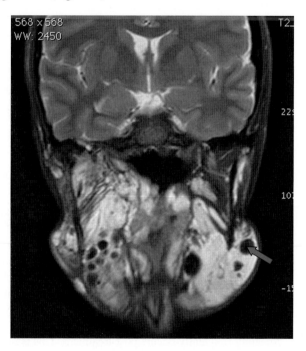

Fig. 14.2 T2-weighted coronal MRI of the head and neck demonstrating a large high-signal cervical venous malformation causing pharyngeal narrowing. There are multiple low-signal phleboliths within the lesion (*arrow*)

- Useful MRI sequences include T1 for anatomical detail, and fat-suppressed T2 that allows excellent visualization of the lesion, which is of high signal intensity compared with the lower signal of surrounding tissue. Intravenous contrast is rarely required.

Indications for Embolization

- If the patient is having pain, swelling, hemorrhage, or finds the lesion aesthetically intolerable, then it is reasonable to proceed after a risk benefit analysis.

- Platelet consumption.
- A significant proportion of patients do not require any intervention.

Alternative Therapies

- Conservative management: if the patient is relatively asymptomatic.
- Surgical resection: best for small superficial lesions. Frequent recurrence is a problem.
- Laser: effective in treating capillary vascular malformations such as the "port wine stain."
- Radiotherapy: rarely used due to limited effectiveness and post-radiotherapy skin changes.

Cautions/Contraindications

- Patent foramen ovale or other right-to-left shunts are relative contraindications. When injecting the sclerosant, you must be sure not to fill a draining vein.

Specific Complications

- Superficial skin ulceration can rarely occur if the sclerosant tracks into the subcutaneous tissues. This is seen more commonly with alcohol than with sodium tetradecyl sulfate (STD).
- Nerve damage rarely occurs if alcohol sclerosant is injected immediately adjacent to a nerve. This should be discussed specifically in the consent process. Temporary facial nerve palsy is a rare complication of sclerotherapy of facial lesions and is due to direct pressure of a swollen vascular mass on the facial nerve.
- Swelling frequently occurs post-treatment. This is rarely a problem and resolves in a few days. However, when treating a lesion in the head and neck, prophylactic steroids are given to prevent obstruction of the airway.

Anatomy

- Dependent on site.
- It is crucial to understand the normal vascular anatomy and to recognize adjacent structures that may be damaged.

Equipment

- 21-G butterfly needle for superficial lesions.
- A 20-G spinal needle can be used with ultrasound guidance for deeper lesions.

Embolic agents: low-flow malformations are treated using sclerosant agents.

- STD 1% or 3%, either in liquid or foam.
- Absolute alcohol.

Medication

- *Pain control*: simple analgesics as required post-procedure.
- *Steroids*: if head and neck lesion. 8 mg of dexamethosone IV during procedure and a 5-day course of 40 mg oral prednisolone. Use with caution in diabetics.

Angiography

The procedure is often performed under general anesthetic due to discomfort during sclerotherapy. This is usually required if a head and neck lesion is treated.

Access

- Ultrasound-guided percutaneous puncture using a 21-G butterfly or 20-G spinal needle under aseptic conditions. Once venous backflow is achieved, then angiography can be performed.

Angiography

- Magnified DSA, usually at two frames per second. Continue until a draining vein fills.
- It is important to note the volume and rate of contrast injection, as this guides the injection of sclerosant.

Assessing the Lesion

Angiographic Appearance

- Angiography reveals abnormal filling of dilated vascular structures. A draining vein or veins are often seen (see Fig. 14.3).

Fig. 14.3 (**a**) DSA via a 21-G butterfly needle demonstrating a venous malformation, (**b**) early filling of a draining vein via alternative puncture site in the same patient

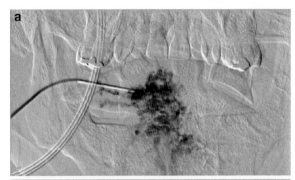

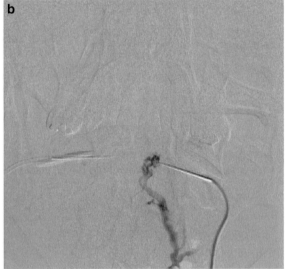

Treatment Plan and Technique

- The ultimate aim is to fill the entire lesion with sclerosant.
- Small areas of the lesion (two or three sites) are treated at each procedure to avoid excessive swelling and the risk of tissue ulceration.
- Several sessions may be needed to treat the entire lesion.
- The sclerosant is mixed with contrast and injected under DSA guidance until a draining vein is seen. As a guide, the volume and injection rate should be similar to that injected in the initial DSA run.
- In low-flow lesions contrast often remains pooled in the lesion from the initial angiogram. If this has washed out then consider diluting the sclerosant with contrast.
- Occasionally a tourniquet is applied to control venous outflow by temporally occluding a draining vein.

Post-embolization

- Compression of the puncture site post-sclerotherapy until hemostasis achieved.
- The patient is reviewed 1 h post-treatment, and can generally then be discharged.
- Normal post-GA discharge protocol if applicable.
- A short course of steroids are given if a head and neck lesion is treated.

Follow-Up

- Follow-up and repeat treatments are carried out every 6–8 weeks to allow any post-sclerotherapy inflammatory reaction to settle.

High-Flow Lesions

Diagnostic Evaluation

Clinical Review

- Clinical evaluation combines history, clinical examination, and ultrasound assessment.

Laboratory

- It is important to check the platelet count in patients with very large vascular malformations as they can be consumptive and are associated with a thrombocytopenia.
- Hemoglobin and clotting parameters are important if intervention is planned.

Imaging

- Ultrasound Doppler can demonstrate arterialized flow with abnormal veins in an arteriovenous malformation, differentiating it from a venous malformation.
- MRI is used to demonstrate the lesion, including the arterial and venous anatomy.

Indications for Embolization

- Significant pain, swelling, or aesthetic appearance.
- Cardiac failure (generally in pelvic AVMs) and peripheral ischemia due to shunting can occur in high-flow lesions and are indications for treatment.
- Platelet consumption.

Alternative Therapies

- Conservative management: if the patient is relatively asymptomatic.
- Surgical resection: best for small superficial lesions. Frequent recurrence is a problem.

Cautions/Contraindications

- Patent foramen ovale or other right-to-left shunts are relative contraindications.
- Non-target embolization: this can result in limb loss when treating digits.

Anatomy

- Dependent on site.

Equipment

Catheters

- *Non-selective catheters:* standard angiographic catheters.
- *Selective catheters:* including a microcatheter for selective embolization.
- Guide catheter as needed.
- Occlusion balloons for venous outflow.

Embolic Agents

- *Coils:* sized appropriately for the target vessel
- Glue
- Particles (polyvinyl alcohol 350–500 μm)
- Onyx

Medication

- *Pain control*: simple analgesia as required post-procedure.

Angiography

Access

- Usually arterial approach, commonly via the common femoral artery.
- Percutaneous direct puncture.
- Venous approach in arteriovenous lesions. This may also be necessary to occlude the venous outflow during transarterial embolization.

Angiography

- Multiple non-selective, selective, and superselective angiograms are performed in different planes to find the nidus of the AVM. High frame rates and multiple projections are often needed for the accurate identification of the nidus. This is crucial to successful treatment.

Assessing the Lesion

Angiographic Appearance

- Selective angiography via the feeding arteries reveals the nidus of the AVM. Rapid filling of the draining veins is seen (see Fig. 14.4).

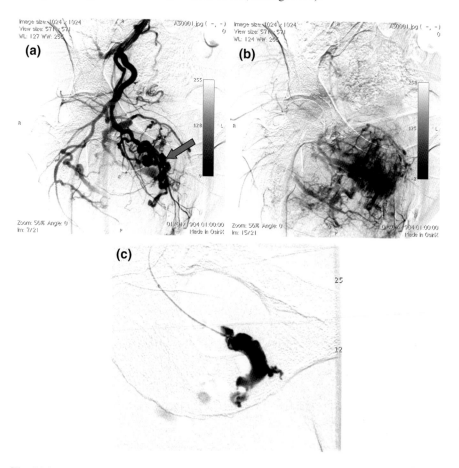

Fig. 14.4 (**a**) Selective angiogram of a pelvic AVM demonstrating the feeding vessels and nidus (*arrow*), (**b**) venous phase of the angiogram and (**c**) the nidus being treated with Onyx

Treatment Plan and Technique

- Successful treatment requires obliteration of the nidus.

- Liquid/particulate agents are essential for this. Proximal coil embolization will inevitably lead to recurrence.
- The embolic agent is delivered as close as possible to the level of the AV shunt. This must be done accurately to avoid non-target embolization.
- Arteriovenous lesions have a solitary venous component and can be embolized via the draining vein or via direct puncture.
- It is often necessary to occlude the venous outflow to reduce flow and prevent systemic migration of the embolic agent. This can be achieved with an occlusion balloon to transiently occlude the shunt or permanently occlude with coils.
- Particle embolization may be used to devascularize lesions prior to surgical debulking.

Post-embolization

- Standard care post-arterial puncture.
- For direct AVM puncture-wound site observation and regular blood pressure and pulse checks.

Follow-Up

- Repeated treatments may be required as determined by follow-up clinical and imaging assessment.

Keypoints

- Differentiation into high-flow arteriovenous and low-flow venous malformation is vital as treatment is different for each group.
- This can be achieved by clinical examination, ultrasound, and MRI assessment.
- These conditions are rarely life threatening. Therefore a risk/benefit evaluation prior to treatment is important.
- Treatment should be carried out by a specialist in the field working as part of a multidisciplinary team.

Safety

- Accurate deployment of the sclerosant or embolic agent is crucial to minimize the risks of complications.

Chapter 15
Pulmonary Arteriovenous Malformations

Graham Robinson

Clinical Features

Like all arteriovenous malformations, pulmonary arteriovenous malformations (PAVM) "steal, shunt, or bleed." PAVMs are important as systemic venous blood can bypass the lungs, leading to hypoxia or paradoxical embolism. PAVMs tend to increase in size with time.

Clinical Presentation

- Transient ischemic attack (TIA)/stroke or cerebral abscess from paradoxical embolization.
- Shortness of breath if large shunt.
- Incidental "mass" on chest radiograph.
- Screening in hereditary hemorrhagic telangiectasia (HHT) (Fig. 15.1).
- Hemoptysis

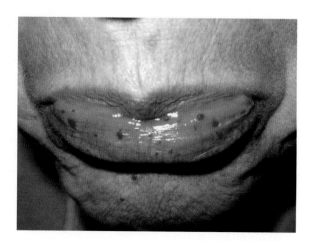

Fig. 15.1 Typical telangectasia on the lips of a lady with HHT and PAVM

Transcatheter Embolization and Therapy,
Techniques in Interventional Radiology, DOI 10.1007/978-1-84800-897-7_15,
© Springer-Verlag London Limited 2010

Clinical Relevance

- Untreated PAVMs carry a 1% stroke and 0.5% brain abscess risk *per annum*. Risk does not correlate well with the size of the shunt. Most patients have a small number of localized pulmonary AVMs; up to 5% of patients have a diffuse pattern with multiple lesions (Fig. 15.2).

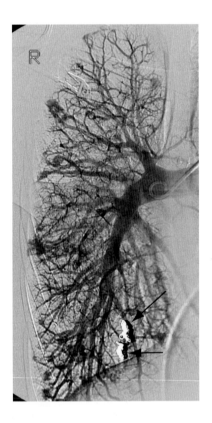

Fig. 15.2 Twenty-one-year-old man with diffuse PAVMs. There are extensive PAVMs throughout the right lung. Note coils in lower lobe from previous embolization (*black arrows*)

- 70–90% of patients with pulmonary AVMs have underlying HHT; relatives should be screened for HHT (and pulmonary AVMs if positive for HHT).
- HHT is an autosomal dominant condition with variable penetrance, and an incidence of 1 in 6,000–10,000. There are five types described, with type 1 having the highest association with pulmonary AVMs (approximately 30%). Pulmonary AVMs do tend to run in families.

Diagnostic Evaluation

Clinical

Multidisciplinary team with chest physician, ENT, neurologist, gastroenterologist, and clinical genetecist. The importance of screening family members cannot be overemphasized.

Laboratory

Hemoglobin, routine biochemistry.
  Oxygen saturation/blood gas analysis if breathless.
  Blood cultures if cerebral or paradoxical abscess.

Imaging

Non-contrast chest CT. There is a risk of paradoxical air embolus in untreated pulmonary AVMs, so *no cannulae or intravenous injections* unless absolutely necessary.

Reformatted multislice CT gives a good appreciation of pulmonary AVM anatomy.

Contrast-enhanced CT (performed under supervision) or pulmonary angiography may be helpful in complex lesions and in planning embolization (Fig. 15.3).

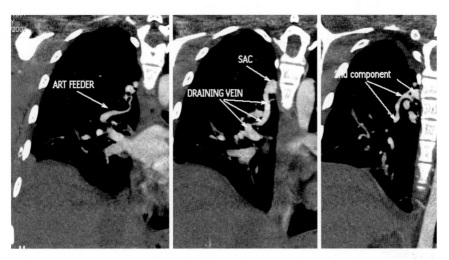

Fig. 15.3 CECT was helpful for planning intervention in this 25-year-old lady presented with life-threatening hemothorax. The reformats show feeding and draining vessels and an unsuspected second component

Indications

- Any symptomatic PAVM regardless of size of feeding vessel
  - o Feeding arteries as small as 2–2.5 mm have caused symptoms.
- Asymptomatic PAVM
  - o There is no published evidence correlating the size of the feeding artery with stroke risk.
  - o Many authors recommend treating lesions with feeding arteries of >3 mm.
  - o If treating smaller lesions, use common sense—the risk of treating small lesions that are technically challenging to catheterize may well be greater than leaving them for a later day when they will be a little larger.

Alternative Therapies

Surgical resection was all that was available until 1977, but has been largely replaced by embolotherapy.

Contraindications

- Severe pulmonary arterial hypertension is a relative contraindication. Recent work shows no consistent response to embolization, with increased pressures in some patients post-procedure and decreases in others. Involvement of a chest physician with an appropriate interest is advisable.
- Usual relative contraindications of contrast allergy, inability to lie still/cooperate with breathing instructions.

Specific Complications

- *Stroke*: the risk of stroke must be discussed and recorded. This is particularly sensitive in asymptomatic patients. It is often helpful to involve both the patients and their relatives.
- *Pleuritic pain*: in some patients, it may be almost impossible to avoid some pulmonary infarction during embolization of PAVM, with a risk of post-procedural pleuritic pain.

Anatomy

A comprehensive knowledge of pulmonary vascular anatomy is a vital pre-requisite for undertaking this procedure.

Equipment

Catheters

- *Non-selective catheters:* 100-cm pigtail catheter, capable of flow rates of 20 ml/s for pulmonary angiography. (There are angled pigtails such as the Grollman catheter specifically designed for pulmonary angiography.)

 Remember always to straighten out the pigtail with a guidewire before removing the catheter after pulmonary angiography. This prevents engagement of the valves and chordae tendinae.

Selective Catheters

- Shaped catheter of choice to negotiate through right heart (e.g., angled pigtail, Berenstein, Cobra). Catheters should be at least 80 cm long.
  Guide catheter
- Personal preference is important. Make sure that it is at least 80 cm long and of suitable diameter.
- Lumax (Cook) coaxial catheter with 7F 80 cm outer and 5F 100 cm hydrophilic Berenstein-type shaped inner, or 8F 90 cm outer with 110 cm inner. The 8F is stiffer and less easy to manipulate—only used when large Amplatzer vascular plugs (AVPs) are to be utilized.
- Some operators use a sheath rather than guide catheter. Use whatever you are most familiar and comfortable with.

Embolic Agents

- Coils—regular/micro, pushable/detachable. Fibered coils are more thrombogenic and usually preferred over non-fibered.
- Amplatzer vascular plugs of appropriate size assessed from pre-procedure imaging (types 1, 2).
- Guglielmi or other detachable coils.

Medication

- *Pain control:* not usually necessary. Symptomatic therapy in case of pleuritic chest pain. Non-steriodal anti-inflammatory drugs are usually all that are required.
- *Infection control:* no routine antibiotics.
- *Sickness control:* not routinely.
- *Hydration:* not routinely.

Angiography

Access

- Right femoral vein.
- Can use jugular approach if required (e.g., IVC thrombus) or preferred.
- Can go through a patent IVC filter, if well incorporated into the IVC wall.

Angiography

- Measure main pulmonary artery pressures (PAP) prior to injecting contrast. *Do not perform pump runs if PAP >40 mmHg.*
- The catheter passes into the left pulmonary artery in most patients, since this vessel courses more posteriorly (this is akin to catheters passing into the splenic artery in preference to the hepatic artery).
- A variety of techniques can be used to select the right pulmonary artery, including prolapse of the floppy end of a Bentson wire, use of a hydrophilic wire, the stiff end of a regular wire to open out the pigtail of a pulmonary pigtail catheter, use of a tip-deflecting wire, or exchange for a multipurpose shape.
- High frame rates (6/sec or more) may be needed to visualize the feeding vessels accurately.

Assessing the Lesion

Non-selective main or lobar injections initially, if no prior angiography.
    Proximal (pulmonary trunk) injections risk missing peripheral lesions (Fig. 15.4)

Angiographic Appearance

Localizing precise anatomy of feeding vessel(s) vital. This may require patience and multiple oblique projections. Biplane angiography is sometimes helpful.

Treatment Plan and Technique

- Aim to occlude the feeding artery as close to the aneurysm sac as possible, as this reduces the risk of reperfusion by collateral feeders and minimizes the risk of pulmonary infarction.
- Aim for a tight coil pack and cross-sectional occlusion.
- The selected embolic device needs to be large enough to occlude the target vessel. If too small, there is a risk of paradoxical embolization into the systemic circulation. Having a team member ready to apply bilateral carotid compression if a

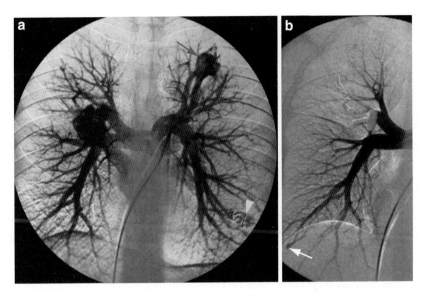

Fig. 15.4 (**a**) Non-selective pulmonary trunk injection showing recanalization of left lower lobe PAVM embolized 10 years before(*yellow arrowhead*), new left and right upper lobe PAVMs (*red arrows*). Despite maximum field of view, there is exclusion of peripheral lung. (**b**) Rt UL lesions occluded with detachable silicone balloons and pushable fibered coils. Non-selective completion angiogram reveals small Rt LL lesion (*white arrow*) excluded from previous non-selective image

device does embolize is potentially useful in preventing the device lodging in the carotid.

- This risk can lead to selection of too large a device, which then creates a risk of coils stringing back and not coiling—this is not good as it prevents distal occlusion and restricts access for subsequent treatment.
- Detachable coils may be useful, since appropriate coil size can be confirmed before final deployment.
- Coil deployment technique is very important (Fig. 15.5) (see Chapter 2).
- Do NON-SELECTIVE completion angiogram to detect other vessels supplying the PAVM.
- The risk of paradoxical embolization has led to the development of detachable devices which do reduce the risk of this complication at the cost of increased complexity and higher costs. The recently introduced Amplatzer vascular plug devices are screw-detachable plugs that are safe and easy to use, but do not yet have the proven long-term efficacy of coils.
- The risk of paradoxical emboli remains until all lesions are treated. Meticulous technique is important to avoid ANY air or blood clot entering the system during the procedure. Wire withdrawal with the catheter tip abutting a vessel sidewall produces a vacuum that fills with air if the catheter hub is open to air. Since superselective catheterization almost always requires the use of a shaped catheter, this situation is difficult to avoid in smaller vessels; having to torque and withdraw

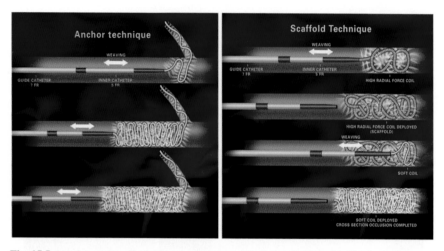

Fig. 15.5 (Anchor and scaffold diagrams courtesy of Dr Robert I White Jr) (**a**) The anchor technique involves deploying the first few centimeters of coil into a side branch and then weaving the remainder of the coil as shown. A coaxial guide catheter or sheath is important to allow sufficient forward pushability of the inner catheter. (**b**) The scaffold technique involves deployment of a high radial force initial coil (typically 2 mm oversized to the vessel), with a softer platinum coil then woven in

the catheter to free the tip can be time-consuming and ultimately unsuccessful in allowing sufficiently distal canulation of small vessels. Various techniques can be used to exclude air including wire exchanges with the catheter hub held beneath the surface in a bowl of saline (simple but can be messy, and difficult to see with backbleeding of blood into the saline) or using a closed system (Fig. 15.6) with pressurized saline, which is more cumbersome but secure.

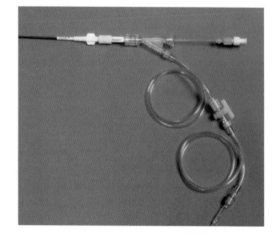

Fig. 15.6 Closed system comprising: coaxial catheters, clear tubing (allows air bubbles to be seen), Tuohy Borst adapter, two-way taps, and obturator for the coil. The tubing is connected to a pressurized bag of heparinized normal saline running at about two drips/second

- *Clot formation* and paradoxical embolization are potential risks during treatment of PAVM. Heparinization during the procedure may help reduce this; the author favors heparinization but the evidence is only anecdotal.

Aftercare

- There is a small incidence of pleuritic chest pain when the aneurysm sac thromboses. This can occur shortly after the embolization (up to 48 h) or may be delayed and typically occurs at 4–6 weeks. This can be severe but rarely requires more than non-steroidal analgesia and reassurance. Some operators advocate treating only one lung at a time because of the potential risk of bilateral pleuritic pain. Geography of patient's travel time to hospital may override this consideration.

Post-embolization

Day case or overnight stay.
  Clinic visit, phone call, or email contact a few days later.

Follow-Up

- Annual clinical review and clinical assessment for continued occlusion of PAVM and to follow any known untreated small PAVMs.
- Radiation dose is clearly an issue, particularly with the potential for multiple follow-up imaging studies. Contrast-enhanced echocardiography and oxygen saturations are preferable for solitary lesions.
- Contrast-enhanced CT is necessary if there are untreated PAVMs.
- Pulmonary angiography every 5-years, should be performed more frequently if
  - Large lesion(s) treated, as recanalization is more likely with large or complex feeding vessels.
  - Return of symptoms.
  - Reduction in oxygen saturation.
- Screen relatives.

Keypoints

Screen family for HHT and PAVMs.
  No air introduction during angiography/embolization!

Embolize as close to the sac as possible.

Correct device size is crucial—do not oversize coils too much, since they will misplace the catheter.

Non-selective completion angiogram.

Safety

If you have not done one before, discussing a case with someone who has may be helpful:

http://www.hht.org/living-with-hht/treatment-centers/ is a good place for contact details.

Suggested Reading

1. Pollak JS, Saluja S, Thabet A, Henderson KJ, Denbow N, White RI Jr. Clinical and anatomic outcomes after embolotherapy of pulmonary arteriovenous malformations. J Vasc Interv Radiol. 2006 Jan;17(1):35–44

2. Lee WL, Graham AF, Pugash RA, Hutchison SJ, Grande P, Hyland RH, Faughnan ME. Contrast echocardiography remains positive after treatment of pulmonary arteriovenous malformations. Chest. 2003 Feb;123(2):351–8.

Chapter 16
Systemic Arteriovenous Fistulae

Robert Rosen

Clinical Features

- An arteriovenous fistula (AVF) is a direct connection between an artery and vein.
- AVFs are not the same as arteriovenous malformations (Chapters 14 and 15).
- AVF can be considered according to etiology, site, and symptoms.
- AVF can be congenital or acquired (e.g., iatrogenic for dialysis or following trauma or biopsy).
- Local effects include dilation and tortuosity of the afferent artery and draining vein, ischemia distal to the AVF, and venous hypertension with secondary degenerative changes in the vein wall and overlying skin.
- Physical examination demonstrates increased pulsation and a thrill; marked dilation and tortuosity of the draining veins; and hyperpigmentation, thickening, and eventual ulceration of the skin distally (Fig. 16.1).

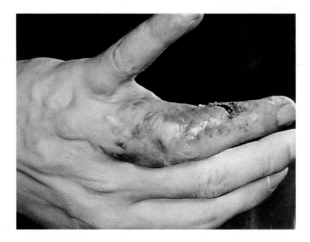

Fig. 16.1 Photograph of a patient with extensive skin changes resulting from an AVF of her fourth digit

- The distal ischemia may be severe and be the patient's primary complaint, with atrophy of the distal soft tissues, cyanosis, rest pain, and ischemic ulceration.
- Reversal of flow in the distal artery (steal) is common.
- Venous hypertension may also occur with time and exacerbate distal ischemia.

Transcatheter Embolization and Therapy,
Techniques in Interventional Radiology, DOI 10.1007/978-1-84800-897-7_16,
© Springer-Verlag London Limited 2010

- Generalized cardiovascular effects are related to both the shunt and the decrease in peripheral vascular resistance, and include increased circulating blood volume, increased cardiac output, and in severe cases, cardiac dilation and eventual high-output failure.
- High-output states are much more common in arteriovenous fistulae (AVF) than in arteriovenous malformations, which generally have a complex nidus rather than a direct arteriovenous connection, resulting in higher resistance to flow. In fact, clinically apparent high-output failure in complex AVMs is relatively uncommon.
- Resting tachycardia may be present in patients with large fistulae, and slowing of the pulse with compression of the feeding artery (Branham–Nicoladoni sign) is a classic physical finding which confirms the presence of a high-output state.
- Most fistulae increase in size and flow over time and will require treatment. It is preferable to treat them prior to the development of secondary pathologic changes, and particularly before secondary irreversible cardiac dilation occurs.

Diagnostic Evaluation

Laboratory

- Standard pre-angiography laboratory evaluation should be undertaken, including the following.
  - Serum creatinine
  - Complete blood count
  - Coagulation profile
  - Liver panel (if embolization of AVF within the liver)

Imaging

- Imaging studies of value include ultrasound, computed tomography, magnetic resonance angiography, catheter angiography, and echocardiography for evaluation of the cardiac changes.
- Ultrasound examination will demonstrate enlargement of the feeding arteries and draining veins, turbulence with mixed arterial and venous signals at the site of the fistula, and high venous velocities.
- CTA, particularly with 3D reconstruction, can provide a detailed anatomic view of the location and size of the actual arteriovenous connection and be helpful in choosing the type and size of embolic device (Fig. 16.2).
- MRA studies will show increased flow and dilation of the involved vessels, but generally lack the temporal and spatial resolution to permit treatment planning.

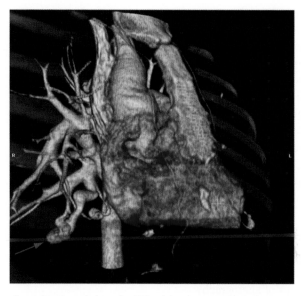

Fig. 16.2 Three-dimensional rendering of a CTA of the chest demonstrating a pulmonary AVM of the right lower lobe (*arrow*)

- Catheter angiography is usually reserved for treatment or instances when non-invasive imaging does not reveal sufficient anatomical detail to plan therapy.

Indications for Embolization

- *Symptomatic AVF:* nearly all will require embolization, especially if there is venous hypertension, symptomatic arterial "steal" syndrome, high-output congestive heart failure or organ insufficiency due to venous hypertension or arterial steal.
- *Asymptomatic AVF*: early embolization should be considered to prevent secondary changes due to venous hypertension or arterial compromise.

Alternative Therapies

- Surgical interventions may be possible in superficial AVF (e.g., in the extremities) and simple AVFs (e.g., those with few feeding and draining vessels).
- Surgical interventions are CONTRAINDICATED in lesions that are complex; these lesions should be treated as one would treat an AVM, with endovascular means only. Surgical interventions in such complex lesions can lead to recruitment of more feeding vessels and a much more difficult endovascular intervention.

Contraindications for Embolization

- *All contraindications are relative, and the risk of doing the procedure must be weighed against the risk of not doing the procedure!*
- Contraindications to angiography
  - o Contrast allergy
  - o Uncorrectable coagulopathy or thrombocytopenia
  - o Renal insufficiency
- Contraindications to embolization
  - o Inability to safely reach target vessel
  - o High risk of embolization of agent through AVF and into pulmonary circulation

Specific Complications

- Complications of angiography.
- Occlusion of draining vein (may be required as part of embolization procedure).
- Pulmonary embolism—may occur due to migration of agent through AVF or may occur in delayed fashion from outflow vein thrombosis.
- Paradoxical systemic embolism—may occur if the patient has a concurrent right to left shunt (e.g., pulmonary AVM).

Anatomy

- Anatomical considerations depend on organ being embolized.
- AVFs, particularly if long-standing, can recruit new vessels similar to an AVM. Proximal angiography to assess for any unsuspected vessel inflow is vital to a successful embolization procedure.
- Variant anatomy for any specific organ undergoing embolization should also be recognized.

Equipment

Catheters

- *Non-selective catheters:* Pigtail, Omni Flush.
- *Selective catheters:* variety of according to the anatomy of the target vessels.
- *Guide catheter:* guide catheters or long sheaths may be particularly helpful to perform check angiograms and roadmaps during selective catheterization.

Embolic Agents

Coils: Coils are suitable if the afferent artery can be safely sacrificed and the size and flow rate of the fistula permit them to be securely deployed without risk of migration.

Other occlusion devices: detachable plugs such as the Amplatzer device offer many of the same advantages as coils and are simple to use.

Liquid agents: adhesives (n-butyl cyanoacrylate) and polymers (Onyx) may be useful in certain types of fistulae where achieving a complete seal is difficult.

The choice of agent is determined by the following:

- The size of the feeding and draining vessels.
- The anatomy of the fistula itself (side-to-side, end-to-side, associated aneurysmal dilation).
- Rapidity of flow.
- The need to preserve flow in the involved artery or vein.
- The consequences of losing the embolic device or agent through the venous side of the fistula.
- In some cases a combination of devices, agents, and techniques will be required.

Medications

Pain Control

- Intraprocedural sedation and analgesia, typically with midazolam and fentanyl
- Post-procedural anti-inflammatory medications (ketoralac, ibuprofen) and pain medications (opiods) as needed

Infection Control

- Antibiotics not often needed.

Sickness Control

- Anti-nausea medications not often needed.

Hydration

- IV normal saline or D5W as needed.
- These procedures may be very lengthy, in which case more aggressive fluid management may be necessary.

Angiography

Arterial and/or venous access may be required for effective treatment. In some instances additional access is required to allow the use of an occlusion balloon to reduce flow through the AVF and decrease the risk of systemic embolization.

Arterial Access

- Plan according to the anatomy and location of the AVF.

Venous Access

- Required in some anatomic situations, particularly
  o When there is aneurysmal dilation of the draining vein
  o When direct trans-arterial access has been sacrificed
  o When venous embolization alone will lead to thrombosis of the AVF

Assessing the Lesion

- Angiography remains the gold standard for evaluating arteriovenous fistulae, demonstrating flow patterns, the precise site of communication, and regional collateral vessels.
- In order to define the anatomy of the fistula, highly selective studies must be performed and will probably require high-frame rates. If this does not give the answer, then some form of occlusion of the inflow artery or outflow vein will be needed.
- If there has been prior unsuccessful intervention, either surgically or with embolization, then the collateral flow may be so extensive that it is virtually impossible to define the original site of AV communication. The angiographic picture may then be indistinguishable from a complex congenital AVM (Fig. 16.3).

Angiographic Appearance

- Appearance depends on the degree of shunting with the AVF.
- Long-standing or large AVF may have a very dilated feeding artery and a very dilated draining vein.
- Multiple feeding arteries may be present—proximal, non-selective angiography is mandatory to evaluate these arteries.
- The artery distal to the AVF is often normal in size or very small.
- Arterial steal may be present with flow reversal. This is readily demonstrated on ultrasound. To demonstrate steal angiographically may require the following:

Fig. 16.3 Unsubtracted
angiogram of a large AVF of
the extremity. Note how the
AVF is indistinguishable
angiographically from an
extensive AVM

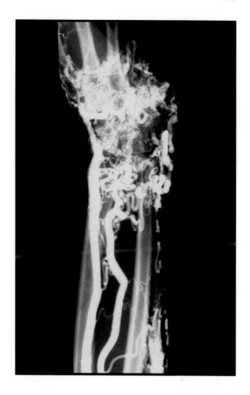

- o The catheter to be passed beyond the AVF.
- o Injection into a collateral vessel that supplies the territory beyond the AVF.
- o Use of a tourniquet or occlusion balloon to reduce venous outflow.

Clinical Scenarios

Etiology of Arteriovenous Fistulae

Congenital arteriovenous fistulae

- These are less common than true arteriovenous malformations, which tend to have more complex anatomic patterns.
- Examples of true congenital fistulae include those occurring in the central nervous system (dural, carotid-cavernous), pulmonary AVMs (which typically resemble fistulas more than true malformations), coronary artery fistulae, and those in the kidney.

Traumatic arteriovenous fistulae can occur anywhere in the body after a penetrating injury, and they were historically the first type of AVF described.

- These lesions are often not apparent until some time after the acute event, when secondary changes such as abnormal pulsation, a palpable thrill, swelling, enlarged regional arteries and veins, and distal ischemia may be noted.
- When the lesion is deep seated, the first sign may be that of a high-output cardiac state.

Iatrogenic arteriovenous fistulae are occurring more frequently with the increasing use of minimally invasive techniques, where a vascular injury may not be immediately apparent.

AVF in Specific Locations

Renal AVF

- Manifest clinically with renal impairment, hypertension, hematuria, flank pain, or asymptomatic bruit.
- Acquired fistulae may result from penetrating trauma or iatrogenic injuries such as renal biopsy, nephrostomy, or percutaneous stone removal.

Small Post-biopsy Renal AVF

- Often resolve without specific treatment; larger fistulae often show progressive enlargement, related to the high flow rate in the renal circulation.
- Require treatment if symptomatic, especially if associated with reduction in renal function in a renal transplant.
- Embolization is usually straightforward and should be as selective as possible to minimize renal parenchymal loss.

Congenital and Large Renal Arteriovenous Fistulae

- These lesions are generally supplied by a single very dilated renal artery branch with a massive draining vein.
- The flow through these lesions is so high that there is often dilation of the inferior vena cava, and there may be associated high-output heart failure.
- Massive renal AVF can be problematic to treat due to the size of the AV communication and the torrential flow.
- There is a significant risk of loss of the embolic device through the fistula and into the pulmonary circulation.
- A combination of inflow and outflow occlusion balloon flow control, oversized coils, vascular plugs, and in some cases liquid agents (nBCA, Onyx) may be necessary to completely close these lesions.

Arterioportal Fistuale

- Generally present with gastrointestinal bleeding due to arterialization of portal flow (Fig. 16.4).

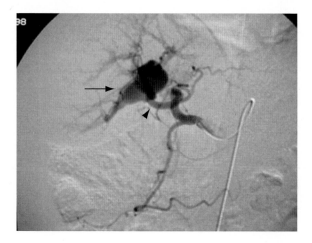

Fig. 16.4 Digital subtraction angiogram of the common hepatic artery (*arrowhead*) demonstrating early filling of the portal vein (*arrows*) as a result of an arterioportal fistula

- This type of arterialization is also sometimes encountered in aggressive hepatocellular carcinoma with rapid arteriovenous shunting through the tumor.
- Care must be taken to avoid loss of embolic materials or devices through the fistula and into the portal vein.
- An additional risk is acute thrombosis of the portal system shortly after closing the fistula, presumably due to the acute decrease in pressure in the portal system.

Aortocaval Fistulae

- Uncommon, usually related to erosion of an aortic aneurysm through the caval wall, penetrating trauma, or iatrogenic injury (particularly during lumbar disc surgery).
- Clinically these patients present with abdominal bruit, pulsatile abdominal mass, widened pulse pressure, and in some cases, renal failure.
- Flow through this type of fistula is extremely high and often results in high-output cardiac failure.
- In the vast majority of these cases, the fistula is side-to-side, and embolization plays little role.
- Endoluminal aortic stent grafts have recently been used to successfully manage this problem while avoiding the risk of free hemorrhage during open repair (Fig. 16.5).

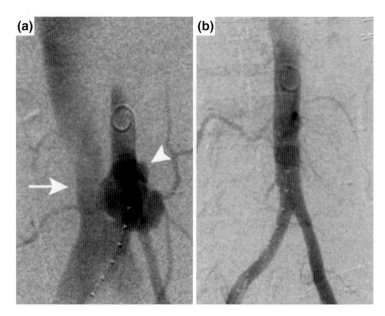

Fig. 16.5 **a)** Digital subtraction aortic angiogram demonstrating an early draining IVC (*arrow*), due to fistula formation between an aortic aneurysm (*arrowhead*) and the IVC. **b)** Angiogram following stent-graft placement, demonstrating complete resolution of the fistula

Treatment Plan and Technique

- The key to successful treatment of an arteriovenous fistula is finding and closing the point of communication between the artery and the vein.
- Choose the correct embolic agent before starting the embolization.

Coil embolization is suitable if the afferent artery can be safely sacrificed and the size and flow rate of the fistula permit them to be securely deployed without risk of migration.

- The initial coils should generally be oversized to create a baffle or nest that will allow the subsequent coils to be safely packed to achieve complete occlusion.
- In larger or higher flow fistulae, the use of detachable coils allows for trial sizing and coil placement prior to release in order to avoid escape of the device through the draining vein.
- An "anchor" approach has been described by White et al., consisting of placing the end of the coil in a more proximal branch to anchor it in place and prevent migration.
- While coil retrieval is an interesting and challenging procedure, it is better avoided by careful planning!

Other occlusion devices

- Detachable plugs such as the Amplatzer device offer many of the same advantages as coils and are simple to use (Fig. 16.6).
- In very large side-to-side fistulae, occluding devices primarily designed for cardiac use (ASD and VSD closure) have also been used successfully.
- Detachable occlusion balloons were used extensively in the past, but are currently not commercially available in the United States.

Liquid agents: adhesives (n-butyl cyanoacrylate) and polymers (Onyx) may be useful in certain types of fistulae where achieving a complete seal is difficult.

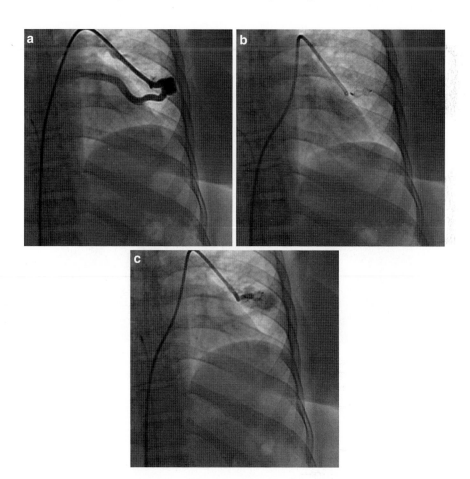

Fig. 16.6 a) Unsubtracted angiogram demonstrating a pulmonary AVM (AVF) with a single feeding artery and a single draining vein. **b)** Unsubtracted image demonstrating a single Amplatzer device in the feeding artery. **c)** Unsubtracted image from the post-embolization angiogram demonstrating complete resolution of the AVM

- Even though the acrylic adhesives can be prepared to form an almost instantaneous cast, they are best used after flow has been diminished somewhat by the initial placement of coils or other devices, or alternatively by using a proximal balloon to control inflow during the embolization process.

Covered stents: if the fistula is side-to-side or if flow through the involved artery and vein must be preserved, the use of covered stents or stent-grafts may be an effective solution (Fig. 16.7).

- As in surgical ligation, they should only be used when there are no branches that could recanalize the fistula over time.
- The long-term patency of a covered stent must also be taken into consideration, particularly in younger patients.

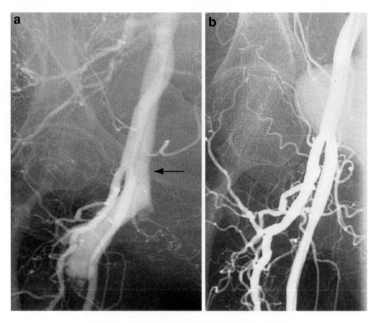

Fig. 16.7 a) Unsubtracted pelvic angiogram demonstrating an early draining iliac vein (*arrow*) during a common iliac artery injection. **b)** Angiogram following deployment of a stent-graft demonstrates complete resolution of the AVF

Approach

Artery

- Most AVF will be approached from the arterial end; this also allows access into the draining vein (through the fistula) if necessary.

Vein

- The venous approach has been described in
  - Carotid-cavernous fistulae
  - Vein of Galen "aneurysms"
  - Certain peripheral arteriovenous fistulae and fistula-like malformations
- If the draining vein can be completely occluded, the arterial feeders will have no low-pressure sump to empty into, resulting in immediate cessation of flow.
- This approach can be performed via transvenous catheterization or by direct puncture of the draining vein if it is accessible, and usually involves completely packing the venous structure with coils and/or liquid agents.

Both

- In high-flow AVF where the risk of systemic embolization is high, consider using balloons to occlude the inflow and/or outflow vessels.

Technical Points

- *The first treatment should be carefully planned and executed, as it represents the best chance for a permanent cure.*
- Simply occluding the feeding artery proximal to the fistula will generally result in long-term failure due to recruitment and enlargement of collateral branches closer to the point of arteriovenous communication. Thus, there is not only recurrence of the fistula, but it is now supplied by multiple smaller branches, making subsequent treatment much more difficult.
- A distinct advantage of endovascular therapy is the ability to obtain detailed, dynamic images of the point of communication.
- In classic "H"-type AVF, four vessels must be considered: the inflow artery, the outflow artery, and the outflow veins upstream and downstream of the AVF. Each of these segments will undergo significant morphologic change.
- The tendency of fistulae to persist or recur suggests that the procedure should not be considered finished until flow has been completely arrested angiographically.
- Although the goal should always be occlusion of the actual fistula site, this may prove impossible in some situations, and reducing flow through collateral feeders may be the only therapeutic option, knowing that further collateral recruitment is inevitable over time.

Aftercare

- In the setting of embolization of a very large AVF, immediate changes in the patients hemodynamic status can occur.

- This is particularly true of patients who present with high-output cardiac failure. *Close evaluation of such patients in the immediate post-embolization period is vital!*
- Consideration should be given for ICU admissions with close hemodynamic monitoring.

Arterial Puncture Site

- Normal post-angiography care.

Post-embolization

- Post-procedure pain medications and anti-inflammatory medications, as outlined above, should be considered.

Follow-Up

- Routine clinical follow-up within a week is recommended.
- Imaging follow-up with cross-sectional imaging within several weeks is recommended to evaluate for incomplete embolization or recurrence of the AVF.
- Non-invasive imaging is generally adequate; the imaging modality used prior to embolization would allow direct comparison of pre- and post-intervention studies.

Keypoints

- Arteriovenous fistulae are, by definition, direct anatomic connections between artery and vein that should be completely curable, unlike some more complex malformations.
- Endovascular techniques are particularly well suited for managing this type of clinical problem, whether by embolization or by stent grafting.
- The best opportunity for complete cure is the initial procedure.
- Careful delineation of the pathologic anatomy and the correct choice of endovascular device are essential.
- Failure to occlude the actual site of connection between artery and vein is likely to lead to rapid recurrence with a much more complex pattern of collateral supply, at which point cure becomes difficult or impossible to achieve.

> ## *Safety*
>
> - Correct sizing of embolic materials such as coils is vital to decrease the likelihood of migration of embolic agent.
> - Rapid changes in hemodynamic status can occur following complete occlusion of high-flow arteriovenous fistulae.

Suggested Readings

Holman, E., *Arteriovenous aneurism: clinical evidence correlating size of fistula with changes in the heart and proximal vessels.* Ann Surg, 1924. 80(6): 801–16.

Early, S.A., et al., *Coronary artery fistula; coronary computed topography—the diagnostic modality of choice.* J Cardiothorac Surg, 2008. 3: 41.

Burchell, H.B., *Observations on bradycardia produced by occlusion of an artery proximal to an arteriovenous fistula (Nicoladoni-Branham sign).* Med Clin North Am, 1958. 42(4): 1029–35.

Iloreta, A.T. and M.D. Blaufox, *Natural history of post-biopsy renal arteriovenous fistula: a 10-year follow-up.* Nephron, 1979. 24(5): 250–3.

Criado, E., et al., *Endovascular repair of peripheral aneurysms, pseudoaneurysms, and arteriovenous fistulas.* Ann Vasc Surg, 1997. 11(3): 256–63.

Halabi, A.R. and D.E. Kandzari, *The thrill is gone: catheter-based exclusion of a posttraumatic arteriovenous fistula with a covered stent graft.* Catheter Cardiovasc Interv, 2005. 66(1): 27–33.

Hart, J.P., et al., *Endovascular exclusion of iliac artery to iliac vein fistula after lumbar disk surgery.* J Vasc Surg, 2003. 37(5): 1091–3.

Donmez, H., et al., *Use of a balloon and N-butyl-2-cyanoacrylate for treatment of arteriovenous fistula.* Cardiovasc Intervent Radiol, 2008. 31(Suppl 2): S111–4.

Peynircioglu, B., et al., *Transvenous embolization of a spontaneous femoral AVF 5 years after an incomplete treatment with arterial stent-grafts.* Cardiovasc Intervent Radiol, 2008. 31(2): 407–10.

Casasco, A., et al., *Percutaneous transvenous catheterization and embolization of vein of galen aneurysms.* Neurosurgery, 1991. 28(2): 260–6.

White, R.I., Jr., *Pulmonary arteriovenous malformations: how do I embolize?* Tech Vasc Interv Radiol, 2007. 10(4): 283–90.

Chivate, J.G. and R.W. Blewitt, *Congenital renal arteriovenous fistula.* Br J Urol, 1993. 71(3): 358–9.

Guzman, E.A., McCahill, L.E., and F.B. Rogers, *Arterioportal fistulas: introduction of a novel classification with therapeutic implications.* J Gastrointest Surg, 2006. 10(4): 543–50.

Kashyap V.S. et al., *Aortocaval fistula.* J Am Coll Surg, 2006. 203(5): 780–86.

Mitchell, M.E., McDaniel, H.B., and F.W. Rushton, *Endovascular repair of a chronic aortocaval fistula using a thoracic aortic endoprosthesis.* Ann Vasc Surg 2008. 22: 742–9.

Barley, F., Kessel. DO., Nicholson, AA and I. Robertson *Technical report: balloon occlusion to reduce flow during selective embolization of large symptomatic iatrogenic renal transplant arteriovenous fistula.* Cardiovasc Intervent Radiol. 2006;29: 1084–7.

Chapter 17
Klippel-Trenaunay Syndrome

Peter Gaines

Klippel-Trenaunay syndrome has been included in this book since those involved with treating vascular malformations are likely to encounter such cases. The importance is in recognizing the condition and avoiding the temptation to embark on embolization therapy unless focal symptoms demand.

Diagnosis

- Klippel-Trenaunay syndrome is a clinical diagnosis.
- Only very rarely is the syndrome inherited.
- Two of the following three features are required for diagnosis of the syndrome.

  1. Capillary malformation of the skin (98% of cases) (Fig. 17.1).
  2. Venous malformation (72% of cases) (Fig. 17.2).
  3. Hypertrophy of bone and soft tissues (67% of cases) (Fig. 17.1).

Clinical Features

The syndrome principally affects a single limb, most commonly the legs (90%), but it may affect the arms (10%) or be bilateral.

Capillary Malformation (Fig. 17.1)

- Typically referred to as a "port wine stain."
- Most commonly affects the limb affected by the other features.
- When it extends to the trunk it extends to, or just over, the midline.
- Only rarely complicated by bleeding, infection, or ulceration.

Transcatheter Embolization and Therapy,
Techniques in Interventional Radiology, DOI 10.1007/978-1-84800-897-7_17,
© Springer-Verlag London Limited 2010

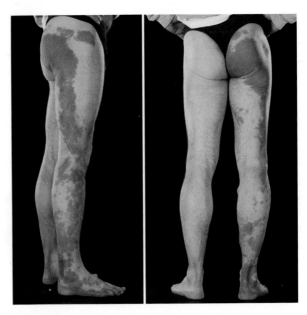

Fig. 17.1 Clinical photograph showing typical port wine stain manifestation of capillary malformation and limb hypertrophy

Hypertrophy of Bone and Soft Tissues (Fig. 17.1)

- Commonly detected as a difference in shoe size.
- When limb discrepancy is likely to affect gait (projected limb length discrepancy of 2 cm or greater), orthopedic correction is necessary.
- Other orthopedic abnormalities include polydactyly, syndactyly, and contractures. When these interrupt normal function, surgical correction is indicated.

Venous Abnormality (Fig. 17.2)

- Typically large and extensive.
- Normally occurs in childhood, and should not be misdiagnosed as simple varicose veins when identified in an adult.
- The classical large lateral "vein of Servelle" only occurs in 30–55% of affected limbs. The vein may drain into internal iliac, external iliac, profunda femoris, superficial femoral, or popliteal veins.
- There may be hypoplasia, aplasia, or aneurysmal dilatation of the deep veins.
- The veins do not function normally. There is always superficial reflux that is accompanied by deep vein reflux and perforator reflux in the majority of affected legs.

Fig. 17.2 Venous malformation in KTS, a port wine stain is just visible

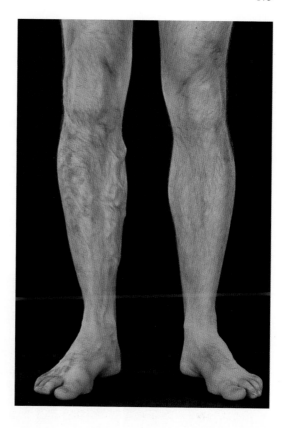

- Such morphological and functional abnormalities result in the following:
    - Superficial thrombophlebitis
    - Deep venous thrombosis
    - Cellulitis
    - Chronic venous insufficiency with lipodermatosclerosis and frank ulceration.

- Large abnormalities may have an associated coagulopathy, which rarely has resulted in significant hemorrhage.

Other Features

- 10% of patients also have a lymphatic vascular malformation.
- Associated nonvascular abnormalities have been described in most organ systems.
- Up to 23% of patients have imaging evidence of involvement of the genito-urinary tract, sometimes clinically evident as bleeding or problems with labor.
- Gastrointestinal involvement occasionally results in bleeding and anemia.

Assessment

- Thorough history and clinical examination is the essential foundation of management.
- Absence of clinically evident high-flow abnormality separates this from Parkes Weber syndrome.
- Examination with a hand-held Doppler device will confirm the lack of high flow in the vascular abnormality.
- Clinical photographs are very helpful to document clinical progression.
- If invasive treatment is considered, an MR examination (including T1 and T2 fat saturated) will demonstrate the extent of the venous abnormality (Fig. 17.3).
- Ultrasound will identify functional venous abnormalities.
- Coagulopathy in large abnormalities can be diagnosed and assessed by measuring platelet count, serum fibrinogen, and fibrin degradation products.

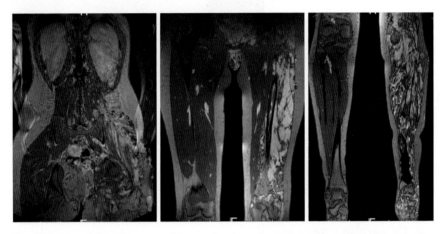

Fig. 17.3 T-2 weighted fat-saturated image showing extensive venous malformation extending from the foot into the buttock

Management

- Patients should be educated regarding the syndrome. Emphasis includes a lack of cure, lack of inheritance, and unlikely impact upon life expectancy.
- Orthopedic correction of functional bone abnormalities should be considered when the patient is a child.
- Invasive management of the venous malformation is largely futile and likely to be associated with recurrence and complications.
- Very occasionally a focal aspect of the venous malformation can be treated by percutaneous embolisation techniques to manage local complications, e.g. pain, bleeding, etc. (see Chapter 2.1.1).

- Before performing embolotherapy/sclerotherapy, it is essential to establish the condition of the deep veins. If the deep veins are abnormal, then treating the superficial veins can lead to worsening edema.
- Recurrence rates following treatment of varicosities are high.
- Care should be directed towards preventing complications and treating disabling symptoms.
- The cosmetic implications of the capillary malformation can be underestimated. Care can include camouflage cosmetics and occasionally laser therapy.
- All patients with leg venous malformation should wear a compression stocking to prevent the complications of venous hypertension.
- Patients with a venous malformation are at increased risk of DVT and PE and therefore should be treated as high risk for this complication through hospital admissions, pregnancy, and on long flights. Female patients may be advised to avoid oral contraceptives.
- Pelvic venous abnormalities may obstruct and complicate labor. Imaging should preferably precede labor and consideration given to elective caesarean section.

Keypoints

- Patients with Klippel-Trenaunay syndrome will seldom require embolotherapy.
- Invasive therapy is indicated for local problems such as pain and bleeding.
- It is essential to remember that the deep veins are frequently abnormal and that this will increase the risks of therapy.
- Patients requiring treatment should be referred for specialist opinion.

Chapter 18
Biologic Effects of Tumor Embolization

Erik Cressman

Introduction

The biological effects of tumor embolization are complex. Effects can be classified as *local* which are a direct consequence of ischemia in the target organ and *systemic* due to the release of chemical mediators by the target organ and the embolic agent/chemotherapy. The biological effects will depend on many interrelated factors including the target tissue, the goal of the embolization, and the choice of the embolic agent and technique used.

The Target Tissue

This depends on susceptibility of both the tumor and the associated organ to embolotherapy. In particular

- Will organ dysfunction following embolization be clinically important?
- Will the tumor respond to treatment?

The Goal of the Embolization Procedure

- Temporary blockage to simplify surgery
- Local chemotherapy
- Infarction of the tumor.

The choice of agent and technique: this will depend on the following:

- The goal of the procedure
- The level of occlusion to be achieved

The following discussion is divided into issues related to the target organ, the local effects, and complications, that are influenced by (and in turn will influence) the biologic effects of embolotherapy.

Transcatheter Embolization and Therapy,
Techniques in Interventional Radiology, DOI 10.1007/978-1-84800-897-7_18,
© Springer-Verlag London Limited 2010

Biological Effects on the Embolized Tissue/Organ

Short Term

- *Ischemia*: blockage of the arterial supply will render the tumor and surrounding tissue ischemic.
- *Inflammation:* the degree varies with embolic agent. Some agents cause an arteritis.
- *Post-embolization syndrome:* This is dealt with in Chapter 13.
- *Necrosis:* cell death due to ischemia or the effects of adjunctive agents such as chemotherapy.

Hypoxia Inducible Factor 1 (HIF-1)

The mechanism underlying many of the local effects is upregulation of HIF-1.

- It is one of the main regulatory substances and is present in every cell.
- Regulates many genes (Table 18.1).
- Allows a cell to rapidly respond to changes in the oxygen environment, although the exact effects differ in each cell type.

Table 18.1 Examples of genes affected by Hypoxia Inducible Factor

Gene	Up ($\uparrow$) or down ($\downarrow$) regulated	Consequence
ABC (ATP-binding cassette), GLUT1 (glucose transporter 1), LDHA (Lactate dehydrogenase A), and PDK1 (Pyruvate dehydrogenase kinase 1)	$\uparrow$	Promote glycolysis
VEGF—vascular endothelial growth factor	$\uparrow$	Promotes angiogenesis
HGF—hepatocyte growth factor	$\uparrow$	Promotes hepatocyte proliferation
TGF-a—transforming growth factor alpha	$\uparrow$	Promotes hepatocyte proliferation in *remnant* liver following portal vein embolization promoting hypertrophy
TGF-b—transforming growth factor beta	$\uparrow$	Promotes hepatocyte proliferation in embolized liver
Ki-67	$\downarrow$	Reduces hepatocyte proliferation, Ki-67 is absent in G0 or quiescent cells
PCNA—proliferating cell nuclear antigen	$\downarrow$	Reduces hepatocyte proliferation, nuclear protein seen in late G1 and S phase

Long-Term Effects of Embolization

- Fibrosis
- Neovascularization
- Recanalization

Tumor Lysis Syndrome (TLS)

This is seen most commonly with leukemias and lymphomas treated with IV chemotherapy, in which large numbers of tumor cells die simultaneously following exposure to cytotoxic drugs.

- TLS phenomenon occurs only rarely with embolization procedures.
- Tumors that are particularly susceptible undergo massive necrosis or apoptosis at a rate faster than the body can dispose of the released intracellular contents.
- Elevated serum levels of potassium, uric acid, and phosphorus and a compensatory lowering of serum of calcium can result.
- Uric acid precipitation in the kidneys may lead to renal failure. One possible treatment strategy is neutralization or very mild alkalinization of the urine, which will decrease the precipitation of uric acid in the kidneys. It must also be remembered that patients vary in their ability to respond to the embolization procedure, with greater risk of renal failure and other complications in advancing age.

Target of Embolization

The Patient

The first question to be addressed is the overall fitness of the patient.

- If the patient is severely compromised already, then any adverse biological effects may be amplified.
- The ability of the patient to tolerate or survive side effects must be taken into account. This is particularly true with chemoembolization of liver cancer patients.

The Target Organ

The function of the target organ may be compromised as a result of the underlying disease process. This will modify the tolerance to and clinical sequelae of embolization. This may limit the amount or degree of treatment that can be safely performed.

Liver

- A patient with a cirrhotic liver and advanced local disease will have less-functional reserve and will not tolerate chemoembolization, as well as a patient with good synthetic function.
- A patient with an occluded portal vein may not tolerate embolization at all.
- Staged and/or superselective procedures may be appropriate to avoid a systemic effect or fulminant iatrogenic liver failure.

Kidney

- A patient with impaired renal function will have less ability to tolerate renal embolization procedures or the sequelae of embolization of other targets.

The Disease Process

The prognosis of the target condition and other co-morbidity will also affect the risk/benefit ratio of the procedure. This entails a thorough knowledge of the prognosis of the patient and also the severity of the symptoms. In general terms:

- *In patients with benign disease/good long-term prognosis/mild symptoms,* a very low-risk profile and excellent long-term outcome are required.
- *In patients with malignant disease with a potential for a good prognosis,* more aggressive intervention with a greater degree of risk may be warranted.
- *In patients with malignant disease with poor prognosis or undergoing palliative procedures,* the short-term outcome is most important.
- *The nature of the treatment* will depend on the severity of the symptoms and the patient's feelings regarding intervention. It is likely that therapy with less risk involved will be appropriate.

Keypoints

The overall effect of embolization at the local level always involves some degree of ischemia, but to assume factors such as VEGF and HIF1 are upregulated in all cases is an oversimplification.

Most embolic agents also result in some degree of inflammation, more so when chemotherapy is coadministered.

Few temporary agents are permanent, whereas there are many cases where a presumably permanent agent was in fact temporary.

Controversy persists over whether or not permanent occlusion is desirable in tumors, and whether ischemia without chemotherapy (as in uterine fibroid embolization) is sufficient to cause tumor degradation. Further work in relevant animal models would help shed light on these issues and is much needed.

Recommended Reading

1. S Baum, MJ Pentecost (eds.) Abrams' Angiography Interventional Radiology 2nd ed, Chapters 10 and 11 Lippincott, Williams, and Wilkins Philadelphia PA, 2006
2. S Stampfl, N Bellemann, U Stampfl et al. Inflammation and Recanalization of Four Different Spherical Embolization Agents in the Porcine Kidney Model. JVIR 2008 19(4): 577–586
3. GP Siskin, A Beck, M Schuster et al. Leiomyoma Infarction After Uterin Artery Embolization: A Prospective Randomized Study Comparing Tris-acryl Gelatin Microspheres Versus Polyvinyl Alcohol Microspheres JVIR 2008 19(1): 58–65
4. BJ Moeller, Y Cao, Z Vujaskovic et al. The Relationship Between Hypoxia and Angiogenesis. Sem Rad Onc 2004 14(3): 215–221
5. S Gupta, S Kobayashi, S Phongkitkarun et al. Effect of Transcatheter Hepatic Arterial Embolization on Angiogenesis in an Animal Model. Invest Rad 2006 41(6):516–521
6. TY Patel, DM Hovsepian, JR Duncan Measurement of Blood Flow Before and After Embolization with Use of Fluorescent Microspheres in an Animal Model. JVIR 2006 17:103–111
7. GL Semenza Hypoxia-inducible Factor 1 and Human Cancer. ASCO Educational Book 2008 548–551

Chapter 19
Liver Tumors (Hepatocellular Cancer)

Jai Patel

This section covers embolic therapy for the treatment of hepatocellular carcinoma (HCC) only. Liver embolization for neuroendocrine tumors and other metastatic tumors is covered elsewhere.

Epidemiology of HCC

- Fifth commonest malignancy world-wide, third commonest cause of cancer-related death.
- Predisposing factors include cirrhosis, chronic hepatitis, aflatoxin.
- Incidence rising due to high prevalence of hepatitis B virus (HBV) in Asia/Africa and hepatitis C virus (HCV) in Europe/United States.
- 90% occur in cirrhotics—common causes include alcohol and HCV in Europe/United States and HBV in Asia/Africa. Other risk factors—hemochromatosis, primary biliary cirrhosis (PBC).

Diagnosis

Based on the European Association for the Study of the Liver (EASL) criteria.

For tumors >2 cm in a patient with cirrhosis, diagnosis is confirmed on the basis of one of the following:

- Two imaging modalities showing arterial hypervascularity in the liver mass.
- One imaging modality showing arterial hypervascularity with alpha-fetoprotein (AFP) > 400 μg/mL.
- Biopsy confirmation of HCC.

Imaging

- CT—hypervascular liver mass enhancing in arterial phase, with washout in the portal phase.

Transcatheter Embolization and Therapy,
Techniques in Interventional Radiology, DOI 10.1007/978-1-84800-897-7_19,
© Springer-Verlag London Limited 2010

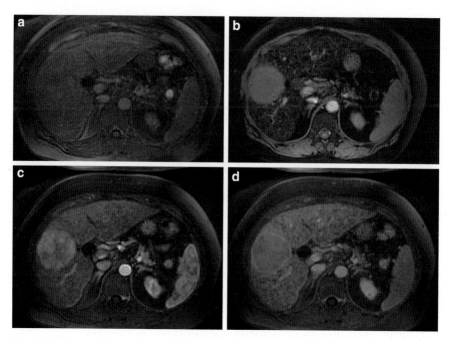

Fig. 19.1 MRI—most commonly mass with decreased signal on T1W, moderately increased signal on T2W (**a**), lack of uptake of super-paramagnetic iron oxide (SPIO) (**b**), arterial-phase enhancement with gadolinium (**c**), and washout in the portal phase (**d**)

- MRI—mass with decreased signal on T1W, moderately increased signal on T2W, lack of uptake of super-paramagnetic iron oxide (SPIO), arterial-phase enhancement with gadolinium and washout in the portal phase (Fig. 19.1).

Differential Diagnosis Includes

- Dysplastic nodules—these require differentiation from HCC in patients with underlying cirrhosis (look for lack of uptake of SPIO and absence of washout in the portal phase).
- Other benign hypervascular lesions, e.g., focal nodular hyperplasia, hemangioma, adenoma (although most of these will have their own specific imaging features).

Laboratory/Other Investigations

- Define the degree of liver dysfunction (LFTs, prothrombin time, AFP). This is important in any form of therapy that might adversely affect function.

- Assess renal function as there is potential for nephrotoxicity from contrast and chemotherapeutic agents.
- Assess left ventricular ejection fraction if using cardiotoxic drugs, e.g., doxorubicin.

General Considerations

Transarterial chemoembolization (TACE) should currently be considered as palliative and not curative. Indications for TACE will vary from institution to institution. TACE is currently indicated for intermediate stage HCC (i.e. patients unsuitable for potentially curative surgical resection, liver transplantation or local ablative therapies) with relatively well-preserved liver function. TACE may also be of value in combination therapy for downstaging focal lesions which are just beyond the size limits for local ablative therapies or as a bridge to transplantation.

Prognosis is affected by both the stage of the tumor and the degree of liver dysfunction at the time of presentation. A number of scoring/staging systems have been developed for prognostic and management purposes (Okuda, Cancer of the Liver Italian Program—CLIP, Barcelona Clinic Liver Cancer—BCLC these include factors such as tumor size, Child-Pugh score, AFP level, presence of vascular invasion, performance status, etc.

Contraindications

No absolute contraindications, but relative contraindications include the following:

- Child-Pugh score ≥ 8
- Bilirubin $> 50 \, \mu mol/L$
- Portal vein (PV) thrombosis (arterial embolization will lead to infarction)
- Hepatofugal PV flow (increased risk of infarction)
- Large-volume tumors (occupying >50% of liver mass)
- Extrahepatic disease

Pre-procedure Evaluation

- Review previous imaging and laboratory results to assess suitability for TACE.
- Determine number, distribution and vascularity of lesions, patency of PV, presence of extrahepatic disease.
- Identify factors that will influence approach or complexity of procedure, e.g., morphology of celiac axis, variant arterial anatomy, arterial stenosis.
- Decide whether selective or lobar embolization is appropriate.

Anatomic Considerations

Normal Anatomy

- Normal liver supplied by portal vein (PV) = 75% and hepatic artery (HA) = 25%.
- HCC supplied by HA = 90% and PV = 10%.
  HA divides into right and left branches; right HA artery sub-divides further into anterior and posterior branches supplying segments 5/8 and 6/7, respectively. This "normal" arrangement is seen in approximately 50% patients.
- Cystic artery usually arises from the proximal right HA.
- Right gastric artery may also arise from the right HA.

Variant Anatomy: (See also Table 33.1) (Fig. 19.2)

Considerable variability in the anatomy of the hepatic artery exists.
  Commonest variants are as follows:

- Replaced (14%) or accessory (6%) right HA arising from superior mesenteric artery
- Replaced (12%) or accessory (8%) left HA arising from the left gastric artery
- Proper hepatic artery arising from the superior mesenteric artery (2.5%).

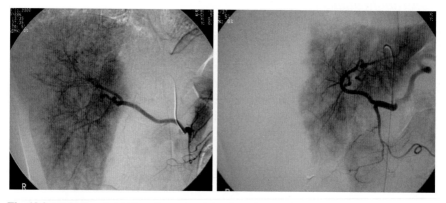

Fig. 19.2 (**a**) Replaced right hepatic artery arising from the superior mesenteric artery. (**b**) The left hepatic artery arises from the common hepatic artery

Extra-hepatic Supply (Fig. 19.3)

Liver tumors may have additional supply from non-hepatic vessels depending on their location (e.g., tumors located in the dome of the liver may be partly supplied

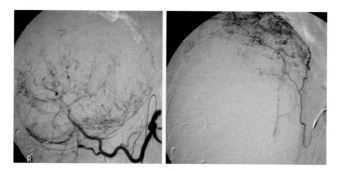

Fig. 19.3 (**a**) Large hepatoma supplied predominantly from the right hepatic artery. (**b**) The superomedial aspect of the tumor is supplied by the right inferior phrenic artery

by the right internal mammary artery when located anteriorly or by the inferior phrenic artery when located posteriorly).

Consent

Important things to explain to the patient during consent are as follows:

- TACE is a palliative procedure and not curative.
- Approximately 50% increase in survival at 2 years compared to conservative therapy.
- Post-embolization syndrome (pain, sickness, flu-like symptoms) is common.
- General feeling of fatigue (usually lasting 2 weeks).
- Complications:
  - Puncture site (<5%)—hematoma, bleeding, thrombosis.
  - Treatment related (1–5%)—infection/abscess, acute liver failure, neutropenia.

Equipment

Catheters

- 4-French sidewinder or cobra catheter (dependent on personal preference) to catheterize celiac axis and hepatic artery.
- Coaxial microcatheter for selective catheterization of segmental vessels as necessary.
- Remember to use catheters without sideholes.

Chemotherapeutic Agents

- Drugs have to be ordered in advance and in accordance with hospital regulations.
- Cisplatin, doxorubicin, mitomycin C or a combination of these have been used.
- There is no absolute evidence for the superiority of any particular agent.
- All staff in the angio room should wear protective masks and visors while handling cytotoxic drugs.

Embolic Agent

Lipiodol

- Drug carrier and partial embolic agent
- Used to create an emulsion with the chemotherapeutic agent prior to infusion into the catheter

Particulate Agents

- Polyvinyl alcohol (PVA)
- Gelfoam

Drug-Eluting Beads

- DC/LC Beads (Biocompatibles UK Ltd) and Hepasphere/Quadrasphere (Biosphere Medical, Rockland, MA, USA) are the main agents.
- Function as both the drug carrier and embolic agent.
- Embolic microspheres loaded with chemotherapeutic agent (usually doxorubicin).
- Subsequent drug elution gives a more sustained concentration of drug within the tumor and much reduced systemic concentration compared with lipiodol-based treatment.
- Only suitable for patients in whom selective TACE (right or left lobe) can be performed.
- Hepasphere/Quadrasphere is slightly different to DC Beads in that they swell within several minutes after contact with aqueous solutions, blocking the embolized artery.
- These are exciting developments in localized chemoembolization of HCC and results are promising.

Bland Embolization Versus TACE

- Note that controversy exists between bland embolization and embolization with chemotherapeutic agents.
- The endpoint of bland embolization is cessation of flow to the tumor and consequent ischemia; this is a different endpoint to TACE.

- However, most IRs continue to use a chemotherapeutic agent as part of TACE, although there is no level-1 evidence to support either approach.

Radioembolization

- Embolization using radioactive particles containing usually yttrium-90.
- Main agents are Therasphere (MDS, Nordion, Canada) and SIR spheres (Sirtex, Sydney, Australia).
- Yttrium-90 is a beta-emitter that irradiates tissue with path length of 2.5 mm (maximum 10 mm) and half-life of 64.2 h.
- Theraspheres are glass yttrium-90 beads and SIR spheres are resin beads containing yttrium-90.
- The technique is much more involved than TACE with embolization of all extra-hepatic collaterals required ("skeletonizing the hepatic artery") and technetium scanning to exclude shunting to the lung beforehand.
- More results from this exciting technology are awaited.

Selective Versus Non-selective TACE

Perform TACE as selectively as possible to reduce post-embolization syndrome and complications. As general principles

- Superselective/sub-segmental—if focal lesion ≤5 cm or up to three lesions ≤3 cm.
- Selective/segmental—if large lesion or several lesions confined to one or two segments.
- Non-selective/lobar—if multifocal lesions scattered diffusely.
- Consider dividing into two to three treatment sessions (right anterior, right posterior, and left lobe) to reduce the risk of significant liver dysfunction.
- Remember to place catheter beyond the cystic artery and/or right gastric artery origins to prevent embolization of the gallbladder or stomach.

Leave 4 weeks between treatment sessions to allow for recovery of liver function.

Procedure

Pre-procedure Preparation

- Fast patient for 4 h (allow clear fluids).
- Ensure hydration: clear fluids and intravenous (IV) hydration.
- IV broad-spectrum antibiotics (e.g., cefuroxime and metronidazole).
- Opiate analgesia—consider patient-controlled analgesia as it is often easier to manage pain control with this, once the patient returns to the ward.
- Antiemetic—nausea can originate from both the opiate analgesia and post-embolization syndrome.

Access

- Femoral artery access is usual.
- Brachial artery access may occasionally be required in cases of difficult anatomy or severe atherosclerotic disease of the iliac arteries.

Initial Diagnostic Study

- Start with angiography of the celiac axis ± superior mesenteric artery.
- Inject 24 ml at 6 ml/second.
- Start imaging at two frames per second for the arterial phase, reducing to one frame per second for the portal phase.
- Consider 8 s injection delay to allow for multimasking.
- Identify any variants in the vascular anatomy.
- Confirm patency/direction of flow in the portal vein.

Selective Angiography

After non-selective angiography, specific feeding segmental arteries can be selected.

- 20 ml at 4 ml/s, 2 s injection delay; two frames/s, arterial and parenchymal phase.
- Projection: AP ± oblique views.
- Localize lesions and identify vessels feeding the tumor.
- The tumor supply will show neovascularity (tortuous vessels with abnormal branching pattern), vascular lakes, arterio-portal or arterio-venous shunting, localized parenchymal blush (Fig. 19.4).

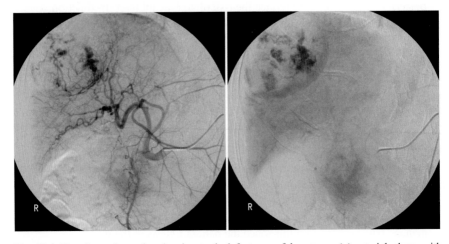

Fig. 19.4 Hepatic angiography showing typical features of hepatoma (**a**) arterial phase with abnormal vessels, venous lakes (**b**) late phase showing peripheral parenchymal enhancement

Catheterize the feeding vessel with a co-axial microcatheter.
- Confirm position with angiography.
- Either, hand injection using a 2–3 mL syringe, or pump injection (6 mL at a maximum of 3 mL/s, maximum 700 psi pressure).

Perform Chemoembolization

Technique: Lipiodol

- Form emulsion of cytotoxic drug and lipiodol by passing between two syringes connected via a three-way tap (Fig. 19.5).
- Infuse through microcatheter until forward flow slows. If necessary, follow lipiodol infusion with particulate embolization using either PVA 300–500 μm particles or gelfoam.
- The maximum dose of chemotherapeutic agent is limited per session.

Fig. 19.5 Technique for mixing lipiodol and cisplatin using two syringes and a three-way tap. The mixture is forced back and forth until it becomes an emulsion at which point there is a notable drop in resistance

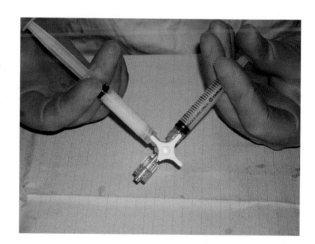

Technique: Drug-Eluting Beads

- DC beads are loaded with doxorubicin in pharmacy and mixed with contrast several hours pre-procedure. For Hepaspheres, doxorubicin is mixed with 10 mL of normal saline and left to stand for 1 h before use.
- Inject down the microcatheter like any other particulate embolic agent until forward flow slows and peripheral side-branch vessels are pruned.

Endpoints: Two Procedural Endpoints Should be Considered

1. Forward flow slows and no further chemoembolic agent can be given without producing non-target embolization.

2. All the chemoembolic agent has been given—consider finishing off with bland particulate embolization or, if there is still significant tumour vascularity, repeating the procedure after a 1-month interval.

Post-procedure

- Remove catheter and achieve hemostasis.
- Reiterate the importance of symptomatic management of post-embolization syndrome to the ward staff and patient.
- Explain the symptoms/signs of delayed infection to the patient (increasing pain and/or pyrexia) and the importance of seeking prompt medical review.
- Patient can usually be discharged at 24–48 h post-procedure.
- Check liver function, prothrombin time, and renal function prior to discharge and repeat again 1 week prior to any further planned treatment.
- Check clinical status of the patient prior to repeat treatment.

Post-procedure Follow-Up

Once there is no residual tumor vascularity on completion angiography or after 3 treatment sessions, re-evaluate the patient with follow-up imaging after 4–6 weeks. RECIST criteria or EASL criteria used for follow-up.

Assess

- Tumor volume
- Amount of lipiodol retention
- Residual viable (enhancing) tumor
- Disease progression: increase in size or enhancement, new lesions, spread to other organs, portal vein thrombosis

Consider further treatment if imaging shows residual tumor enhancement.

Keypoints

- TACE is a palliative procedure for intermediate-stage HCC and early-stage disease unsuitable for potentially curative treatment.
- It is important to select patients carefully, based on both tumor morphology and liver function as both these have prognostic implications for patient survival.

- Treat as selectively as possible to minimize side-effects and complications, especially if patients are in Child-Pugh class B.
- Avoid non-target chemoembolization to the gallbladder or stomach.
- If considering a repeat procedure, ensure that the patient has recovered both clinically and biochemically following the preceding procedure.
- Results of DC-bead/LC bead studies and radioembolization studies are awaited.
- In future, combinations of therapies with Sorafenib may be very promising.

Suggested Reading

Llovet JM, Bruix J. Systematic review of randomised trials for unresectable hepatocellular carcinoma: chemoembolization improves survival. Hepatology 2003; 37:429–42.

Kettenbach J, Stadler A, Katzler I, Schernthaner R, Blum M, Lammer J, Rand T. Drug-loaded microspheres for the treatment of liver cancer: review of current results. Cardiovasc Intervent Radiol 2008; 31:468–76.

Lee KH, Sung KB, Lee DY, Park SJ, Kim KW, Yu JS. Chemoembolization for hepatocellular carcinoma: anatomic and haemodynamic considerations in the hepatic artery and portal vein. RadioGraphics 2002; 22:1077–91.

Kim CH, Chung JW, Lee W, Jae HJ, Park JH. Recognising extrahepatic collaterals vessels that supply hepatocellular carcinoma to avoid complications of transcatheter arterial chemoembolization. RadioGraphics 2005; 25:S25–39.

Clark HP, Carson WF, Kavanagh PV, Ho CPH, Shen P, Zagoria RJ. Staging and current treatment of hepatocellular carcinoma. RadioGraphics 2005; 25:S3–23.

Chapter 20
Liver Tumors: Metastases

Ahsun Riaz and Riad Salem

Clinical Features

- Secondary liver tumors are more common than primary liver tumors.
- Embolization in these cases is performed as an elective procedure.
- Tumors that commonly metastasize to the liver are
  - Colorectal carcinoma (CRC)
  - Neuroendocrine tumors (NET)
  - Other: breast cancer, sarcoma, melanoma

Available Embolic Therapies

- Following are the embolic therapeutic options available in the management of secondary live tumors
  - Bland embolization
  - Transarterial chemoembolization (TACE)
  - Yttrium-90 radioembolization (Y-90)
  - Drug-eluting bead-transarterial chemoembolization (DEB-TACE)

Diagnostic Evaluation

- *Clinical*

  - Secondary liver lesions rarely lead to signs and symptoms of liver decompensation (e.g., encephalopathy). However, evidence of liver dysfunction in cases of metastatic liver lesions indicates a poor prognosis.

- **Laboratory**
  - The laboratory tests include the following:
    - Liver function tests (LFT)
    - Complete blood count (CBC)
    - Carcinoembryonic agent (for colorectal carcinoma)
  - Urinary 5-HIAA (for carcinoid)

- **Imaging**
  - The imaging characteristics of metastatic lesions to the liver are assessed using contrast-enhanced CT or MRI. Biopsy may be required if the diagnosis is uncertain.
    - Colorectal carcinoma: moderately hypervascular lesions
    - Neuroendocrine tumors: very hypervascular tumors

- Pre-treatment angiography is performed to assess vascular anatomy prior to all embolic therapies.
- Technetium-99m macroaggregated albumin (Tc-99m MAA) scan is a nuclear scan that is performed before Y-90 to assess the following:
  - Lung shunt fraction (LSF)
  - Splanchnic flow

Indications

- Unresectable metastatic liver lesions.

Relative Contraindications

- Poor performance status (Eastern Cooperative Oncology Group performance status >1).
- Deranged liver function (bilirubin > 2 mg/dL).
- Y-90: LSF allowing >30 Gy dose delivery to the lungs in one session.

Anatomy

The aorta, iliac arteries, and portal vein are usually assessed on cross-sectional imaging. Pre-treatment angiography is performed to assess vascular anatomy, in particular the cystic artery, anatomical variations, extrahepaatic tumor supply, and communications with the gastrointestinal and systemic circulations. The following are typically performed.

  - *Superior mesenteric angiogram*: for replaced hepatic arteries.

○ *Celiac arteriogram*: for left gastric supply to liver (replaced left hepatic) and inferior phrenic arteries.

○ *Common hepatic arteriogram*: for communications between hepatic and gastrointestinal vasculature (right gastric, dorsal pancreatic, and gastroduodenal artery).

○ *Gastroduodenal arteriogram*: for cystic, superior pancreaticoduodenal, and accessory hepatic arteries. Parasitization of flow to liver from GDA or its branches is also assessed.

○ *Proper hepatic arteriogram*: for right gastric artery communication between hepatic and gastrointestinal vasculature.

○ *Right hepatic arteriogram*: vascular supply of tumor is assessed. Vessels of interest include the cystic, supraduodenal, and middle hepatic arteries.

○ *Left hepatic arteriogram*: vascular supply of tumor is assessed. Vessels sought include the accessory left gastric inferior esophageal, right gastric, falciform, and left inferior phrenic arteries. Delayed imaging is recommended to confirm that the coronary vein does not opacify as this indicates splanchnic flow.

Patient Preparation

• Coil embolization of arterial communications with non-hepatic tissue is recommended to prevent aberrant flow of embolic particles (the threshold for coil embolization prior to radioembolization should be low). Arterial communications with non-hepatic tissue are meticulously sought during pre-treatment angiography and embolized with coils.

Pre-procedure Medications

• The pre-procedure medications include anti-emetics, anti-histamines, proton pump inhibitors, and antibiotics.

Equipment

• Catheters: once the vascular anatomy has been studied, microcatheters are recommended. The vessels may be fragile due to previous exposure to systemic chemotherapeutics and are prone to spasm and dissection anyway.
• Bland embolization: Gelfoam or PVA particles.
• Y-90: TheraSphere (glass) or SIR-Sphere (resin). Specific equipment is provided for radioembolization.
• TACE: chemotherapeutic agent mixed with lipiodol. This is followed by injection of bland embolic particles as above.
• DEB-TACE: chemotherapeutic agent-loaded microspheres.

Procedure

- **Access**
  - ○ The femoral artery is used in most cases, but access from the arm may be necessary in some cases.
- **Performing the Procedure**
  - ○ The angiogram is performed on the same day of the procedure in cases of bland embolization, TACE, and DEB-TACE.
  - ○ Y-90: The pre-treatment angiography and Tc-99m MAA scan are performed approximately 1 week prior to the actual procedure.
- **Technique**
  - ○ It is recommended to be as selective as possible, as secondary lesions (with the exception of NET) may not be very hypervascular relative to surrounding normal tissue.
  - ○ Whole liver infusions are not recommended (a "bilobar lobar" approach is recommended if the whole liver is to be treated—separate injection of the left and right hepatic arteries to minimize aberrant flow of embolic material and hence incidence of toxicities.)
- **Endpoints**
  - ○ Bland embolization: stasis.
  - ○ Y-90: the particles are minimally embolic; hence flow is maintained post-radioembolization.
  - ○ TACE: stasis or sub-stasis of flow.
  - ○ DEB-TACE: the particles are minimally embolic; so flow is maintained.
- **Immediate Post-procedure Care**
  - ○ Access puncture site is closed.
  - ○ Y-90: radiation safety protocols are followed; catheters and equipment are disposed appropriately.

Post-procedure Medications

- Supportive management of the post-embolization syndrome (pain, fatigue, nausea, vomiting).
- Patients are discharged on the same day in the case of Y-90.

Follow-Up

- Two week phone call (to assess general patient well being)
- One month follow-up
  - ○ Cross-sectional Imaging: to assess tumor response to therapy using size (RECIST)/necrosis (EASL) guidelines
  - ○ Laboratory work-up: this includes LFTs, CBC, and tumor markers

- After the first follow-up visit, radiologic evaluation is recommended every 3 months

Current Data

- **Bland Embolization**
  - It has also been used for pain relief and control of symptoms in hepatic metastases from neuroendocrine tumors and sarcomas [1].
- **Y-90**
  - CRC: the combination of radioembolization with systemic chemotherapy has been shown to have a significantly better tumor response, a longer time to progression, survival benefit, and an acceptable safety profile than chemotherapy alone [2]. Dose escalation studies have shown a better response with increasing doses [3].
  - NET: radioembolization of metastatic disease to the liver from a neuroendocrine neoplasia has been shown to be effective and safe. A prolonged response to treatment, i.e., greater than 2 years has been seen [4, 5].
  - Breast cancer: radioembolization is an efficacious treatment for unresectable reast cancer metastases to the liver [6]. There is a significant radiologic response after radioembolization, but the survival benefit of this treatment in these patients has not been established.
- **TACE**
  - CRC: Geschwind *et al.* demonstrated that TACE can prolong survival of patients with colorectal metastases even in patients who had not responded to systemic chemotherapy [7].
  - NET: Liapi *et al.* analyzed imaging responses and determined outcomes of 26 patients with neuroendocrine metastases treated with TACE and showed a mean patient survival of 78 months [8].
  - Breast cancer: patients with breast metastasis to the liver unresponsive to standard of care chemotherapy have been treated with TACE and the survival benefit seen is not impressive as most patients develop extrahepatic metastases [9, 10].
- **DEB-TACE**
  - DEBs loaded with irinotecan are being investigated for the treatment of patients with colorectal hepatic metastases [11].

Alternative Therapies

- Surgical resection
- Thermal ablation (e.g., radiofrequency ablation)

Complications

- Post-embolization syndrome is managed supportively.
- Biliary complications: biliary strictures, abscesses, etc are seen more often in non-cirrhotic livers (metastatic) [12]. Cholecystitis due to aberrant deposition of embolic material into the gall bladder wall may be seen.
- Hepatic dysfunction: whole liver chemoembolization and radioembolization may lead to liver dysfunction.
- Gastrointestinal (GI) complications: GI ulcers may be seen. The vascular communications of hepatic vasculature with the GI tract should be studied in detail and prophylactic proximal coil embolization should be performed to prevent particulate agent bowel embolization.
- Vascular injury: Vessels may be fragile due to previous history of exposure to chemotherapeutic agents. Careful wire/catheter manipulation and use of microcatheters are recommended.

Keypoints

- Limited options available for unresectable liver metastases.
- Embolization techniques (Bland, Y-90, TACE, DEB-TACE) present safe and efficacious methods of management for some of these tumors.
- The decision to use a treatment modality should be made after consensus of a multi-disciplinary team.
- Meticulous assessment of the pre-treatment angiography and the prophylactic coil embolization of vessels prevent the occurrence of serious complications following these procedures.

Suggested Reading

1. Maluccio MA, Covey AM, Schubert J, et al. Treatment of metastatic sarcoma to the liver with bland embolization. Cancer 2006; 107:1617–1623.
2. Gray B, Van Hazel G, Hope M, et al. Randomised trial of SIR-spheres plus chemotherapy vs. chemotherapy alone for treating patients with liver metastases from primary large bowel cancer. Ann Oncol 2001; 12:1711–1720.
3. Goin JE, Dancey JE, Hermann GA, Sickles CJ, Roberts CA, MacDonald JS. Treatment of unresectable metastatic colorectal carcinoma to the liver with intrahepatic Y-90 microspheres: a dose-ranging study. World J Nucl Med 2003; 2:216–225.
4. Rhee TK, Lewandowski RJ, Liu DM, et al. 90Y Radioembolization for metastatic neuroendocrine liver tumors: preliminary results from a multi-institutional experience. Ann Surg 2008; 247:1029–1035.

5. Kennedy AS, Dezarn WA, McNeillie P, et al. Radioembolization for unresectable neuroendocrine hepatic metastases using resin 90Y-microspheres: early results in 148 patients. Am J Clin Oncol 2008; 31:271–279.

6. Coldwell D, Nutting C, Kennedy AK. Treatment of hepatic metastases from breast cancer with Yttrium-90 SIR-Spheres radioembolization. In: Society of Interventional Radiology Annual Meeting. New Orleans, LA, 2005.

7. Hong K, McBride JD, Georgiades CS, et al. Salvage therapy for liver-dominant colorectal metastatic adenocarcinoma: comparison between transcatheter arterial chemoembolization versus yttrium-90 radioembolization. J Vasc Interv Radiol 2009; 20:360–367.

8. Liapi E, Geschwind J-F, Vossen JA, et al. Functional MRI evaluation of tumor response in patients with neuroendocrine hepatic metastasis treated with transcatheter arterial chemoembolization. Am J Roentgenol 2008; 190:67–73.

9. Giroux MF, Baum RA, Soulen MC. Chemoembolization of liver metastasis from breast carcinoma. J Vasc Interv Radiol 2004; 15:289–291.

10. Buijs M, Kamel IR, Vossen JA, Georgiades CS, Hong K, Geschwind JF. Assessment of metastatic breast cancer response to chemoembolization with contrast agent enhanced and diffusion-weighted MR imaging. J Vasc Interv Radiol 2007; 18:957–963.

11. Taylor RR, Tang Y, Gonzalez MV, Stratford PW, Lewis AL. Irinotecan drug eluting beads for use in chemoembolization: in vitro and in vivo evaluation of drug release properties. Eur J Pharm Sci 2007; 30:7–14.

12. Yu JS, Kim KW, Jeong MG, Lee DH, Park MS, Yoon SW. Predisposing factors of bile duct injury after transcatheter arterial chemoembolization (TACE) for hepatic malignancy. Cardiovasc Intervent Radiol 2002; 25:270–274.

Chapter 21
Liver Tumors: Neuroendocrine Hepatic Metastases

Kenneth J. Kolbeck and John A. Kaufman

Clinical Features

- Historically less aggressive than gastrointestinal adenocarcinoma, thus the term *carcinoid*.
- Primary tumor can be from many locations: foregut (lungs, bronchi, and stomach), midgut (small intestine, appendix, and proximal colon), or hindgut (distal colon, rectum).
- Majority of cell types originate from neural crest during fetal development.
- Secretory/functional tumors release physiologically active compounds; non-secretory/non-functional tumors do not.
- Symptoms frequently related to hormone (peptides, steroids, and neuroamines) production and release.
- Hormones produced include insulin, glucagon, gastrin, vasoactive intestinal peptide, pancreatic polypeptide, somatostatin, calcitonin, neurotensin, ACTH, growth hormone releasing factor, corticotrophin, histamine, dopamine, substance P, neurotensin, prostaglandins, kallikrein, as well as serotonin and its precursor 5-hydroxytryptophan and metabolite 5-hydroxyindoleacetic acid (5-HIAA).
- Carcinoid lesions (primarily neuroamine producers) present with carcinoid syndrome in approximately 10% of cases. Pancreatic endocrine tumors (primarily peptide producers) secrete functioning peptides in approximately 75% of cases and present with symptoms related to the specific peptide.
- Carcinoid syndrome is a constellation of symptoms including diarrhea, frequent bowel movements, weight changes, heart palpitations, hypotension, hypertension, wheezing/asthma, intermittent skin flushing, acromegaly, Cushing's syndrome, and right heart valvular disease/heart failure.
- Carcinoid crisis (sudden release of active agents and abrupt onset of severe symptoms) can be induced with surgery, chemotherapy, emotional stressors, and iodinated contrast injection (can be confused with contrast allergy).
- Patients with secretory lesions present with symptoms related to the agent released, while those with non-secretory lesions present late with bulk symptoms.
- Many neuroendocrine lesions over-express somatostatin receptors on the cell surface (which can assist in diagnosis and monitoring response to therapy).
- Non-specific symptoms frequently delay an accurate diagnosis.
- The majority of patients present with hepatic metastases; the primary lesion may never be identified.

Transcatheter Embolization and Therapy,
Techniques in Interventional Radiology, DOI 10.1007/978-1-84800-897-7_21,
© Springer-Verlag London Limited 2010

Diagnostic Evaluation

Laboratory

- Several secreted neuroamines and peptides have specific serum/urine tests that assist in diagnosis and evaluation of response to therapy.
- Twenty four hour urine serotonin/5-HIAA results in false negatives in up to 50% of cases.
- Serum serotonin, tryptophan, and Chromogranin A commonly assist in the diagnosis in the appropriate patient population.

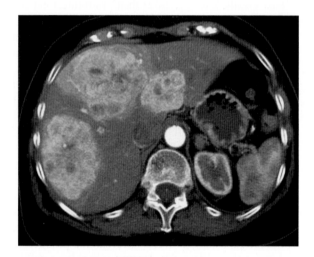

Fig. 21.1 An axial image from a contrast-enhanced CT scan in a patient with symptomatic metastatic neuroendocrine tumor demonstrates multiple, large, hypervascular lesions within the liver

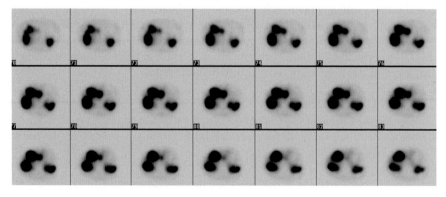

Fig. 21.2 An Octreoscan from the same patient demonstrates the high concentration of somatostatin receptors within the hepatic metastases. The primary lesion was not identified in this patient; however, an isolated bone metastases was also identified

Imaging

- Ultrasound, CT, and MRI are used frequently in diagnosis of hepatic metastases (lesions are primarily hypervascular compared to adjacent liver parenchyma).
- Endoscopy and colonoscopy may assist in identifying the primary lesion.
- An Octreoscan (radiolabeled somatostatin analog) may assist in identifying primary and metastatic lesions.

Indications for Embolization

- Uncontrolled symptoms of hormone release in spite of adequate subcutaneous octreotide therapy.
- Tumor bulk with mass effect symptoms (i.e. early satiety and weight loss)
- Clinical concern for residual liver function being overwhelmed by hepatic metastases

Alternative Therapies

- Observation: for asymptomatic patients with small metastatic liver tumor burden.
- Systemic administration of octreotide (long acting ± short acting): can lead to tumor regression and sympton control in some cases.
- Resection of primary and/or dominant metastases: goal of reducing the overall number of metastases and tumor bulk.
- Chemoinfusion liver metastases: 5 day infusion from intra-arterial delivery of 5-fluorouracil.
- Ablation of liver metastases: radiofrequency ablation and cryoablation have been utilized.
- Bland embolization: usually particle embolization.
- Routine chemoembolization: frequently with three drug combination (cisplatin, doxorubicin, and mitomycin C).
- Drug-eluting bead chemoembolization: primarily doxorubicin.
- Y-90 radiotherapy with arterial delivery of glass/resin microspheres: increasing in popularity, less overall embolic effect per treatment. Expensive.
- Intravenous delivery of Y-90 radiotherapy-labeled octreotide peptide analog.

Contraindications

- Contraindications to arteriography: bleeding/coagulopathy, poor arterial access, unstable catheter position, diminished renal function.
- Contraindications to chemotherapy: agent/dose specific, rare cardiac and renal toxicity with doxorubicin/cisplatin.

- Contraindications to embolization: limited residual liver function, risk of inducing liver failure.
- Relative contraindications: portal vein thrombosis, biliary obstruction, and tumor burden greater than 50% of the functioning liver.

Specific Complications

- Arterial access: as previously described in this book.
- Non-target embolization: symptoms depend upon embolic material as well as organ embolized.
- Complex/distorted hepatic arterial anatomy: can severely limit catheter access and make catheterization extremely difficult.
- Carcinoid reaction/crisis: sudden hormone/neurotransmitter release during contrast injections, embolization, or with tumor necrosis.
- Premedication with 500 µg octeotide IV helps block receptors, reducing side effects.
- Steroids, anti-histamines, anti-asthmatic agents, anti-hypertensives, as well as adrenergic blockers (alpha and beta), may be required pending individual patient reactions.

Vascular Anatomy

- All the variations of hepatic arterial anatomy are possible.
- Bulky liver disease frequently results in extremely distorted anatomy.
- Hypervascular lesions occasionally parasitize adjacent, non-hepatic arteries (e.g., phrenic artery).

Equipment

Catheters

- *Non-selective catheters:* aortic flush run rarely used to identify aberrant vessels. Vessel origins for selective catheterization and evaluation can frequently be identified on previous cross-sectional imaging.
- *Selective catheters:* anatomy dependent, frequently able to selectively catheterize target vessels with 5Fr celiac catheter and microcatheter. Other selective catheters include cobra, Simmons, Omni Select, with superselection via microcatheters.
- *High-flow microcatheters:* often used to diminish risk of catheter occlusion with particulate embolics.
- *Guide catheter/sheath:* if catheter changes are expected a 5 Fr common femoral sheath is recommended.

Embolic Agents

- Bland embolization (iodinated oil emulsion or particles)
- Chemoembolization (oil emulsions mixed with doxorubicin alone or the three drug combination—cisplatin, doxorubicin, and mitomycin C)
- Multiple embolic agents (gel foam slurry, polyvinyl alcohol suspensions, as well as engineered copolymer embolic agents)
- Drug-eluting bead co-polymers
- Resin and glass Yttrium-90 microspheres

Medications

- Routine chemoembolization premedication regimen include an anti-inflammatory (e.g., ketorolac, 30 mg IV), steroid (e.g., 20 mg dexamethasone), antibiotic (e.g., 1 g cefotaxime), and anti-emetic (e.g., ondansetron 8 mg IV).
- Intra-procedural medications include midazolam and fentanyl for moderate sedation.
- Intravenous octreotide (500 μg) prior to treatment/infusion of iodinated contrast is recommended to reduce the risk of carcinoid crisis.
- In the event of carcinoid crisis, additional doses of octreotide as well as symptomatic control (oxygen, volume support for hypotension, anti-hypertensives, anti-emetics, and anti-histamines) may be required. Note that epinephrine may induce/provoke attacks rather than alleviate symptoms. Dopamine infusion is recommended as the primary vasopressor in the event of a hemodynamic collapse.
- Bolus administration of an additional 500 μg IV octreotide and/or a titrated continuous IV infusion of octreotide may be required for symptom control. Infusion doses of 100–500 μg/hour may be required. Monitoring for bradycardia and arrhythmias is recommended with octreotide infusions.

IR Evaluation

Access

- Common femoral artery, most commonly right, related to physician preference.

Arteriography

- Frequently, hypervascular tumors require high volume injections and high flow rates to adequately assess the vasculature.

Assessing the Lesions

- Due to hypervascular tendencies, evaluation with a 4–5Fr catheter is recommended. Microcatheters frequently do not allow enough contrast volume/flow to adequately asses the entire vascular distribution.
- Once adequate arteriographic evaluation has been obtained, further selection and embolization with a microcatheter is frequently required.

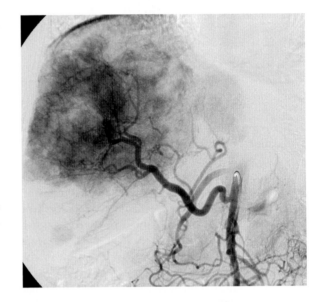

Fig. 21.3 The Superior mesentric arteriogram (from the same patient in Fig. 21.1 and 21.2) demonstrates a replaced right hepatic artery with multiple hypervascular lesions in an enlarged right lobe of the liver

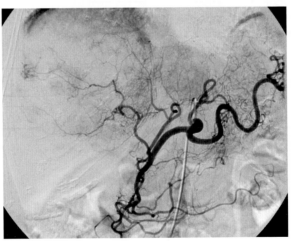

Fig. 21.4 Celiac axis arteriogram in the same patient as Fig. 21.3 demonstrates a steep caudal shift to the common and proper hepatic arteries with a significant (approximately 150° reversal in direction) change of both medial and lateral segmental left lobe arterial supply

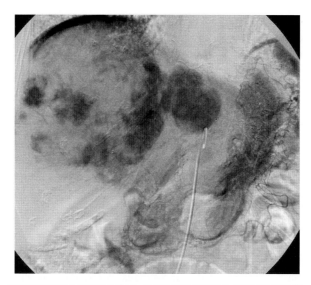

Fig. 21.5 Parenchymal phase arteriogram of the same patient as Figs. 21.3 and 21.4 demonstrates hypervascular lesions from the celiac axis injection. Note the right lobe lesions are partially supplied via intrahepatic collaterals from the left lobe arterial supply

Angiographic Appearance

- The majority of neuroendocrine tumors are hypervascular with an intense arterial blush and slow washout relative to the hepatic parenchymal phase.

Clinical Scenarios

Treatment Plan and Technique

- Primary goal is usually symptomatic relief or control of bulk disease. These patient populations frequently require multiple treatments to multiple liver lesions prior to attaining symptom control. Due to the number of treatments required, embolization goals/endpoints should allow for multiple treatments of the same area of the liver.
- Note that symptom control is likely related to hormone release. Unfortunately, hormone release is not necessarily related to lesion size. Once adequately treated, the active hormone should no longer be released, and the clinical symptoms should improve.
- Plan to treat the liver lesions in stages. Start with a specific lesion if it is suspected of releasing the majority of the active hormone (by Octreoscan, PET, or biopsy characteristics). Otherwise treat the large/dominant lesions first, followed

by secondary lesions after a 4–6-week recovery period. Each lesion may require two to three treatments prior to symptom control.

- Embolization to stasis may reduce the ability to treat future lesions in the same area of the liver and is *not* recommended.

Aftercare

Usually admitted to the hospital for overnight observation for both intravenous nausea and pain control. Majority of patients are discharged on post procedure day 1.

Arterial Access Site

Given the high probability of multiple procedures in this patient population, manual compression is recommended in most cases. Arterial access with a 5Fr sheath requires bed rest for a 4–6 h period. If closure devices are used, then the bedrest time may be shortened.

Post-embolization

Post-embolization syndrome (pain, nausea, vomiting, fatigue, low-grade fevers, mild/moderate elevation of white blood cell count, and other liver-specific blood tests) may occur and frequently subsides within 7–10 days.

Follow-Up

Post-procedure (7–14 days) clinic visit: to evaluate arterial access site, assess degree of post-embolization syndrome, and discuss the results of the procedure and plan upcoming procedures. After all liver lesions have been treated and symptoms have improved, clinic visits every 6–12 months assist in planning future treatments.

Keypoints

1. Diffuse hepatic metastases frequently alter/distort hepatic arterial supply. Understanding the arterial anatomy assists in complete therapy.
2. Symptomatic control is the dominant goal of embolization therapy.

3. Multiple treatments will likely be required; therefore, attempt to preserve patency of dominant hepatic arterial vessels and minimize impact at common femoral arterial access site.
4. Carcinoid crisis may require urgent/emergent control even with preprocedure prophylactic IV octreotide.

Suggested Reading/References

Clancy TE, Sengupta TP, Paulus J, Ahmed F, Duh MS, Kulke, MH. Alkaline Phosphatase Predicts Survival I Patients with Metastatic Neuroendocrine Tumors. Dig Dis Sci 2006; 51:877–884.

de Baere T. Interventional Radiology for the Treatment of Liver Metastases from Neuroendocrine Tumors. In: Geschwind JFH and Soulen MC, eds. Interventional Oncology Principles and Practice, pp. 301–310. New York, NY: Cambridge University Press, 2008.

Garrot C, Stuart K. Liver-Directed Therapies for Metastatic Neuroendocrine Tumors. Hematol Oncol Clin N Am 2007; 21:545–560.

Ho AS, Picus J, Darcy MD et al. Long-Term Outcome After Chemoembolization and Embolization of Hepatic Metastatic Lesions from Neuroendocrine Tumors. Am J Roentgenol 2007; 188: 1201–1207.

Kulke MH, Mayer RJ. Carcinoid Tumors. N Engl J Med 1999; 340:858–868.

Murthy R, Kamat P, Nunez R, et al. Yttrium-90 Microsphere Radioembolotherapy of Hepatic Metastastic Neuroendocrine Carcinomas after Hepatic Arterial Embolization. J Vasc Interv Radiol 2008; 19:145–151.

Ruutianen AT, Soulen MC, Tuite CM, et al. Chemoembolization and Bland Embolization of Neuroendocrine Tumor Metastases to the Liver. J Vasc Interv Radiol 2007; 18:847–855.

Rhee TK, Lewandowski RJ, Liu DM, et al. [90]Y Radioembolization for Metastatic Neuroendocrine Liver Tumors: Preliminary Results from a Multi-Institutional Experience. Ann Surg 2008; 247:1029–1035.

Warner RRP, Kim MK. Carcinoid and Related Neuroendocrine Tumors. In: Geschwind JFH and Soulen MC, eds. Interventional Oncology Principles and Practice, pp. 290–300. New York, NY: Cambridge University Press, 2008.

Chapter 22
Embolization of Benign and Malignant Renal Tumors

David O. Kessel

Clinical Features

- Renal tumor embolization can be required as an elective or emergency procedure. It is essential to understand the implications of treatment of such an important end organ.
- Renal cell cancer (RCC): 80–90% of malignant renal tumors, peaks in 6th–7th decade, mean age 55, hypervascular with AV shunting.
- Angiomyolipoma (AML): contains blood vessels, smooth muscle and fat, 60% asymptomatic, F:M, 4:1 in isolated AML, 20% are associated with tuberous sclerosis. AMLs are prone to aneurysm formation and hemorrhage.

Diagnostic Evaluation

Laboratory

Beware of renal impairment and ensure adequate hydration; consult renal physicians if necessary.

Imaging: never start renal embolization until you have formally reviewed the pre-procedure imaging.

Use contrast-enhanced CT/MRI (Fig. 22.1) for the following:

- To verify the condition of the contralateral kidney.
- To demonstrate the location of the tumor and any local and distant spread that may affect treatment.
- To identify renal blood supply.
- To assess tumor vascularity and look for the presence of arteriovenous shunting.
- Target treatment.
- In angiomyolipoma, target the largest tumor or the one with the hematoma.
- Extension of tumor to renal vein/IVC.

Transcatheter Embolization and Therapy,
Techniques in Interventional Radiology, DOI 10.1007/978-1-84800-897-7_22,
© Springer-Verlag London Limited 2010

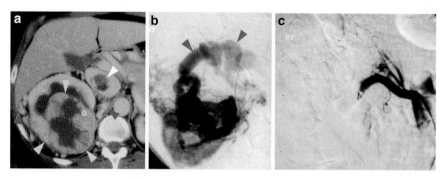

Fig. 22.1 (**a**) Pre-embolization CT. (**b**) Angiogram showing vascular large right renal cancer (*yellow arrowheads*) with IVC tumor thrombus (*white arrowhead*). Note extensive shunting through multiple large retroperitoneal veins (*red arrowheads*). (**c**) Post-embolization with spongestan: the arterial and venous flow has been abolished. Coils were subsequently deployed distal to the adrenal artery

Indications

These include the following:

- Symptomatic relief for inoperable or hemorrhagic RCC.
- Reduced blood loss at nephrectomy for RCC.
- Definitive therapy for hemorrhagic AML.
- Prophylactic treatment for AMLs >4 cm.

Contraindications

- As always, the contraindications are relative and relate to the indication; thus there is little that will prevent emergency embolization for hemorrhage from a tumor.
- Renal insufficiency. Patients with tuberous sclerosis will often have diffuse involvement of both kidneys and preservation of renal function can be an issue.
- Extensive collateral supply increases the risk of non-target embolization and may limit effectiveness of proximal embolization. Beware supply to spinal cord and bowel.
- Massive arteriovenous shunts increase risk of pulmonary embolization.

Anatomy

Assess the vascular supply on the pre-procedural imaging. Multiple vessels supplying the tumor indicate that the case will take longer to perform.

Normal Anatomy

- Accessory renal arteries arise from a variety of positions on the aorta and iliac arteries.
- Inferior adrenal artery typically arises from the proximal renal artery.
- Capsular arteries typically arise from the proximal renal artery.

Aberrant Anatomy

Collateral supply (Fig. 22.2) arises from the following:

- Lumbar arteries.
- Adrenal arteries.
- Capsular arteries.
- Phrenic arteries.
- Occasionally mesenteric vessels.
- Ectopic kidneys and horseshoe kidneys may have very unusual arterial supplies.
- Large tumors may be very vascular with extensive abnormal draining veins; this can be associated with arteriovenous shunting which affects the choice of embolic agent.

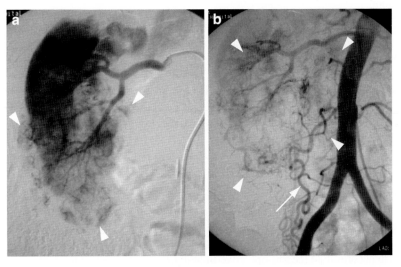

Fig. 22.2 (**a**) Large right renal tumor supplied from the right renal artery (*white arrowheads*). (**b**) Flush aortography reveals the true extent of the tumor (*white arrowheads*) with extensive collateral supply from the L2–L4 lumbar arteries and also a large unnamed collateral vessel (*white arrow*)

Equipment

- *Non-selective catheters:* pigtail or straight catheter if flush aortogram is necessary.
- *Selective catheters:* cobra, renal double curve, sidewinder. Microcatheter for selective embolization.
- *Guide catheter with detachable hemostatic valve* if using Amplatzer vascular plugs (AVP).

Embolic Agents

The choice of agent depends on the clinical context.

- *Pre-operative*: gelfoam and coils or AVP
- *Selective*: polyvinyl alcohol particles 350–500 μm unless shunting or very large vascular tumor; microcoils
- *Hemorrhage*: PVA (350–700 μm)/coils

Medication

Renal tumor embolization is often painful and post-embolization syndrome is common.

- *Pain control*: prophylactic anti-inflammatory strong analgesia is often needed and should be given early. Patient-controlled analgesia should be established.
- *Infection control:* broad spectrum antibiotics are recommended as tissue necrosis is likely.
- *Sickness control:* anti-emetics should be given prophylactically.
- *Hydration*: intravenous normal saline.

Procedure

Access

- Plan according to the pre-operative imaging.
- >90% approached from the femoral artery.
- The approach may have to be altered with ectopic kidneys.

Angiography

Flush aortography can be helpful in patients with large tumors when the blood supply may not derive exclusively from the renal artery.

- Either perform initial flush aortogram to obtain an overview and identify the position of the renal arteries before embolization.
- Or reserve flush aortography for after-embolization of the main renal artery to identify alternative tumor supply.
- If in doubt, perform selective angiography of all potential vessels of supply.
- Pre-nephrectomy angiography is solely intended to demonstrate the entire tumor and renal supply and its subsequent occlusion.

Assessing the Lesion

Location: the location of the tumor should be known from the pre-operative imaging.

Angiographic Appearance

- The tumor is identified by chaotic neovascularization replacing the typical branching pattern of the normal renal artery.
- Look for aneurysms and vascular displacement in AML.

Treatment Plan and Technique

The treatment plan and embolic agent depend on the indication.

Pre-operative Embolization

- Goal is to prevent venous bleeding from extensive collaterals and in patients with extensive renal vein or IVC tumor involvement embolization can lead to marked retraction of the "tumor thrombus" thus reducing the need for caval/atrial clamping and cardiopulmonary bypass.
- Performed immediately before surgery if possible. This minimizes post-embolization syndrome and complications due to local inflammation.
- Main renal artery.
- Use gelfoam/particles to slow the flow before occluding the main renal artery. Note a guiding catheter allows gelfoam to be injected very readily but has a

large dead space with high potential for non-target embolization if flushed. Either remove the hemostatic valve and aspirate or remove the catheter and flush.
- AVP is ideal to occlude the main renal artery especially when hypertrophied.
- Coils or AVP are deployed close to the bifurcation of the renal artery rather than at the origin of the vessel as this allows the surgeon to clamp and ligate the artery.
- Embolization is complete when the vast majority of tumor flow has been obliterated—remember that you are trying to make the surgery simpler with less bleeding from collateral veins.
- Leave any tumor supply arising from the mesenteric vessels. You will cause more harm than good.
- Inform the surgeon what you have done, especially if significant supply persists.

Embolization in Patients with Inoperable Cancer

- Aim to devascularize the tumor alone in order to relieve symptoms.
- May be performed selectively if desire to preserve renal function equivalent to partial nephrectomy.
- Permanent agent such as PVA should be used to occlude the tumor circulation.
- Alternative agents: 50:50 mixture of alcohol/lipiodol, Glue or Ethibloc. Liquid agents are most often given through an occlusion balloon to prevent reflux.
- The inflow vessel is spared to allow access in future if needed.

Embolization in AML

- Goal is permanent embolization of AML with preservation of normal renal tissue.
- Performed as selectively as possible.
- Occlude tumor circulation with permanent agent, e.g., PVA. Alternative agents: 50:50 mixture of alcohol/lipiodol, Glue or Ethibloc.
- Coils should be used to occlude the inflow as there is a risk of post-embolization aneurysm rupture.
- Look for additional supply to the tumor after the principal supply has been treated.
- AML should be treated as part tumor and part aneurysm; hence it is necessary to occlude both the tumor circulation **and** the arterial inflow.

Arterial Puncture Site

- Use a closure device if patient is in pain or agitated as less likely to lie still.
- It is essential in patients who are going to the operating theatre, as the groin will not be observed during surgery.

Post-embolization Syndrome

- Ensure that the patient is prepared for this and knows that pain and sickness can be treated effectively.
- Treatment is supportive.
- Ensure that the ward staff know what to look for and do.

Follow-Up

- Embolotherapy is usually effective in all of the above situations.
- Patients require follow-up imaging if symptoms recur.
- Following embolization of large AML, it is helpful to demonstrate tumor devascularization and shrinkage.
- Patients with multifocal AML are managed expectantly and only treated when symptomatic as the loss of renal tissue would otherwise be too great.

Alternative Therapies

The indications for embolization are well established and should be offered according to local expertise.

Specific Complications

Renal failure should be managed by a renal physician.

Keypoints

Review the pre-procedural imaging to plan the procedure.
Ensure you understand the rationale for treating each patient; this will ensure the following:

- Correct choice of embolic agent
- Correct endpoints
- Appropriate consent

Consider the possibility of extensive arterial supply to renal cancers.
Ensure adequate supportive therapy before, during, and after the procedure.
Perform pre-operative embolization as close to surgery as is practicable.

Safety

Never start embolization until you have personally reviewed the imaging.
Stick to the indications for the procedure, use appropriate agents, and
remember the endpoints depend on the indication.
Stop if uncertain, especially if there is risk of non-target embolization.

Suggested Reading

Kothary N, Soulen M, Clark T, Wein A, Shlansky-Goldberg R, Crino P, Stavropoulos W.
    Renal angiomyolipoma: long-term results after arterial embolization. J Vasc Interv Radiol
    2005;16:45–50
Rimon U, Duvdevani, Garniek A, Golan G, Bensaid P, Ramon J, Morag B. Large renal angiomy-
    olipomas: digital subtraction angiographic grading and presentation with bleeding. Clin Rad
    2006;61(6):520–526

Chapter 23
Embolization of Bone Tumors

Eric J. Hohenwalter, William S. Rilling, and David M. King

Clinical Features

- Bone tumor embolizations can be performed for palliation of pain/symptoms, or pre-operatively to reduce blood loss during surgery.
- Embolization has been described as definitive treatment for aneurysmal bone cyst, osteosarcoma, and giant cell tumors refractory to conventional treatment.
- The most common hypervascular metastatic bone tumors include hepatocellular carcinoma, renal cell carcinoma, thyroid carcinoma, neuroendocrine malignancies, multiple myeloma, lung cancer, leiomyosarcoma, and angiosarcoma.
- Typically performed in conjunction with an orthopedic surgeon or musculoskeletal oncologist in order to optimize care.

Diagnostic Evaluation

Laboratory

Evaluate renal function prior to embolization procedure. Ensure adequate hydration pre- and post-procedure.

Imaging (Fig. 23.1)

Use contrast-enhanced computed tomography (CT) or magnetic resonance imaging (MRI) for the following

- To demonstrate location of tumor and to evaluate for any satellite lesions.
- To assess tumor vascularity and surrounding anatomy.
- Dedicated CT or MR angiography may demonstrate feeding vessels.
- To form treatment plan and approach.

Transcatheter Embolization and Therapy,
Techniques in Interventional Radiology, DOI 10.1007/978-1-84800-897-7_23,
© Springer-Verlag London Limited 2010

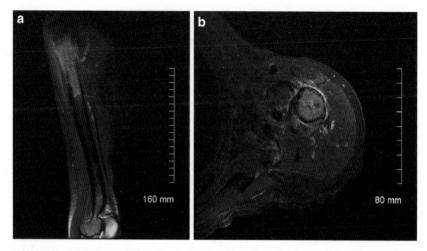

Fig. 23.1 Pre-procedure imaging. (**a** and **b**) Coronal and axial MR with contrast demonstrating a hypervascular mass in the proximal humerus

Indications

- Facilitation of subsequent surgical excision/spinal stabilization
- Symptomatic relief from painful bone metastasis
- Inhibition of tumor growth
- Control of hemorrhage

Alternative Therapies

- Cementoplasty
- Radiofrequency ablation

Contraindications (Relative)

- Renal insufficiency
- Patient unable to be positioned for embolization procedure
- Massive arteriovenous shunting (rare)
- Severe contrast allergy
- Uncorrectable coagulopathy

Specific Complications

- These relate to the vascular territory from which the tumor supply arises.
- Damage to the spinal cord is the most feared complication.

Anatomy

- Assess vascularity of the tumor on pre-procedural imaging. Vascular anatomy will vary depending on location of tumor.
- Evaluate for associated soft tissue mass.
- Evaluate extent and potential involvement of adjacent structures.
- Must assess proximity to significant vessels, such as the spinal artery in cases of vertebral metastases.

Equipment

Catheters

- *Non-selective catheters:* Pigtail or flush catheter for arterial mapping.
- *Selective catheters:* cobra, angled catheter, or guide catheter.
- *Microcatheters*: high-flow microcatheters allow for power injection and improved angiographic visualization, as well as less clumping of embolic agents.

Embolic Agents

- PVA or Embospheres (Biosphere Medical, Rockland, MA, USA): usually 300–500 μm, but particle size depends on size of artery and A-V shunting.
- Gelfoam (Upjohn, Kalamazoo, MI, USA).
- Microcoils—especially for coil protection of non-target branches.
- Liquid embolic agents.

Medication

Bone tumor embolization can be painful and induces post-embolization syndrome.

- *Post-operative pain control:* patient-controlled analgesia and anti-inflammatory medications as needed.
- *Infection control:* pre-procedure antibiotics (usually Cefazolin or Clindamycin).
- *Hydration:* intravenous normal saline.
- *Post-embolization syndrome:* supportive therapy. Anti-emetics, anti-inflammatory, and oral pain medications as needed.

Procedure

Access

- Plan according to pre-procedure imaging.
- Vast majority will be common femoral artery approach.

Angiography

- Initial flush arteriogram to map out arterial anatomy. For spinal and pelvic tumors, an aortagram is performed initially. For peripheral tumors, an arteriogram of the main extremity artery is performed.
- Selective arteriogram. In tumors of the spine, this must include visualization of the arteries at levels above and below the tumor.
- When stable selective catheter position is achieved, a microcatheter is usually used to select the arteries directly supplying the tumor.
- Evaluate for significant non-target branches and consider coil protection depending on size and distribution of vessels.
- Non-selective arteriography post-embolization to assess for residual tumor blush, collateral arterial feeders, and adequacy of embolization.
- Frequent control angiography as pressure/flow relationships change during embolization. This may increase the risk of non-target embolization.

Assessing the Lesion

Location: determined from pre-operative imaging.

Angiographic Appearance

- Evaluate number and origin of tumor feeding vessels.
- Identify arteriovenous shunts.
- Evaluate for collateralization to or from adjacent healthy tissue especially spinal supply.

Treatment Plan and Technique

The treatment plan and embolic agent depend on the indication.

Pre-operative Embolization (Fig. 23.2)

- The goal is to exclude all of the capillary bed in order to prevent excessive blood loss at surgery. Lack of tumor blush is the angiographic endpoint; however, any decrease in flow is helpful to the surgeon.
- Should be performed within 24 h of surgery. This prevents significant collateral vessels from forming between the embolization and surgery.
- Generally use small (100–200 μm) or medium (300–500 μm) particles or Gelfoam slurry.
- For larger tumors of the spine, it may be necessary to coil-embolize the feeding artery distal to the target, prior to subselective embolization. This will help prevent non-target embolization of the adjacent tissues as well as prevent any retrograde filling of the tumor.

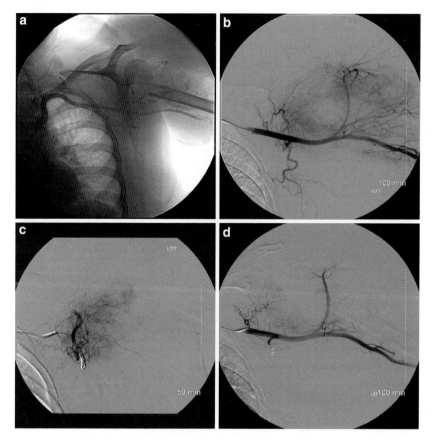

Fig. 23.2 Pre-operative embolization with coil protection. (**a** and **b**) LUE arteriogram demonstrating a hypervascular mass in the proximal L. Humerus and associated pathologic fracture. (**c**) Selective arteriogram through a high-flow microcatheter after coil protection of arteries supplying normal tissue. (**d**) Post-particle embolization demonstrating a significant decrease in tumor blush

Palliative Embolization

- The goal is to inhibit tumor growth or decrease the size of the tumor, resulting in a reduction in tumor-associated pain.
- Particles are the embolic agent of choice. Size depends on the size of the feeding artery (typically 300–500 μm).
- Some studies have reported increased effectiveness when a chemotherapeutic agent (most frequently carboplatin) is mixed with the particles.
- The combination of embolization with radiation therapy may further increase the efficacy of palliative embolization.

Embolization as a Primary Treatment

- Most frequently used in aneurysmal bone cysts and giant cell tumors.
- Advantageous in treatment of tumors of the spine and long bones, so as to avoid radical excision and rigid fixation.
- Treatment goal is to exclude capillary bed.
- Particle embolization is the agent of choice, with sizing according to vessel diameter.

Complications

- Non-target embolization
- Renal failure

Post-embolization Syndrome

- Treatment is supportive (intravenous fluids, anti-inflammatory medications, anti-emetics).
- Ensure the patient and nursing staff are aware of post-embolization syndrome, and know what to expect.

Follow-Up

- Should be done in conjunction with a musculoskeletal oncologist/surgeon.

Keypoints

1. Use pre-operative imaging to guide embolization.
2. Base embolic agent choice on indication and size of feeding artery.
3. Always be aware of the potential for non-target embolization (coil protection may be necessary).
4. Perform pre-operative embolization as close to surgery as possible.
5. Ensure adequate pre- and post-procedure supportive care.
6. Consult with a musculoskeletal oncologist/surgeon regarding specific treatment goals and follow-up.

Suggested Readings

1. Huddleston JR, Johnson SP. Embolization of painful neoplasms. In Ray CE Jr (ed), *Pain Management in Interventional Radiology*: New York, NY, Cambridge University Press, 2008, pp.199–216.
2. Liapi E, Geschwind JF. Transcatheter and ablative therapeutic approaches for solid malignancies. J Clin Oncol 2007;25(8):978–986.
3. Tegtmeyer CJ, Spinosa DJ, Matsumoto AH. Angiography of bones, joints, and soft tissues. In Baum S (ed), *Abrams' Angiography*: Boston, Little Brown and Company, 1997, pp.1813–1820.

Chapter 24
Uterine Fibroid Embolization

Sriharsha Athreya and Jon G. Moss

Clinical Features

- Uterine leimyoma (fibroids) are the most common benign tumor in the female pelvis.
- Heavy menstrual bleeding (HMB), pelvic pain, and pressure are the most common symptoms.
- There is an association with infertility and early pregnancy loss.

Diagnostic Evaluation

Before undergoing uterine artery embolization (UAE), the patient should be seen by a gynecologist and an interventional radiologist.

Gynecologic Examination

- Appropriate measures taken before UAE to exclude cervical cancer, endometrial carcinoma, or endometrial hyperplasia as a cause of bleeding.
- Pregnancy test to exclude pregnancy.

Laboratory

- *Full blood count*—to screen for anemia.
- *Coagulation screen*—optional but essential if any history of liver disease or anticoagulant therapy.
- *Renal function*—serum creatinine.
- *Hormone profile* —optional, may be useful as a baseline indicator of pituitary–ovarian function.

   Imaging: pre-procedure imaging (Figs. 24.1a and 24.2a) is essential to
- Confirm diagnosis of fibroids
- Assess the size, location, and number of fibroids

Transcatheter Embolization and Therapy,
Techniques in Interventional Radiology, DOI 10.1007/978-1-84800-897-7_24,
© Springer-Verlag London Limited 2010

- Assess vascularity
- Detect other pathology, e.g., adenomyosis

Note that no imaging can reliably differentiate leiomyosarcoma from leiomyoma.

Contrast-enhanced MRI (CEMRI): CEMRI is the imaging modality of choice. CEMRI

- Characterizes fibroids better than ultrasound.
- Enhancement reflects vascularity (Figs. 24.1b and 24.2b).

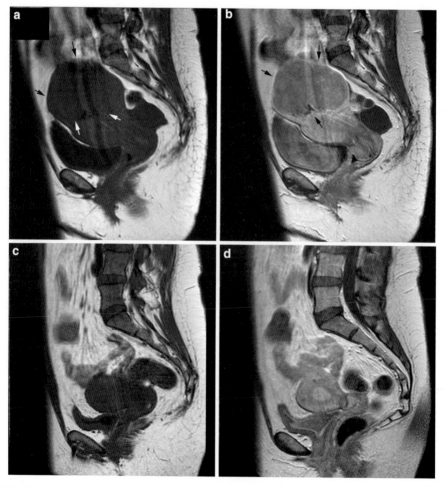

Fig. 24.1 (a) Pre-UAE T1 sagittal showing a large intramural fibroid (*arrows*). (b) Pre-UAE T1 sagittal post-gadolinium showing enhancement of the fibroid (*arrows*). (c) Post-UAE T1 sagittal showing the fibroid to have completely involuted. (d) Post-UAE T1 sagittal post-gadolinium showing complete fibroid involution with no enhancement

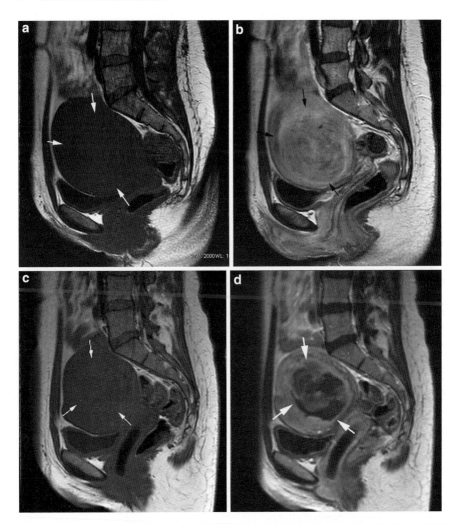

Fig. 24.2 (**a**) Pre-UAE T1 sagittal showing a large intramural fibroid (*arrowheads*). (**b**) Pre-UAE T1 sagittal post-gadolinium showing enhancement of the fibroid (*arrowheads*). (**c**) Post-UAE T1 sagittal showing the fibroid (*arrowheads*). (**d**) Post-UAE T1 sagittal post-gadolinium showing partial enhancement and incomplete fibroid involution (*arrowheads*)

- Devascularization demonstrates fibroid infarction (Figs. 24.1d and 24.2d).
- Is excellent for establishing anatomical location.
- Is good for detecting adenomyosis.

Pelvic ultrasound (US): US is readily available and cheap but is operator dependent. Compared to CEMRI ultrasound is

- Less able to provide anatomical definition

- Poor at detecting adenomyosis
- Less able to assess vascularity

Transvaginal Ultrasound (TVUS)

- Easily available, cheap
- Slightly intrusive examination for some women
- Less good for large-volume uterus and multiple fibroids

Indications

These include the following:

- Symptomatic leimyoma—asymptomatic fibroids are common and require no treatment.
- Patient prefers a minimally invasive intervention to surgery.
- Patient wishes to conserve uterus for either fertility or cultural reasons.
- Not suitable for or unwilling to have a myomectomy.

Contraindications

Absolute

- Recent or ongoing pelvic infection.
- Diagnosis of fibroids is in doubt.
- Post-radiotherapy to pelvis—risk of tissue necrosis with embolization.
- General contraindications to angiography such as uncorrectable coagulopathy, severe iodinated contrast allergy.

Relative

- Pedunculated and intraligamentous fibroids—risk of peritoneal adhesions following UAE.
- Fibroids extending into the endometrial canal. This may lead to fibroid expulsion into the endometrial canal, leading to cervical os obstruction.
- Concomitant adenomyosis—controversial area. Adenomyosis can respond to UAE but less well than fibroids.
- Wishing to preserve fertility and is suitable for a myomectomy—some weak evidence of superior reproductive outcomes with myomectomy.
- Renal insufficiency.

Normal Anatomy

- The uterine arteries typically arise from the anterior division of the internal iliac artery.

Aberrant Anatomy

Collateral supply can arise from the following:

- Ovarian arteries
- Lumbar arteries
- External iliac arteries (rarely)
- Artery of the round ligament

Pre-treatment Patient Information

It is advisable to have an initial consultation in a clinic environment (ideally a radiology clinic) to explain the following:

- The procedure, complications, and expectations
- Alternatives to UAE
- Periprocedural medication, pain relief
- Post-embolization syndrome symptoms
- Follow-up regime

Equipment

- *Non-selective catheters:* Pigtail catheter for flush aortogram to assess the arterial supply in recurrent embolization procedures. Aortagrams are not typically needed for all UAE procedures.
- *Selective catheters:* personal preference is important. 5Fr hydrophilic cobra (Terumo, Europe), 5Fr Vanschie 1,11,111 catheters (COOK, Europe), and occasionally other shapes may be useful.
- **Microcatheters** for selective embolization are useful to prevent arterial spasm and are becoming increasingly standard.

Embolic Agents

- Variety of embolic agents, with little evidence to support one over the other. Poly vinyl alcohol (PVA) (Cook, Europe), Beadblock (Terumo, Europe), Embospheres (BVM Medical, UK), Gelatin sponge (Johnson & Johnson, Europe). Commonest size used is in the range 500–700 μ. 700–1000 μ size is often used with the newer

agents. Larger agents are also useful following initial embolization with smaller particles, e.g., after 3–4 units of 500–700 size.
- *Coils should not be employed* as they do not provide distal embolization and prevent repeat embolization.

Medication

Uterine artery embolization is itself not a painful procedure but post-embolization pain is almost universal and requires active management.

- *Pain control*: adequate pain relief is a must during the pre-, peri-, and post-UAE period. Usually a combination of non-steroidal anti-inflammatory analgesia and opioids are needed. Some centers use patient-controlled analgesia. It may be helpful to establish a pain-control protocol involving the anesthetic department.
- *Sedation:* a short-acting benzodiapine such as midozolam is administered intravenously. An intraprocedural short-acting narcotic such as fentanyl is typically used in conjunction with a benzodiazepine.
- *Infection control:* broad spectrum antibiotics are administered in many centers, though there is no good evidence to support their use.
- *Sickness control:* antiemetics should be routinely administered.

Procedure

Access

- Almost always the femoral artery.
- Bilateral femoral arterial approach is employed in some centers. Requires two operators and it probably reduces the radiation dose if the procedure is performed simultaneously.

Angiography

Low-dose pulsed fluoroscopy should be used whenever possible. Angiographic runs should also be limited in order to reduce radiation dose. The uterine artery is usually hypertrophied and easy to recognize (Fig. 24.3).

- Following femoral arterial access, the contralateral iliac artery is selected.
- Using a contralateral oblique projection, road map, the internal iliac artery is selected.
- Using an ipsilateral oblique, the anterior division of the internal iliac artery is selected.

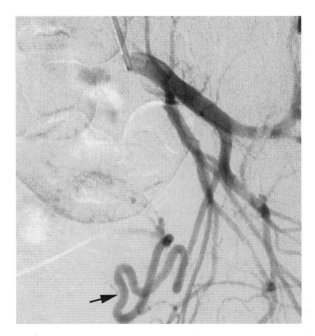

Fig. 24.3 Left internal iliac artery angiogram showing an enlarged and tortuous left uterine artery (*arrows*)

- A microcatheter is then used to access the uterine artery. This helps prevent spasm and allows effective free flow directed embolization
- The uterine artery is embolized to an angiographic end point (see below).
- The procedure is then repeated on the ipsilateral uterine artery—it is essential to embolize both sides to produce satisfactory infarction.

Flush aortography is usually not required but can be helpful in patients with abnormal arterial anatomy and in patients undergoing repeat UAE, to identify any non-uterine blood supply.

Angiographic Appearance

- The uterine arteries are usually hypertrophied, tortuous, and laterally displaced. A hypervascular delayed phase is also visualized.

The angiographic end point: the exact end point of embolization remains controversial. Commonly employed end points are as follows:

- Complete stasis over either five or ten cardiac beats.
- Complete stasis with reflux back along the angiographic catheter.

- A "pruned-tree" appearance with maintained forward flow in the main uterine artery.

Re-embolization of Uterine Artery

- Useful option in patients with persistent or recurrent symptoms who do not wish surgery.
- A CEMRI should be done first to confirm either incomplete infarction or new fibroid formation.
- If the ovarian arteries are to be embolized, then the risk of ovarian failure must be discussed with the patient in advance.

Arterial Puncture Site

- Manual compression is adequate and a closure device is not usually required.

Post-embolization Syndrome

- Almost inevitable following UAE.
- Ensure that the patient and ward staff are appropriately briefed and aware that it can be treated effectively.
- Treatment is supportive and consists of fluids, analgesia, and anti-inflammatory medication (see chapter on post-embolization syndrome).

Follow-Up

- Follow-up is essential and, a local post-procedure protocol agreed and written down.
- A common protocol is 1, 6, and 12 monthly clinical assessment.
- Repeat imaging within first 6 months is highly desirable; CEMRI is the ideal imaging modality.

Treatment Failures

- 20–25% at 2–5 years.
- Usually due to incomplete fibroid infarction or rarely new fibroid formation.
- Best assessed with CE MRI.
- Treatment options for initial failures include myomectomy, hysterectomy, and repeat UAE.

Specific Complications

Immediate—occurring during the procedure or in first few days.

- Groin hematoma, arterial dissection, pseudoaneurysm formation.
- Non-target embolization typically to the other pelvic organs. Should not occur with good technique.
  Early (first 30 days)
- Post-embolization syndrome—flu-like symptoms, with pain, nausea, and fever. Raised white cell count and inflammatory markers.
  Late (after first 30 days)
- Infection: may present with non-specific flu-like symptoms, fever, purulent discharge. Requires prompt investigation and may necessitate hysterectomy. Infection should be considered in cases where post-embolization syndrome persists beyond 10 days.
- Vaginal discharge.
- Fibroid expulsion: in up to 10% (more common with submucosal fibroids).
- Ovarian failure leading to amenorrhea.
- Endometritis: treated with antibiotics and usually responds well. Occasionally hysterectomy is required.
- Ischemic vaginal or uterine damage.
- Sexual dysfunction—may be due to embolization of the cervicovaginal arterial branches.

Suggested Reading

1. Edwards RD, Moss JG, Lumsden MA, Wu O Murray LS, Twaddle S, Murray GD. Committee of the Randomised Trial of Embolisation versus Surgical Treatment of Fibroids. Uterine artery embolisation versus surgery for symptomatic fibroids. NEJM 2007;356:360–70
2. Dutton S, Hirst A, McPherson K, Nicholson T, Maresh M. A UK multicentre retrospective cohort study comparing hysterectomy and uterine artery embolisation for the treatment of symptomatic uterine fibroids (HOPEFUL study): main results on medium-term safety and efficacy. BJOG 2007;114: 1340–51.
3. Pelage J-P, Cazejust J, Pluot E, Le Dref O, Laurent A, Spies JB, Chagnon S, Lacombe P. Uterine Fibroid Vascularization and Clinical Relevance to Uterine Fibroid Embolization. RadioGraphics 2005;25(Special Issue): S99–117

Appendix

UAE—uterine artery embolization
INR—international normalized ratio
PVA—poly vinyl alcohol
CE MRI—contrast-enhanced magnetic resonance imaging
USS—ultrasonography

Chapter 25
Embolization of Hemorrhage Due to Pelvic Fractures

Douglas Coldwell and Clayton Trimmer

Clinical Features

- Due to disruption of the pelvic ring due to blunt trauma.
  Types of pelvic fractures are as follows:

  - *Lateral compression*—causes vertical compression fracture in sacrum and oblique fractures of the pubic rami anteriorly.
  - *Anterior–posterior*—opens the pelvis with rotation of iliac wings outward and disruption of pubic symphysis and sacral-iliac joints.
  - *Vertical shear*—moves one hemi-pelvis superiorly, tearing the SI joint.
  - *Combination*—mixed features of any of above, usually in much more severe trauma.

- Extent of vascular damage always greater than plain films would suggest due to shearing action of the ligaments in the pelvis.
- The more severe the instability of the pelvic fracture, the more likely it is that life-threatening hemorrhage will occur.
- Bleeding as a result of pelvic injury comes from

  1. Arterial injury—hemodynamic instability and needs embolization immediately.
  2. Venous injury—especially the posterior venous plexus; bleeding normally stops with stabilization of the pelvis with external wrap or external fixators.
  3. Fractured cancellous bone edges—stabilized with external fixators.
  4. Other injuries, e.g., solid organ injury!! This may be overlooked by orthopedic surgeons.

Diagnostic Evaluation

Laboratory

- Many of these patients are hemodynamically unstable and require blood products to maintain their blood pressure with decreasing hemoglobin/hematocrit,

Transcatheter Embolization and Therapy,
Techniques in Interventional Radiology, DOI 10.1007/978-1-84800-897-7_25,
© Springer-Verlag London Limited 2010

increasing lactic acidosis (base deficit), and hypothermia. All procedures must be performed in the most expeditious way possible. *Time is of the essence.*

Imaging (see also Chapter 10)

Clear protocols need to be in place to ensure rapid and appropriate imaging.

- Stable patients with or without fluid resuscitation should undergo a CT scan first in order to assess the state of their injuries; splenic or hepatic injury is common. Additionally, the CT will demonstrate sites of hemorrhage allowing the interventional radiology team to focus their attention directly to the sites of hemorrhage.
- Patients who are unstable despite fluid resuscitation should go straight to interventional radiology where their hemorrhage sites can be embolized. Trauma surgeons may wish to place an external fixator device first so that the pelvic fracture fragments can be stabilized. A pelvic wrap is preferable to an external bone fixator, as it simplifies arterial access and angiography.

Indications

- Any bleeding that results in hemodynamic instability or continued loss of blood over the patient's hospitalization.

Contraindications

- Relative only. If the patient is unstable despite fluid resuscitation, they need immediate surgery or embolization. It may be necessary to go to the operating room to begin the procedure while the surgeon is exploring.
- Not having the interventional radiology team available on a 20-minute call-back time. This does not usually occur at a Level-1 trauma center.

Complications

- Non-target embolization. This is typically avoided if the embolization is performed under continuous monitoring with frequent checks for stasis.
- Impotence has been suggested as a complication but it is most likely due to the disruption of the neural plexus. As Dr. Yorum Ben-Menachem, one of the fathers of trauma angiography, once said, "I would rather have a patient alive and impotent than dead with a massive erection."

Anatomy

- The vessels of the pelvis are reasonably consistent.
- The common iliac artery bifurcates to the following:
  - External iliac artery
    - Inferior epigastric artery—originates at about the level of the inguinal ligament and supplies the anterior abdominal wall, anastomozing with the internal mammary artery at the level of the diaphragm.
    - Pubic symphaseal artery—may originate directly from the external iliac or the inferior epigastric artery.
  - Internal iliac artery—concentrate here as most of the arteries effected will be in this distribution. Bifurcates to
    - Anterior division
      - Obturator artery—passing through the obturator foramen.
      - Inferior gluteal—supplying the buttocks.
      - Umbilical artery/superior vesical artery—feeding the bladder.
      - Uterine artery—may also originate vaginal artery.
      - Inferior vesical artery—supplying bladder.
      - Middle rectal artery.
      - Internal pudendal artery—supplying genitalia.
    - Posterior division
      - Superior gluteal artery—commonly injured.
      - Iliolumbar artery.
      - Sacral arteries.

Equipment

Catheters Required

- Non-selective
  - Pigtail or other flush catheter to be used at the aortic bifurcation.
- Selective catheters
  - Cobra or Headhunter or Berenstein type—simple curve for selection.
  - Reverse curve catheters like the Simmons 1 or Sos selective. Usually 5Fr.
- Vascular sheath
  - 5 or 6Fr

Embolization Agents

- The goal of trauma embolization is to achieve tissue ischemia, *not* tissue necrosis.
- Gelfoam slurry—the mainstay of trauma embolization. Will dissolve in hours to days.
- Coils—stainless steel or platinum. Use in larger vessels when permanent occlusion is necessary, e.g., on-going severe hemorrhage. Use gelfoam suspension first, then place coils in internal iliac or anterior/posterior division of internal iliac artery ("gelfoam-coil sandwhich" technique). Authors preference is not to use coils bilaterally unless absolutely necessary.
- Glue—should only be used by those experienced, with it; it is very expensive and typically requires the use of a microcatheter.

Angiography (See Figs. 25.1 and 25.2)

- Selective or even non-selective arteriography will demonstrate the arterial damage by the following:
  - o Obvious extravasation of contrast into the soft tissues
  - o Blunt ending artery—check for retrograde filling of the more distal arterial distribution via collaterals.
  - o Spasm in the artery.
- Place sheath in groin, as removing it at end of the procedure will take additional time and the patient is likely coagulopathic. Suture sheath in place for removal later.

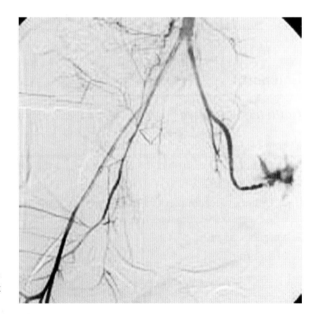

Fig. 25.1 Arteriogram demonstrates the classic appearance of extravasation due to a very significant hemorrhage in the pelvis due to a complete transaction of the external iliac artery at the level of the inguinal ligament

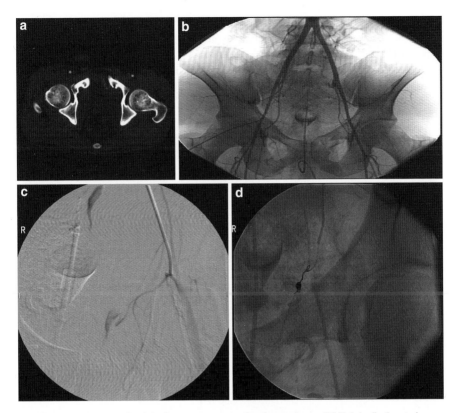

Fig. 25.2 (**a**) CT scan of pelvis demonstrates ongoing hemorrhage. (**b**) Pelvic flush arteriogram does not demonstrate any ongoing hemorrhage. (**c**) Selective external iliac arteriogram shows the extravasating contrast due to the hemorrhage. This originated from the anatomic variant of a replaced obturator artery to the external iliac artery. (**d**) Selective embolization of this artery with coils was performed halting the hemorrhage

- The pelvic aortogram should be performed first to obtain a view of the entire area. Then more selective arteriograms of the internal iliac arteries bilaterally are performed, even in the absence of vascular injury on the flush pelvic angiogram.
- The internal iliac anatomy is reasonably predictable but *time is of the essence*. A more proximal embolization in the internal iliac artery rather than selective embolization is preferred if it is going to require extra time and there is ongoing severe hemorrhage.
- Microcatheters are usually not required, as the selective work necessary can be performed with a 5Fr catheter. Microcatheters may be required if the bleeding artery is small and if microcoils are utilized.
- If the bleeding site is not found within the internal iliac distribution, an external iliac arteriogram should be performed. Branches of the external iliac, e.g., pubic symphaseal branches, also supply the pelvis.

- Very distal embolization should not be performed bilaterally, as the collateral arteries to the same structure would be eliminated, leading to tissue necrosis.
- Place the catheter in position for embolization and slowly inject the Gelfoam, observing under fluoroscopy continuously. Every few milliliters of suspension, check for stasis with a small contrast injection.
- For the final arteriogram before ending the study, use either an internal iliac run if the embolization was unilateral or an aortogram at the aortic bifurcation to check for any untreated sites (Fig. 25.3) .

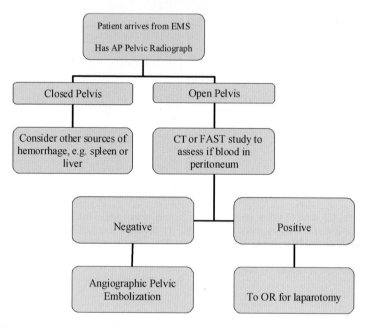

Fig. 25.3 Management of pelvic fractures

Recommendations

Note: Insure that cystography is *not* performed before the arteriogram. It delays the study and, more important, if the bladder is torn, the contrast will obscure the angiographic extravasation of contrast and the study will be compromised.

Keypoints

Venous bleeding will usually stop with external compression.

Arterial bleeding will not stop and needs immediate embolization.

Signs of arterial bleeding include extravasation of CM, spasm, and abrupt arterial cut-off.

Gelfoam slurry is the preferred agent.

Suggested Reading

1. Ben-Menachem Y, Coldwell DM, Young J, Burgess A: Hemorrhage Associated with Pelvic Fractures: Causes, Diagnosis, and Emergency Management. AJR 157:1005, 1991.

Chapter 26
Embolization of Extremity Trauma

Tanya Tivorsak and Catherine Vu

Clinical Features

Management Goals

- Life-saving and resuscitation: direct application of pressure on bleeding site or proximal tourniquet remains first step in control of hemorrhage.
- Limb salvage.
- Preservation of limb function.
- Clinical urgency depends on the presentation.

Mechanisms of Extremity Vascular Injury

- *Penetrating injury:* shooting, stabbing (more common)—causes transection, pseudoaneurysm, or arteriovenous fistula.
- *Blunt injury:* in the setting of fractures and joint dislocation—causes dissection or spasm. Some injuries such as knee dislocation are particularly prone to associated vascular injury.

Clinical Manifestations of Extremity Vascular Trauma

- Hemorrhage
- Ischemia
- Compartment syndromes

Role of Intervention

- Rapid control of hemorrhage
- Definitive therapy
- Pre-operative intervention to temporize bleeding prior to surgery
- Post-operative intervention to control non-operative vascular bleeding

Transcatheter Embolization and Therapy,
Techniques in Interventional Radiology, DOI 10.1007/978-1-84800-897-7_26,
© Springer-Verlag London Limited 2010

Diagnostic Evaluation

This includes clinical and imaging.

Clinical Evaluation

Physical Signs of Vascular Injury

These can be misleading; remember that injuries proximal to the shoulder girdle and hips have variable signs on physical examination. Consider the mechanism of the injury and the possibility of co-existing remote problem, e.g., aortic injury, organ damage.

Hard Signs—Indicate increased likelihood of vascular injury requiring intervention.

- Diminished or absent peripheral pulses or asymmetric limb blood pressures
- Expanding hematoma
- Vascular thrill or bruit
- Active or pulsatile arterial hemorrhage
- Limb ischemia (5Ps = pain, pallor, paresthesias, pulse deficit, paralysis)

Soft Signs—Less useful in predicting vascular injury requiring intervention.

- Hypotension or shock: remember that this may be a manifestation of another more serious injury!
- Adjacent nerve injury
- Adjacent fracture
- Stable/non-pulsatile hematoma
- Delayed capillary refill
- Soft tissue injury

Laboratory: Decreasing hematocrit and hemoglobin are usually present. Coagulopathy may be present in the setting of large volume transfusion.

Imaging

Radiographs

- Initial evaluation in extremity trauma—assess for displaced fractures but do not give information on the blood vessels.

Computed tomography angiography (CTA): CTA is becoming a crucial investigation in trauma.

- Demonstrates signs of arterial injuries including active extravasation of contrast, pseudoaneurysm, occlusion/stenosis/narrowing of an artery, early draining vein in arteriovenous fistula (AVF).
- Identifies collaterals and variant anatomy.
- Identifies other injuries.

Catheter Angiography

- Usually performed in association with intervention to control bleeding or restore flow.
- May be required to demonstrate distal circulation.

Ultrasound with Doppler/Duplex

- Promising but not widely used
- Operator dependent

Magnetic resonance angiography—not commonly used in the acute setting.

Indications

- Bleeding
  o In areas that are difficult to access surgically
  o Control of bleeding prior to surgical repair
  o Ongoing bleeding after surgical operation
  o In poor operative candidates

- Pseudoaneurysm Formation
- Arteriovenous Fistula Formation
- Hemodynamic Instability

Alternative Therapies

- Direct compression and tourniquet first aid. Compression may be therapeutic in minor injury (just like post-angiography).
- Endovascular: balloon tamponade, stent graft.
- Emergent exploration and surgical correction—especially when arterial injury is associated with ischemia of the extremity.
- Ultrasound-guided compression closure and ultrasound-guided thrombin injection for pseudoaneurysms. Seldom used in the context of acute trauma.

Contraindications

- Absolute—None
- Relative
  - Non-salvageable limb—this will require amputation, this may be the best primary therapy.
  - Uncorrectable coagulopathy.
  - Signs of ischemia.
  - Limited collateralization.
  - Dialysis grafts/fistulas.
  - Renal insufficiency.

Anatomy

Injury Can Affect the Major Artery or Small Branch Vessels

Upper extremity arteries—proximal to distal	
Artery	Major branches
Subclavian	Vertebral, internal mammary, thyrocervical trunk, dorsal scapular artery
Axillary	Superior thoracic, thoracoacromial, lateral thoracic, subscapular, anterior and posterior humeral circumflex
Brachial	
Radial	Radial collateral, middle collateral, and radial recurrent arteries
Ulnar	Superior and inferior ulnar collateral arteries, anterior and posterior ulnar recurrent arteries
Interosseous	

The brachial and forearm vessels are the most commonly injured with approximately equal incidence. The subclavian and axillary arteries are the least the frequently injured vessels thought to represent 2–12% of all upper limb arterial injury. Paradoxically interventional radiologists may be needed more frequently in these larger central vessels.

Aberrant Anatomy

- The radial and ulnar arteries frequently arise proximally from the brachial or axillary arteries.
- Arteriography of the upper extremity should include the axillary artery to identify major arterial anomalies.

- Anomalous radial or ulnar arteries in the forearm are typically superficial to the flexor muscles, making them more vulnerable to trauma.

Lower extremity arteries—proximal to distal	
Artery	Major branches
Common femoral artery (CFA)	PFA and SFA, inferior epigastric, lateral circumflex iliac artery
Superficial femoral artery (SFA)	Descending genicular, muscular branches
Profunda femoral artery	Lateral femoral circumflex, medial femoral circumflex, perforating arteries of adductor magnus
Popliteal artery	Genicular arteries, sural branches, ATA, TPT
Anterior tibial artery (ATA)	Muscular, dorsalis pedis
Tibioperoneal trunk (TPT)	PTA, peroneal artery, muscular branches
Posterior tibial artery (PTA)	Muscular branches medial and lateral plantar arches
Peroneal artery	Muscular branches, anterior and posterior terminal divisions

Variant Anatomy of Lower Extremity

- Persistent sciatic artery—less than 0.1%. Normal fetal branch of internal iliac artery that continues into lower extremity as the popliteal artery supplying the runoff vessels.
- High origin of one or more of the tibial arteries—2–8%. Important to identify to prevent unexpected arterial injury during surgery.
- Peroneal origin from anterior tibial artery—1%.
- True popliteal artery trifurcation (no tibioperoneal trunk)—4%.
- Hypoplastic tibial arteries—2%. Peroneal artery supplies foot instead. Identification may prevent false diagnosis of arterial damage in trauma if ankle pulses are absent or diminished.

Equipment

Catheters

Non-selective

- Multi-sidehole pigtail or straight catheters for flush aortic angiography and iliac angiography.

Selective Catheters

- Shapes to catheterize aortic arch vessels, cross aortic bifurcation, and access peripheral vessels: head hunter, Berenstein, Cobra, Sidewinder.
- End-hole catheters for embolization.

- Microcatheters for more selective embolization.
- Occlusion balloon or angioplasty balloon to temporize bleeding from major vessels. An aortic balloon can be lifesaving!

Guide Catheters and Sheaths

- Appropriately sized sheath for primary access.
- Long sheath or guide catheter if necessary for upper limb procedures.

Embolic Agents

For Dispensable Branch Vessels

- Gelfoam.
- Coils/microcoils.
- Coil–Gelfoam sandwich—useful in coagulopathic patients in whom coils are going to be used. Adding Gelfoam allows for mechanical occlusion.
- Glue/Onyx®—risk of ischemia from distal embolization, expensive, and technically challenging to use. May be useful in AVF. Limited utility in extremities.
- Particles—risk of ischemia depends on size; may be useful with redundant vascular supply to decrease risk of retrograde bleeding. Limited utility in extremities.

For Indispensable Vessels

- Stent grafts—not embolic agents but extremity work is where they are often essential to stop bleeding and preserve distal flow!

Medication

- Analgesia and sedation with fentanyl and midazolam. Hemodynamically unstable patients will require resuscitative support.

Angiography

Access

- *Should be chosen according to the clinical scenario*
- Most commonly the common femoral artery
- Consider the contralateral side if there are proximal injuries
- Brachial artery access may sometimes help
  - o If both lower extremities involved
  - o To retrogradely negotiate upper limb vascular injury

Angiography: General Principles

- Higher volumes of contrast and higher injection rates may be required in trauma patients especially due to high cardiac outputs from hypotension and hypovolemia to obtain adequate arterial opacification. ("High, hot, and hell of a lot."—Yorum Ben-Menachum.)
- Angiography should
  - o Delineate injury
  - o Demonstrate inflow and outflow
- Selective branch angiography may be necessary.
- Do not get too close to the site of injury until ready to treat.
- Evaluate collateral vessels and variant anatomy.
- In instances where the anatomy or site of injury is unclear, consider contralateral limb angiography to evaluate for asymmetry.
- Determine treatment plan based on staging angiography.

Angiographic Appearance

Positive Findings of Vascular Injury

- Extravasation in active hemorrhage
- Transection
- Pseudoaneurysm formation
- Arteriovenous fistula
- Occlusion
- Intimal irregularity
- Intraluminal filling defects
- Dissection (Figs. 26.1, 26.2, and 26.3)

Indirect findings may be a sign of a significant vascular injury but are less specific. Selective angiography may reveal the true nature of the injury, which includes the following:

- Spasm, protective spasm
- Luminal narrowing or focal widening,
- Arterial deviation by hematoma,
- Slow flow, e.g., in calf due to high compartment pressures.

Clinical Scenarios

Treatment Plan and Technique

The site of the injury governs the approach and the targets for angiography/intervention.

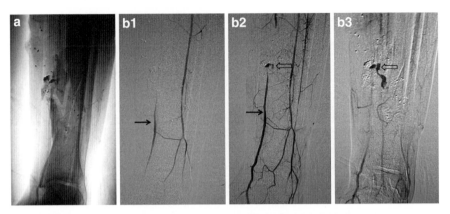

Fig. 26.1 Twenty-two-year-old man status post-gunshot wound to the left lower extremity and continued bleeding from the traumatic injury. (**a**) Unsubtracted left lower extremity angiography demonstrating the severity of the osseous injury. (**b**) Early, mid, and late arterial phase angiography of the left lower extremity demonstrating retrograde filling of the posterior tibial artery (*arrows*), which is the source of the bleeding (*open arrows*). Due to the inability to selectively catheterize the posterior tibial artery in retrograde fashion, the patient was taken to the operating room to control the hemorrhage

Fig. 26.2 Nineteen-year-old man with self-inflicted gunshot wound to the chest. (**a**) Angiography demonstrates a pseudoaneurysm arising from the left midaxillary artery (*arrow*).(**b**) Late arterial phase demonstrates persistence of the contrast in the pseudoaneurysm following washout of the intravascular contrast. Due to the inability to sacrifice downstream flow (the entire brachial artery distribution would have been sacrificed), an embolization procedure was not performed. This patient underwent a surgical procedure, since at the time of the procedure (2000) stent-grafts were not widely available

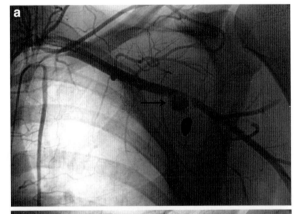

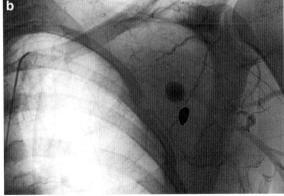

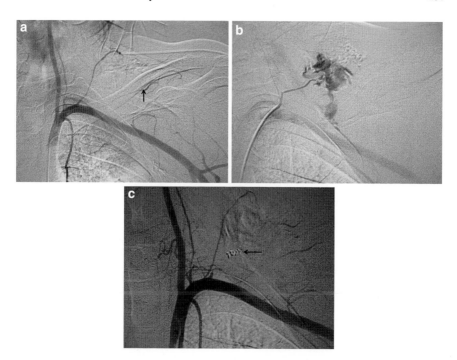

Fig. 26.3 Forty-five-year-old man with a stab wound to his upper chest and an expanding hematoma. (**a**) Angiography of the left subclavian artery fails to demonstrate any active contrast extravasation. Note that there is an underfilled vessel (*black arrows*) an "indirect sign" of arterial injury. (**b**) Superselective angiography of the suprascapular artery demonstrates active contrast extravasation, outlining the importance of pursuing selective angiography in the setting of high clinical suspicion of bleeding and a negative proximal angiogram. (**c**) Angiography post-embolization using both gelfoam slurry and microcoils (*arrow*) demonstrates complete cessation of contrast extravasation

Consider

- Therapeutic options to gain control as rapidly as possible; this may simply be balloon occlusion.
- Whether the damaged vessels can be sacrificed, if not therapy must preserve flow either stent grafting or surgery.

Special Considerations

- Arteriovenous fistulae are often treated differently to other traumatic injuries (e.g., approach from venous side, use of stent grafts, may be preferable to treat in a delayed fashion).
- Avoid embolization of actively bleeding major vessels which are the sole supply to the limb such as axillary artery, brachial artery, SFA, and popliteal artery due

subsequent limb-threatening ischemia. Injuries to these arteries may be treated with a stent-graft or a temporary occlusive balloon may be placed prior to surgical intervention.

- Arteries that may be embolized include those that are surgically inaccessible (e.g., PFA, branch vessels of major arteries).

Specific Blunt Injuries

Upper Limb

Axillary artery injury—anterior and medial to the proximal humerus.

- RARE in anterior dislocation without fracture.
- Severe anterior dislocation injures associated with damage to thoracoacromial trunk, subscapular, and circumflex humeral.
- EXTREMELY RARE in closed humeral neck fractures.
- Severe medial displacement increases risk.

Brachial artery injury—occurs in

- Up to 5–13% of patients with elbow dislocations (open and closed).
- Up to 38% of patients with completely displaced supracondylar fractures (pediatrics, usually in severe posterior lateral displacement).
- RARE in condylar, transcondylar, intercondylar fractures.

Radial and ulnar artery injuries

- Seldom require intervention.
- Most patients have adequate collateral circulation through the palmar arch system.

Lower Limb

- *Knee dislocation*
  - Popliteal artery injury (14–50%).
  - Anterior dislocation tends to stretch the popliteal artery, resulting in intimal disruption or vasospasm.
  - Posterior dislocations may be associated with transection of the popliteal artery and with more severe vascular injury.
  - Ischemia often resolves when the dislocation is reduced.
- Arterial injuries for other fractures are not as common
  - Femoral artery injury in 2% femoral shaft fractures.
  - Popliteal artery injury in 3% of fractures about the knee.

- Tibial artery injury in 12% of tibial shaft fractures.
- Screws and drills used in internal fixation can sometimes result in arterial injury.

Aftercare

Arterial Puncture Site

Routine care.

Post-embolization

Ensure that the patient is closely observed for ischemia and compartment syndrome.

Follow-Up

- o Is not normally necessary following definitive embolization.
- o Repeat imaging if there is any sign of further vascular compromise or bleeding.

Keypoints

- Extremity arterial injury is relatively uncommon.
- Clinical consequences include bleeding, ischemia, and compartment syndrome.
- Consider whether the vessel can be sacrificed.
  - o If so embolization may be the treatment of choice.
  - o If flow must be preserved, then consider balloon tamponade, stent grafting or surgery.
- Use of embolization is limited by ability to sacrifice downstream flow.
- Trauma patients with high cardiac outputs may need higher volumes of contrast and higher injection rates.
- Gelfoam, coils, and coil–gelfoam sandwich are commonly used.
- Emergent exploration with surgery may be required instead of embolization in patients with signs of ischemia and/or hemodynamic instability.

Safety

- Embolization in the upper limb is associated with the risk
  - o of hand ischemia
  - o cerebral embolization via the vertebral artery

Suggested Reading

Aksoy et al. Percutaneous transcatheter embolization in arterial injuries of the lower limbs. Acta
  Radiol 2005;46:471–475.
Bauer JR, Ray CE Jr. Transcatheter arterial embolization in the trauma patient: a review. Semin
  Intervent Radiol 2004;21(1):11–22
Fields, et al. Brachial and forearm vessel injuries. Surg Clin North Am 2002; 82(1):105–14.
Kadir S. Atlas of Normal and Variant Angiographic Anatomy. 1991, Philadelphia: WB Saunders.
Mavili et al. Endovascular treatment of lower limb penetrating arterial traumas. Cardiovasc
  Intervent Radiol 2007; 30:1124–1129.

Chapter 27
Solid Organ Embolization in Trauma

Otto van Delden

Clinical Features

- Blunt abdominal trauma from motor vehicle accidents or a fall from height is a common cause of hemorrhage from liver, spleen or kidney.
- Abdominal injury and significant injury to pelvis and/or chest frequently occur together necessitating accurate pre-procedure assessment of *all* potential bleeding sites.
- Hemodynamic instability or transient response to fluid resuscitation indicates ongoing bleeding and is often associated with arterial hemorrhage.
- Non-operative management is currently the therapy of choice for blunt injuries to liver, spleen, and kidneys in hemodynamically stable patients in most trauma centers. Avoidance of emergency surgery directly after the trauma (the so-called "second hit") leads to a better outcome for the patient.
- Non-operative management of high-grade injuries to the liver is associated with a significant number of late sequelae, such as infected hematomas and bilomas regardless of whether embolization has been performed or not. Most of these can be treated percutaneously.

Diagnostic Evaluation

Clinical

The Importance of Blood Pressure in the Context of Trauma

- *Incorrectable hemodynamic instability* should lead to immediate emergency laparotomy!
  - An exception to this is when arterial hemorrhage is due to pelvic fracture. In this case embolization should be the first step before proceeding to the OR for pelvic fixation.

Transcatheter Embolization and Therapy,
Techniques in Interventional Radiology, DOI 10.1007/978-1-84800-897-7_27,
© Springer-Verlag London Limited 2010

- *The "metastable" patient:* this is the situation when hemodynamic stability can be maintained by continuous fluid resuscitation. "Metastability" is not a contraindication to imaging or intervention when the CT and angiography suites are appropriately equipped to deal with such situations.

Imaging (See Also Chapter 10)

Abdominal Ultrasound (FAST)

- Is often performed in the emergency department by emergency physicians or trauma surgeons.
- First and quickest test for abdominal injury.
- Has reasonable sensitivity for the detection of intraperitoneal blood.
- Has only moderate sensitivity for the detection of solid organ injury, retroperitoneal, and pelvic hematoma.
- Blood can be echogenic and therefore easily missed by inexperienced operator.
- Should be followed by CT in patients who are stable enough to undergo CT.
    o In all patients with a positive FAST.
    o In patients with a negative FAST but ongoing clinical suspicion of injury.
- Some would suggest that there is little logic in performing FAST if CT is available and any other imaging is required.

Contrast-Enhanced CT

- Most accurate and comprehensive test for assessment of abdominal injury, particularly good at grading injuries of liver, spleen, and kidneys. MDCT preferred as thin slices and multi-planar reformats provide a good road-map for angiography.
- IV contrast is mandatory.
- Detects both active arterial hemorrhage and false aneurysm.
- Contrast "blush" indicates arterial hemorrhage and should be followed by angiography in most cases.
- Late phase helpful in patients with renal injury to differentiate perinephric hemorrhage from urinary leakage.
- CT in patients with liver injuries is often helpful in differentiating arterial hemorrhage from hemorrhage from the major liver veins or inferior vena cava (which can be a lethal injury!).
- Has only moderate sensitivity for detecting injuries to pancreas, mesentery, and bowel.

Imaging Findings: The Following Predict the Need for Intervention

- Contrast extravastion or false aneurysm on contrast-enhanced CT. This is the most reliable predictor for the presence of active bleeding on an angiogram and the most practical imaging feature to use.
- High-grade (>grade 3) injury to liver, spleen or kidney.
- Large hemoperitoneum or increasing hemoperitoneum on sequential CTs.

Indications

Indications to perform angiography and embolization are clinical signs of ongoing bleeding, imaging findings consistent with arterial hmorrhage or a combination of clinical signs and imaging findings. The goal of arterial embolization in patients with blunt trauma of liver, spleen or kidney is as follows:

- Treatment of ongoing bleeding of liver, spleen, and kidneys
  - o Reducing the need for blood transfusions
  - o Avoiding surgery altogether
  - o Allowing elective rather than emergency surgery
- Treatment of a false aneurysm or contained hemorrhage, thereby preventing delayed rupture and increasing the splenic salvage rate and the success rate of non-operative management.
- Treatment of perinephric bleeding or hematuria in renal injury.

Alternative Therapies

Surgery

- Operative management is indicated when there is suspicion of injury to mesentery and/or bowel. Laparotomy should be performed in such cases.
- For splenic injury, surgery is usually splenectomy.
- For renal injury, partial or complete nephrectomy.
- For liver injury, packing with gauze. Acute partial hepatectomy is associated with a high mortality and is usually avoided. As bleeding from liver vessels may not be controlled by packing with gauze alone, angiography and embolization should be considered as additional treatment directly following damage-control surgery.

Contraindications

- The only contraindication is incorrectable hemodynamic instability: these patients must have *immediate* laparotomy.

- Renal insufficiency and coagulopathy do not constitute contraindications in an emergency setting.

Complications

All complications that are associated with angiography may occur and are probably more common.

- Systemic complications (allergic reaction, contrast-induced nephropathy)
- Puncture-site complications (groin hematoma, false aneurysm, thrombosis, dissection)

  Specific complications are covered under separate headings for liver, spleen, and kidney.

Anatomy

Most anatomic variants will be apparent on the contrast-enhanced CT, which is preferably obtained prior to angiography.

Normal Anatomy and Common Variations

- Common variations of celiac anatomy such as replaced right hepatic artery from the superior mesenteric artery or left hepatic artery originating from the left gastric artery are frequently seen. Variations such as a common hepatic artery originating from the aorta or superior mesenteric artery are seen much less frequently, but are not exceedingly rare.
- Splenic artery anatomy is usually classic.
- Accessory renal arteries arise from a variety of positions on the aorta and iliac arteries.
- Bleeding may also occur from the adrenal glands or diaphragm; so also assess adrenal branches and inferior phrenic arteries.

Equipment

- *Sheath*: a 5-French sheath suffices in most cases. The sheath may be left in (sutured to the skin) after the procedure when
  - An arterial line is required
  - There is coagulopathy
- *Non-selective catheters:* Pigtail or straight catheter for flush aortogram if CT does not indicate the site of bleeding.
- *Selective catheters:* 5-French cobra and celiac-type catheters will suffice in the vast majority of cases. 4-French hydrophylic catheters may be useful for superselective catheterization.

- *Micro-catheters and appropriate guidewires* are mandatory for selective embolization. When using micro-catheters, the use of a Tuohy Borst adaptor is recommended.
- *Guiding catheters:* not usually required.
- *Closure devices.*

Embolic Agents

The choice of agent depends on the situation, but the vast majority of cases can be performed using the following:

- *Coils* (diameters 3–12 mm): accurate placement is safe and easy. Associated with low risk of ischemic complications in both liver, spleen, and kidneys. Require at least some degree of clotting in order to induce occlusion of a vessel and may therefore be insufficient in patients with severe coagulopathy. In such cases, a combination of coils and gelfoam or gelfoam alone may be used.
- *Micro-coils* (3–8 mm): same as above. Micro-coils usually required when performing selective embolization of the liver, spleen or segmental renal branches. Micro-coils usually not required for proximal splenic artery embolization or large renal branches.
- *Gelfoam*: gelfoam pledgets can be cut to the preferred size and mixed to a slurry using a three-way stop-cock and two 1-ml Luer-lock syringes. Gelfoam pledgets can be used for a more proximal occlusion and can be injected through both regular 5-French diagnostic and micro-catheters.

The availability of both coils and gelfoam are mandatory for trauma embolization.

Rarely Required

- *Amplatzer vascular plug* may be useful in rare instances.
- *Poly-vinyl alcohol particles* 300–500 μ may also be useful in rare instances.

Medication

Patients with major injury require physiological support during imaging and embolization—this is not the role of the interventional radiologist and must be provided by emergency physicians, anesthetists, and other appropriately trained staff.

Angiography

Access

- Almost always approached from the femoral artery.
- In the presence of a pelvic fracture, the sheet wrap or pelvic binder may sometimes need to be displaced somewhat in order to expose the groin. The presence of an external pelvic fixation device usually poses no problem.
- If embolization is required for a pelvic fracture, then it may be practical to puncture the contralateral side. Puncture the side which lends itself to the most rapid catheterization of the target artery.

Angiography

- Flush aortography is usually only helpful to assess for the presence of accessory renal arteries in case of renal injury or when doubt exists about the anatomy of the visceral vasculature (variations of celiac axis or superior mesenteric artery). However, when a good contrast-enhanced CT is performed prior to intervention, a flush aortogram can usually be left out all together. Moreover, a flush aortogram only adds to the contrast load which will often be significant when a contrast-enhanced CT is followed by angiography.
- Selective injections should be performed of all suspected vessels. Cobra or sidewinder type catheters will allow rapid selection of all relevant vessels including the renal arteries in most cases.
- Repeated, forceful hand injections may sometimes be helpful, when extravasation is expected (from the CT) but not seen on the initial angiogram.

Angiographic Appearance

Vascular abnormalities that should actively be sought for and embolized include the following:

- *Extravasation of contrast medium.*
- *False aneurysms*: these represent contained hemorrhage, embolization prevents delayed rupture and free extravasation into the peritoneal space.
- *AV-fistula* (particularly in renal and splenic injuries): these are associated with ongoing hemorrhage and hematuria. AV fistulae often present days or weeks following the initial trauma.
- *Vessel occlusions "cut-offs"*: occlusions represent vessels that have been dissected or completely transected. The vessel is typically occluded by spasm and or superimposed thrombus. When the blood pressure of the patient normalizes during resuscitation, such vessels are prone to start hemorrhaging again. They should be embolized.

Clinical Scenarios

Embolization

- Generally speaking, embolization should be performed as selectively as possible. However, in practice the way embolization is performed is often dictated by the clinical circumstances. Although salvage of the organ involved is desirable, saving the patients life is paramount.
- In most situations, embolization can be performed using coils, particularly when one or at the most a few focal bleeding vessels are identified. When many bleeding points are identified or when there is diffuse bleeding, the use of gelfoam is more appropriate.

Liver

- Due to its dual vascularization (75% of total flow supplied by portal vein, 25% by hepatic artery), the liver is able to tolerate occlusion of part of its arterial inflow. However, the bile ducts and gallbladder are fully dependent on hepatic arterial blood flow. Occlusion of the cystic artery should therefore be avoided. The cystic artery usually originates from the proper hepatic artery, but may also originate from the right hepatic artery. This vessel should always be identified prior to embolization; occlusion of the cystic artery should be avoided if possible (Fig. 13.1).
- Embolizing as selectively as possible is recommended as intra- and extra-hepatic collateral arteries may cause bleeding to persist when embolization has not been performed selectively enough.
- Hepatic vessels are prone to developing spasm during manipulation: for selective catheterization of hepatic vessels, the liberal use of micro-catheters is recommended. Micro-coils are usually adequate for inducing hemostasis of liver hemorrhage.
- When a large subcapsular hematoma has disrupted the liver capsule, torn capsular vessels may cause many bleeding points and this is best treated by more proximal embolization gelfoam or particles ("shotgun embolization").

Complications of Hepatic Embolization

- The biliary system is dependent on arterial blood supply. Bile duct ischemia leading to liver abscess may develop after embolization.
- Abscess can usually be managed with percutaneous drainage.
- Biliary drainage is rarely required.
- Remember that liver abscess, infected hematoma, and infected biloma are frequently seen after high-grade injuries to the liver in both patients who did and who did not undergo embolization.
- Occlusion of the cystic artery may lead to gallbladder necrosis, which should subsequently be treated with cholecystectomy. However, flow to the gallbladder

may also remain preserved as a result of collaterals, and occlusion of the cystic artery should not automatically lead to cholecystectomy.

Figs. 27.1 (a–d) (Liver Case)

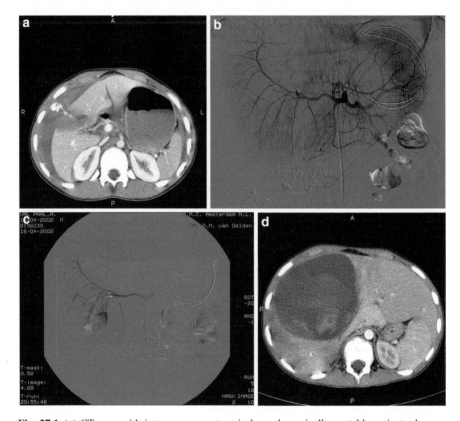

Fig. 27.1 (**a**) CT scan with intravenous contrast in hemodynamically unstable patient who sustained blunt abdominal trauma shows a deep liver laceration with extravasation of contrast medium into the peritoneal cavity. (**b** and **c**) The hypotensive patient was immediately transferred to the angio-suite and a selective angiogram of the common hepatic artery shows a so-called "cut-off" sign of the hepatic artery branch that had been severely bleeding on the preceding CT scan. As there is a high chance for this branch to start bleeding again once normal blood pressure has been restored, coil embolization of this branch was subsequently performed (Fig. 27.3c). (**d**) CT scan performed 2 weeks after the trauma shows large inhomogenous fluid collection in the liver with hyperdense areas consistent with a hematoma. This collection showed no signs of infection and was treated conservatively

Spleen

- Splenic salvage is preferred to splenectomy because it avoids the risk of overwhelming post-splenectomy sepsis.

- For splenic embolization, two different techniques are available; proximal embolization of the splenic artery and distal or selective embolization. Neither of these two techniques has proved superior in the literature.
- Proximal embolization is performed by coil occlusion of the proximal splenic artery. The Amplatzer vascular plug may also be used for this purpose, although it requires a larger delivery system than coils. As a result of this, the pressure in the splenic artery is lowered causing hemorrhage to cease. Splenic perfusion is preserved via collateral flow through the short gastric, gastroepiploic, and pancreatic branches. This technique is especially appropriate when
  - there is diffuse splenic injury with multiple bleeding vessels or when
  - selective embolization is difficult and time-consuming.
- Distal or selective splenic embolization is performed by embolizing a bleeding vessel as selectively as possible. This typically requires the use of microcatheters. This technique is especially appropriate when one focal bleeding vessel is identified.
- Distal embolization is associated with a higher chance for developing splenic infarction compared to proximal embolization, but such infarcts are usually clinically silent.
- Delayed rupture of the spleen and subsequent life-threatening hemorrhage may occur days after the initial trauma and poses the biggest threat to the success of non-operative management.

Figs. 27.2 (a–d) (Splenic Case, Proximal Embolization)

Complications of Splenic Embolization

- Infarcts are commonly seen after distal or selective embolization of splenic injuries. These are often noted on follow-up CT and generally produce no clinical sequelae.
- DO NOT OCCLUDE the distal main splenic artery beyond the short gastric vessels, as this may cause massive splenic infarction!
- Splenic abscesses can usually be treated percutaneously.
- Air in a splenic infarct as seen on follow-up CT is not a specific sign for infection and should not lead to aspiration or drainage unless clinical signs of infection exist.

Figs. 27.3 (a–d) (Splenic Case, Distal Embolization)

Kidney

- Always assess for accessory renal arteries (pre-embolization CT or flush aortogram).

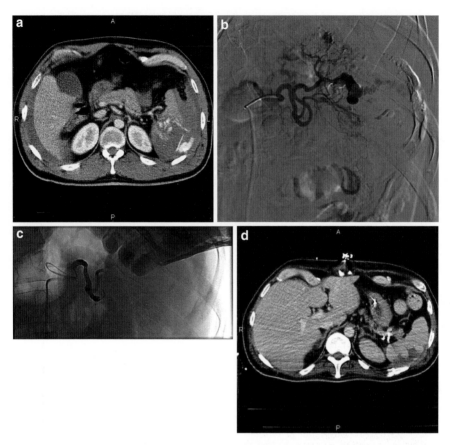

Fig. 27.2 (**a**) CT scan with intravenous contrast in hemodynamically unstable patient who sustained blunt abdominal trauma shows blood around the liver and spleen and active extravasation of contrast medium into the peritoneal cavity from the ruptured spleen. (**b** and **c**) The patient was immediately transferred to the angio-suite and a selective angiogram of the splenic artery shows brisk extravasation of contrast medium from a large branch of the splenic artery at the level of the splenic hilum. As the patient was hemodynamically unstable, no attempt was made to perform superselective catheterization and coil embolization of the proximal splenic artery was done (Fig. 27.1c). (**d**) CT scan performed 1 week after the embolization shows a small peripheral hypodense area in the spleen, caused by the laceration, but no significant area of infarction

- Renal pedicle injury may cause complete occlusion of the proximal renal artery. In such cases, embolization of the proximal renal artery may prevent recurrent hemorrhage when normal blood pressure is restored.
- When superselective embolization is impossible or too time-consuming, embolizing somewhat proximal to the bleeding point may suffice. Renal artery branches are end-arteries and bleeding will not persist or recur, as there is no collateral flow.

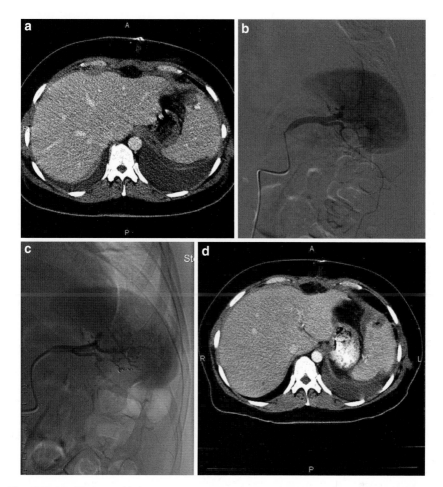

Fig. 27.3 (a) CT scan with intravenous contrast in hemodynamically stable patient who sustained blunt abdominal trauma shows focal area of contrast pooling in the spleen consistent with a pseudoaneurysm. No contrast extravasation outside the spleen is noted. (b and c) The patient was transferred to the angio-suite and a selective angiogram of the splenic artery shows a 1.5-cm pseudoaneurysm in the spleen with an associated traumatic AV fistula (not shown in this image). The small feeding branch was subsequently selected using a co-axial micro-catheter and coil embolization was performed (Fig. 27.2c). (d) CT scan performed 1 week after embolization shows a small splenic infarction in the area, which was embolized. A small air bubble is also noted in the infarcted area, but there were no signs of infection and the patient was asymptomatic

Complications of Renal Embolization

- As renal arteries are end-arteries, embolization of kidney injury will lead to infarction of part of the kidney. This seldomly leads to clinical sequelae.
- Infected hematoma or urinoma may occur and can be treated by percutaneous drainage.

- Renal embolization will result in loss of function in any parenchyma distal to the embolization.

Aftercare

Arterial Puncture Site

Closure device: preferably used in all patients as

o Coagulopathy is frequently present especially if the patient is hypothermic or has received multiple transfusion.
o Agitated patients are unlikely to lie still for a longer period of time.
o The groin will not be observed in patients who proceed to surgery after the embolization.

Post-embolization

- *Continue to monitor the following:*
  o *Complications of embolization*
  o *Further bleeding*
  o *Other injuries:* In the context of major trauma, it is easy to overlook important but non-life-threatening injuries in the heat of the moment.

Follow-Up: No specific follow-up is indicated and the patient should be managed clinically.

Keypoints

Imaging with contrast-enhanced CT is essential for triage of any patient who does not require immediate surgery (the importance of blood pressure!).

Patients with major injury require physiological support during imaging and embolization—this is not the role of the interventional radiologist and must be delivered by other trained providers.

CT with reformats will identify patients with injury to liver, spleen or kidneys, who are candidates for embolization.

Contrast extravasation at CT, the so-called "blush" is the best predictor of arterial hemorrhage as found at angiography. Pseudoaneurysms also mandate emergency embolization.

The goals of solid organ embolization in the trauma setting are as follows:

- To improve outcome by stopping bleeding without the morbidity and mortality associated with emergency major surgery.

- To avoid surgery all together or to delay surgery to a more elective stage.

Embolization materials of choice for trauma embolization of liver, spleen, and kidney are coils and gelfoam.

Embolization should be performed as selectively as time permits. In severely hypotensive patients, saving the patient is more important than saving the organ!

Chapter 28
Post-traumatic Priapism

Peter Littler, Peter Rowlands, and Richard McWilliams

Clinical Features

- Priapism is defined as a sustained, often painful erection unrelated to sexual stimulation.
- Priapism is idiopathic in 50% but other etiologies such as trauma, hyperviscosity syndromes, sickle cell disease, and drugs are recognized causes.
- Priapism can be classified as low flow (common) or high flow (uncommon).

Low-Flow Priapism

- Due to intrinsic or extrinsic venous outflow obstruction.
- Causes tissue ischemia and is painful.
- Treatment is an emergency. Options include aspiration, irrigation, anticoagulation, or shunt formation designed to improve cavernosal outflow.

High Flow or Arterial Priapism

- Usually due to penile or pelvic trauma.
- Due to laceration of a cavernosal artery and arteriocavernosal fistula formation.
- Painless and causes a partially erect penis, which can increase in rigidity on sexual stimulation.
- Patients can present days or even weeks following perineal or penile trauma.
- Treatment of high-flow priapism is not an emergency, unlike in low-flow priapism. However, reduced potency is reported in longstanding cases.
- Treated by embolization.

Transcatheter Embolization and Therapy,
Techniques in Interventional Radiology, DOI 10.1007/978-1-84800-897-7_28,
© Springer-Verlag London Limited 2010

Diagnostic Evaluation

History and examination will usually discriminate between low- and high-flow priapism.

Laboratory

Cavernosal Blood Gas Analysis

- Low pO_2/high pCO_2 in a patient with painful priapism is suggestive of a veno-occlusive low-flow cause. The aspiration of cavernosal blood is often therapeutic.
- High pO_2 in a patient with painless priapism and history of trauma is suggestive of high-flow arterial priapism. The aspiration of cavernosal blood is not therapeutic.

Imaging

Color Doppler Imaging of the Penis

- Axial and parasagittal ultrasound of the penis in greyscale and with optimized color Doppler to detect cavernosal arterial flow and pseudoaneurysms.
- Dilated cavernosal sinuses with increased flow are commonly reported in high-flow priapism, and a turbulence may be seen at the site of the arterio-cavernosal fistula.
- A focal area of reduced echogenicity with flow within it on Doppler may be seen representing a pseudoaneurysm.
- Ultrasound with color Doppler may demonstrate which side the AV fistula is on, although this can be misleading due to collateral supply or variant anatomy.
- Localization of the fistula guides arterial access, as the contralateral femoral artery approach is often preferable for angiography and embolization of the internal iliac artery.

Indications

For Angiography

These include patients with the following:

- Painless priapism
- A history of trauma to the perineum or penis

- A penile ultrasound suggestive of a high-flow etiology
- High pO$_2$ on the blood gas analysis suggestive of arterial blood

For Embolization

- Positive angiography

Alternative Therapies

- Surgical ligation of the internal pudendal artery. This may need to be bilateral.
- Other methods of treatment reported have poor success rates, including perineal compression, intracavernosal phenylephrine injection and topical ice.

Cautions

- Bleeding diathesis (as for any angiographic procedure)
- Renal impairment (caution due to contrast burden)

Specific Complications

- General complications of angiography and embolization.
- Impotence: the incidence is not known but this risk should be discussed and documented during the consent process. The risk is probably greater with highly selective embolization using permanent agents.

Anatomy

Normal Anatomy

The penis is supplied from the following arteries:

- The anterior division of the internal iliac artery.
  - The penile artery arises from the internal pudendal artery (Fig. 28.1).
  - It divides to form the bulbourethral artery to the corpus spongiosum and part of the urethra and the dorsal penile and cavenosal arteries to the corpus cavernosum.

Fig. 28.1 (Courtesy Dr Chuck Ray) Normal internal pudendal artery angiography. *Black arrows*—perineal artery; *large arrowhead*—penile artery; *proximal white arrowhead*—bulbourethral artery; *distal white arrowheads*—cavernosal artery; *black arrowheads*—dorsal penile artery

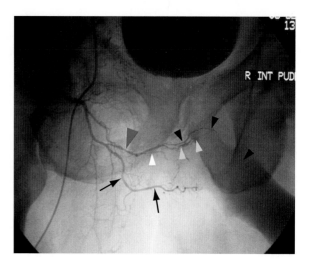

Aberrant Anatomy

- The penile arterial supply can occasionally arise from the contralateral side as a normal variant.

Equipment

Catheters

- *Non-selective catheters*: a pigtail or straight catheter if a flush aortic run is necessary.
- *Selective catheters:* a cobra or sidewinder. A microcatheter for selective embolization.
- *Guide catheter*: a renal double curve or long sheath may be used to gain stable position from the contralateral iliac.

Embolic Agents

- *Autologous clotted blood:* from patient
- *Gelfoam:* plegets or slurry
- *Coils:* small diameter microcatheter compatible coils
- *N-butyl-cyanoacrylate (NBCA)*
- *Onyx*

Medication

- *Pain control*: local analgesia at puncture site. May require analgesia post-procedure.
- *Hydration*: pre-hydration for patients with renal impairment.

Angiography

Access

- Via a contralateral or ipsilateral common femoral approach, dependent on anatomy.
- The likely side of the lesion should be assessed by ultrasound Doppler imaging pre-angiography.
- Access may need to be bilateral.

Angiography

- If necessary, flush aortography to demonstrate and lateralize the fistula.
- Selective catheterization of the internal iliac arteries and angiography with further superselective microcatheter runs of the anterior division/ internal pudendal arteries.

Angiographic Appearance

- Active cavernosal extravasation or pseudoaneurysm may be seen.
- Direct visualization of the arteriovenous fistula or pseudoaneurysm (Fig. 28.2a).
- Persistent staining is abnormal.
- If identified, then you can proceed to embolization (Fig. 28.2b).
- Note a normal cavernosal blush seen at the base of the penis (Fig. 28.3), which could be confused with a bleeding point/AV fistula. Differentiation can be difficult, but in a patient with a painless erection following trauma with a persistent asymmetric cavernosal blush then bleeding is the likely cause.

Aftercare

Post-embolization

- Standard care post-arterial puncture.

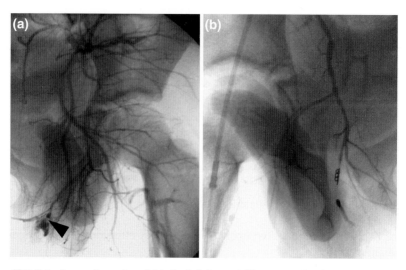

Fig. 28.2 Selective angiography of (**a**) the left internal iliac artery showing cavernosal arteriovenous fistula. (**b**) Successful occlusion of the arteriovenous fistula following selective coil embolization

Fig. 28.3 Normal cavernosal blush (*arrow*) at the base of the penis seen at conventional aortic angiography in a patient investigated for peripheral vascular disease

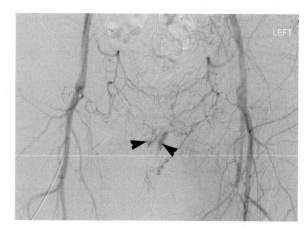

Follow-Up

• Repeat Doppler ultrasound of the penis, if no clinical improvement.
• Most high-flow priapism resolves in the first 24 h post-embolization.

Keypoints

- A painless partial erection following perineal or penile trauma is highly suggestive of high-flow priapism.
- Doppler ultrasound is sensitive for the detection of high-flow arterio-cavernosal fistulae and pseudoaneurysm, can aid in lateralization of the lesion, and is useful in follow-up.
- Superselective angiography of the internal pudendal arteries and embolization of the causative vessel is the mainstay of treatment.

Safety

- Be aware of a normal cavernosal blush on angiography simulating bleeding. In the context of painless post-traumatic priapism, asymmetric persistent cavernosal blush on angiography is likely to represent bleeding and should prompt embolization.
- Document the risk of erectile dysfunction following therapy.

Suggested Reading

Bertolotto M, Quaia E, Mucelli F P et al. Colour doppler imaging of posttraumatic priapism before and after selective embolization. Radiographics 2003; 23: 495–503

Kang B.C, Lee D.Y, Byunt J.Y et al. Post-traumatic arterial priapism: colour doppler examination and superselective arterial embolization. Clin Rad (1998) 53, 830–834

Schrumpf J.D, Sommer G, Jacobs R.P, Bleeding simulated by the distal internal pudendal artery stain. Am J Roengenol (1978) 131, 657–659

Shankar K.R, Babar S, Rowlands et al. Posttraumatic high-flow priapism: treatment with selective embolisation. Pediatr Surg Int (2000) 16: 454–456

Yilmaz T, Parildar M, Oran I et al. High-flow priapism due to cavernosal artery fistula with pseudoaneurysm treated by N-butyl-cyanoacrylate embolization. Eur J Radiol Extra (2003) 46, 56–59

Chapter 29
Embolization for Pancreatic Bleeding

Tony Nicholson

Clinical Features

- Embolization for hemorrhage secondary to pancreatic pathology is usually carried out as an emergency or very urgent procedure.
- Pancreatic bleeding typically occurs in the context of pancreatitis and pancreatic surgery.

Hemorrhage in Pancreatitis

- 10% of patients with acute pancreatitis develop arterial or portal venous vascular complications; these are commonest if there is pseudocyst development.
- Leakage of pancreatic enzymes leads to the development of aneurysms and pseudoaneurysms of the pancreatic vasculature.
- The mortality rate for pancreatic hemorrhage is over 90% if only treated conservatively. The mortality for surgery has been quoted to be as high as 56%.
- Recurrent bleeding occurs in up to 10% of patients surviving surgery.
- Early upper abdominal pain without active bleeding ("herald pain") may precede a bleed.
- Occasionally patients with pancreatitis can develop occult pseudoaneurysms, which manifest as a decreasing hemoglobin on serial full blood counts and/or a pulsatile upper abdominal mass.

Hemorrhage Following Pancreatic Surgery

- Pancreatic hemorrhage can also be iatrogenic secondary to pancreatic surgery for cancer or pancreatitis. The most common location for such hemorrhage is the gastroduodenal artery, but any artery in the pancreatic arcade can be affected.
- Post-pancreatico-duodenectomy hemorrhage occurs in approximately 10%, with 2% occurring from the pancreatic cut surface and 8% from the gastroduodenal artery stump due to infection or poor suture technique.

Transcatheter Embolization and Therapy,
Techniques in Interventional Radiology, DOI 10.1007/978-1-84800-897-7_29,
© Springer-Verlag London Limited 2010

Diagnostic Evaluation

- As the patients usually have acute hematemesis and/or melena, laboratory examinations do not generally help with diagnosis. Clearly a blood count and a cross match are essential in the early phase.
- Clotting studies should be performed if there is liver dysfunction or if there has been transfusion of >4 units of blood.

Imaging

- Contrast-enhanced thin-slice multidetector CT scanning is the initial imaging investigation of choice. Ultrasound is not sensitive or specific enough.
- The scan should cover from the diaphragm to the pelvis.
- Pancreatic calcification may cause confusion with contrast extravasation. To avoid this, perform unenhanced scans in addition to arterial and portal vein phase delayed scans.
- Look for the following:

  - Active contrast extravasation that indicates sites of active hemorrhage.
  - Arterial pseudoaneurysms: these typically have thick walls and show peak enhancement in the arterial phase (Fig. 29.1).
  - Venous or capillary bed pseudoaneurysms show delayed enhancement.
  - True arterial aneurysms are smaller with thin walls (Fig. 29.2(a–c)).
  - In post-surgical patients, try to identify the reconstructed arterial anatomy which may require coronal oblique reconstructions.

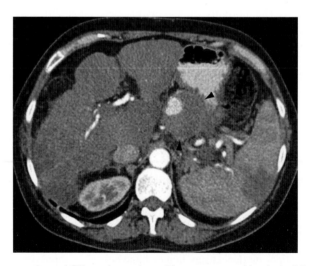

Fig. 29.1 Contrast-enhanced CT scan in a patient with acute pancreatitis who had developed a pulsatile epigastric mass and anemia. It demonstrates a thick-walled pseudoaneurysm (*arrowheads*) of the gastroduodenal artery

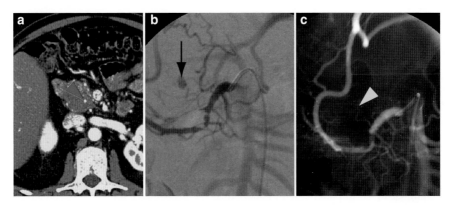

Fig. 29.2 A patient who had hematemesis following recent pancreatitis; endoscopy suggested hemobilia. (**a**) CT scan demonstrates a small contrast-enhanced area in the head of the pancreas (*arrowhead*), not present on non-contrast scans and not continuous with any structure above or below this axial slice. (**b**) Selective inferior pancreatico-duodenal arteriography demonstrates the aneurysm (*black arrow*) arising from a small pancreatic head branch. (**c**) This was successfully embolized by superselective injection of 500 μ PVA (*arrowhead*)

Indications for Imaging and Embolization

- Hematemesis and/or melena in a patient with pancreatitis or a patient who has undergone recent pancreatic surgery.
- Progressive anemia in a patient with pancreatitis.
- Asymptomatic false aneurysm.
- Development of a pulsatile or non-pulsatile mass in a patient with pancreatitis.

Contraindications

- There are no specific contraindications to imaging or intervention in this group of patients.
- A patient with acute massive hemorrhage will be unstable and should be vigorously resuscitated—*do not let this delay life-saving therapy.*
- Consumptive coagulopathies should be treated in the catheter lab either during angiography or beforehand.

Specific Complications

- Rupture of an aneurysm or a pseudoaneurysm is a rare event, but if it happens before the embolization is completed, then it can be catastrophic. Use of a balloon occlusion catheter may prevent exsanguination under these circumstances.

- Non-target embolization leading to infarction and infection of solid organs around the gastroduodenal and splenic arcade.
- Embolization may lead to anastomotic breakdown. Most common, in post-pancreatico-duodenectomy patients, the bleeding is from a suture line. Gelfoam is the agent of choice.

Anatomy

- As stated, the vascular anatomy should be determined from the CT scan prior to angiography. In patients with pancreatitis the most likely sources of hemorrhage are (in order) as follows:

  1. Splenic artery
  2. Gastroduodenal artery
  3. Left gastric artery
  4. Inferior and superior pancreatico-duodenal arteries
  5. Hepatic artery
  6. Jejeunal branches

- There are some pseudoaneurysms that can be seen easily on CT scanning but that are difficult to find at arteriography (Fig. 29.3a and b). It is postulated that many of these aneurysms arise from the venous and capillary bed, which is extensive particularly around the tail of the pancreas and at the foramen of Winslow.

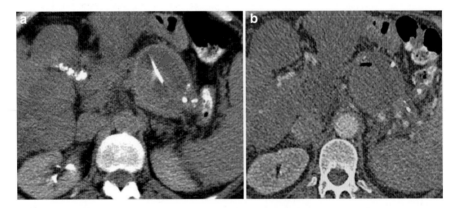

Fig. 29.3 CT scans of a patient with a post-pancreatitis pseudoaneurysm that was not visualized at angiography. It was treated by CT-guided percutanous thrombin injection (*arrowhead*) (**a**). Complete thrombosis of the aneurysm is seen following injection of 2500 units of thrombin (**b**)

Aberrant Anatomy

- Aberrant anatomy of the arteries arising from the celiac trunk is very common. For a full description, the reader is directed to Kadir's textbook of diagnostic angiography (see Selected Reading list).

Angiography and Embolization Equipment

- Non-selective angiography is often unnecessary, if a CT scan has been performed and interpreted correctly. However, a pigtail catheter should be available.
- The choice of selective catheters can often be determined from the CT scan. A variety of 4Fr and 5Fr femoral visceral catheters will be necessary for selective angiography. A co-axial microcatheter will be necessary for superselective angiography and embolization.
- Guide catheters are rarely necessary but should be available.
- Iodinated contrast agents are most often used but CO_2 may be useful.

Embolic Agents

- For post-pancreatitis and post-surgical aneurysms and pseudoaneurysms, coil and histacryl glue are the most useful embolization agents (Fig. 29.4a and b).

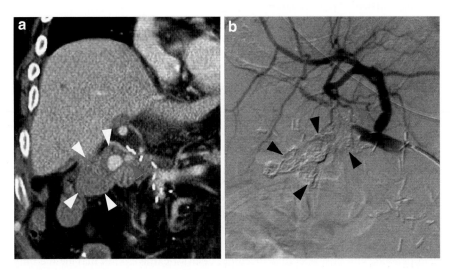

Fig. 29.4 CT scan of a patient presenting with massive hematemesis 7 days after pancreatico-duodenectomy (**a**) CT scan demonstrates a pseudoaneurysm (*white arrowheads*) of the gastroduodenal stump (*arrowhead*). (**b**) This was embolized with a 2:1 lipiodol:histacryl glue mixture (*black arrowheads*). The stump of the GDA (*gray arrowhead*) is seen. The patient made a full recovery

- For pseudoaneurysms that cannot be seen at arteriography and that are probably pseudoaneurysms of the vascular bed, percutaneous injection of thrombin under CT or ultrasound guidance maybe successful (Fig. 29.3a and b).
- For post-operative bleeding from the cut surface of the pancreas, coils and gelfoam are the embolic agents of choice.

Procedure Access

- This can be planned from the pre-procedural imaging.
- In the majority of patients, a common femoral approach is the approach of choice.
- Acute angulation of celiac axis or superior mesenteric arteries, especially in thin patients, may require a left arm approach.

Angiography

- Flush angiography is only of value, if after selective angiography, no aneurysms, pseudoaneurysms, or bleeding can be identified. Selective angiography of all potential arteries as in the list above would then be required.

Angiographic Appearance

- A true aneurysm of an upper GI visceral artery will be seen on CT as a small dot of contrast which has no obvious continuity on slices above and below. At angiography, it will be seen as a small outpouching of a visceral artery that may remain contrast-filled after contrast in the main artery has disappeared (Fig. 29.2(a–c))
- A pseudoaneurysm will generally be seen as a collection of contrast with a thick wall containing thrombus on a CT scan. On angiography, it is difficult to tell the difference between a pseudoaneurysm and a true aneurysm (Fig. 29.5(a–d)).
- A collection of contrast as above that is easily seen at CT, but that appears only in the late phase of an angiogram or does not appear at all, is likely to be a vascular bed pseudoaneurysm. This is unlikely to respond to even the most extensive embolization, and may best be treated by percutaneous thrombin injection (Fig. 29.3a and b).
- In patients with post-operative bleeding, contrast extravasation may be the only sign of the source of bleeding. This should be seen on both the CT scan and the angiogram.

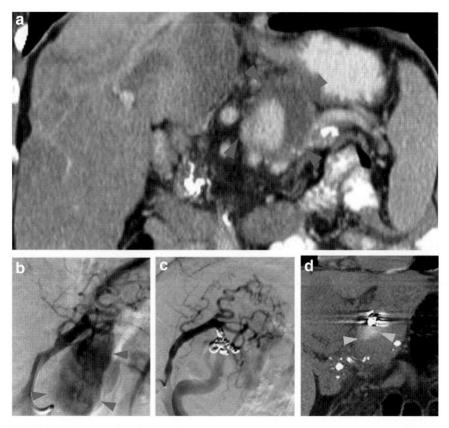

Fig. 29.5 A CT scan and angiogram of a patient with gallstone-induced acute pancreatitis who had a large hematemesis. (**a**) Demonstrates a thick-walled pseudoaneurysm from the left gastric artery (*arrowheads*). (**b**) Selective angiography of the LGA confirms this (*arrowheads*). (**c**) Selective coil embolization. (**d**) A non-contrast CT scan the following day demonstrates artifact from the coils (*red arrowhead*) and retained contrast in the sac (*yellow arrowheads*) indicating thrombus formation

Clinical Scenarios

Embolization for Post-pancreatitis Aneurysm and Pseudoaneurysm

- It is important to occlude both the inflow and the outflow.
- Occlusion of the aneurysm or pseudoaneurysm itself while maintaining patency of the artery invariably does not work and can lead to massive hemorrhage.
- Stent graft insertion should only be used if the artery is essential. Small tortuous arteries are unsuitable for stent grafts.

- Histacryl glue can be useful if the outflow artery cannot be catheterized. In such cases, a 2:1 or 2.5:1 mixture of histacryl and lipiodol will flow across the aneurysm neck (Fig. 29.4a and b). However, great care has to be taken not to embolize a non-target structure such as the spleen.

Embolization for Post-operative Bleeding

- Everything above applies, but occasionally it is sufficient to occlude a small end-artery.

Aftercare

Puncture Site

- Consider leaving sheath in situ, if there are any questions regarding coagulation status.
- Most patients will be on HDU or ITU; so bedrest should not be an issue.

Post-embolization

- Remember that if post-operative hemorrhage is secondary to sepsis, rebleeding is likely if the infection is not controlled.
- Anastomotic dehiscence (due to ischemia) is possible unless embolization is highly selective.

Follow-Up

- Use CT.
- Remember, following successful embolization, contrast is trapped in the aneurysm sac. Initial non-contrast CT scan will demonstrate this and prevents false-positive diagnosis of persistent aneurysm perfusion (Fig. 29.5d).
- If contrast is seen in the sac on the unenhanced scan, no further imaging is necessary! This imaging should take place within 24 h of embolization.
- If there is no residual contrast in the sac, contrast-enhanced CT is required.
- If there is any doubt regarding the patency following embolization, repeat angiography should be performed with repeat embolization as necessary.
- Imaging follow-up is not routinely required after embolization for post-operative bleeding.
- The patient's clinical course will determine whether imaging is required. Only where it has been impossible to access the bleeding artery for embolization, should surgery be necessary.

- Following percutaneous thrombin injection, repeat imaging at 24 h, 1 week, and 1 month are necessary as these pseudoaneurysms can sometime recanalize. They may require repeat thrombin injections; this is particularly so, if the patient's pancreatitis is still active.

Keypoints

Pancreatic hemorrhage occurs in the context of acute pancreatitis and following surgery and can be life threatening.

Selective embolization can be performed in most cases without placing the pancreas at risk.

Some aneurysms may be more amenable to percutaneous thrombin injection than endovascular embolization.

Post-procedure imaging can be misleading. Always start with a non-contrast enhanced CT scan!

Safety

False aneurysms should always be treated without delay as there is a high risk of bleeding.

Bibliography

1. Kivluto T, Givissari L, Kivilaakso D. Pseudocysts in chronic pancreatitis: Surgical results in 102 consecutive patients. Arch Surge 1989; 124: 240–243
2. Sankaran S, WaltAJ. The natural and unnatural history of pancreatic pseudocysts produced J Surg 1975; 62: 37–44.
3. Sessay C, Tinelli G, Porcu P, et al. Treatment of visceral artery aneurysms; description of a retrospective series of 42 aneurysms in 34 patients. Annals Vasc Surg 2004; 18: 695–703
4. Frey CF Pancreatic pseudocyst: Operative strategy. Annals Surg 1978; 188: 652–662.
5. El Hamel A, Parc R, Adda G. Bleeding pseudocysts and psuedoaneurysms in chronic pancreatitis. Brit J Surg 1991; 78: 1059–1063.
6. Billadur P, Christophe M, Tiret E, et al. Bleeding of the pancreatic stump following pancreatic duodenectomy for cancer. Hepatogastroentorology 1996; 43: 268–270.
7. Nicholson AA, Patel J, McPherson S, et al. Endovascular of treatment of visceral aneuryms associated with pancreatitis and the suggested classification with theraputic implications. JDIR 2006; 17: 1279–1285.
8. Kadir S, ed. Atlas of normal and variant angiographic anatomy. Philadelphia: W.B. Saunders Company, 1991; pp. 387–429
9. Cronin P, Patel JV, Kessel DO, et al. Carbon dioxide angiography: a simple and safe system of delivery 2005; 60:123–125
10. Nicholson T, Travis S, Ettles D, et al. Hepatic artery angiography for haemobilia following laporoscopic colecystectomy. CVIR 1999; 22: 20–24

Chapter 30
Embolization in Post-operative Hemorrhage

Kim Wright and Ben English

Clinical Features

- There are many causes of post-operative hemorrhage. The sites of bleeding usually relate to the following:
  - Vessel transaction/ligation
  - Anastomoses
  - Damaged organs
- Bleeding is most common following complex surgery (e.g., pancreatic resection) with the following:
  - Sepsis
  - Leak of bile, pancreatic or gastric fluid
- In the acute setting, there is often bleeding from one of the operative drains. This can help localize the site.
- Iatrogenic injury and subsequent hemorrhage can occur following minimally invasive procedures such as sphincterotomy of the papilla of Vater, central venous line placement, and deep tissue biopsy.
- Intermittent severe bleeding suggests false aneurysm.

Diagnostic Evaluation

Clinical

- It is essential to review the operative notes and discuss the case with the surgeon in order to understand exactly what procedure was performed and whether there were any difficulties. This will help
  - Anticipate the likely source of the bleeding.
  - Anticipate any anatomic problems which may be encountered.
  - Understand the surgical options available. Repeat surgery can have an exceedingly high morbidity and mortality.
- The underlying hemodynamic status and comorbidities (e.g., cardio respiratory problems) should be taken into account when considering therapy. Patients with

Transcatheter Embolization and Therapy,
Techniques in Interventional Radiology, DOI 10.1007/978-1-84800-897-7_30,
© Springer-Verlag London Limited 2010

post-operative bleeding are often on the intensive therapy unit and may have multiorgan failure.

- Make sure that the patient is being actively resuscitated during the procedure.
- Patients who have repeated episodes of bleeding despite embolotherapy and surgery seldom have a good clinical outcome.

Laboratory

- Full blood count.
- Coagulation profile: this is often deranged especially if multiple transfusions have been given.
- Renal function: often deranged; so ensure that renal protection is implemented if possible. It is better to have a live patient on dialysis than a dead patient.

Imaging

- Triple-phase contrast-enhanced computed tomography (CT) examination with image reformats is the investigation of choice. Post-operative patients often have complex anatomy, additional pathology, and may bleed from unexpected sites. Only CT gives information on these factors. CT is more sensitive than angiography at detecting bleeding as well as the site of bleeding. Performed first, it is replacing diagnostic angiography.
- Radionuclide scans with Tc-99m-labeled red blood cells can detect active hemorrhage but this test is normally reserved for more insidious or low-grade intermittent bleeding.
- Ultrasound is useful in detecting large, superficial pseudoaneurysms, and can be used to direct therapy such as thrombin injection.
- Angiography is usually performed if the patient is unstable with obvious ongoing bleeding where there is the intention to go directly to embolization or surgery.

Indications

- Embolization is advocated when
  - There is ongoing bleeding
  - A pseudoaneurysm is discovered as rebleeding is very common.
- Embolization can be
  - Definitive therapy
  - Used to stabilize the patient pre-operatively
  - Or to allow time for natural healing

- o In the presence of sepsis, embolization should be regarded as a temporizing measure
- Embolization is often used in certain post-radiation or post-surgical settings, due to the surgical challenges in such populations.
- The clinical scenario (e.g., hemodynamic stability) largely determines the urgency of the embolization.

Alternative Therapies

Surgical Repair

- Surgery typically is reserved for patients in whom embolization fails or where surgical treatment is less risky than transcatheter therapy (e.g., brachial artery injuries). Remember that repeat surgery can be very difficult in the presence of adhesions and inflammation.
- Emergency surgery may be necessary if there is any delay obtaining angiographic intervention.
- It will also be required if, in addition to bleeding, there are other problems such as sepsis, tissue infarction or anastomotic breakdown.

Alternative Interventional Techniques

- Stents, stent grafts
- Direct puncture with thrombin injection, e.g., common femoral artery pseudoaneurysm

Contraindications

- All contraindications are relative in the context of life-threatening bleeding.
- Incorrectable coagulopathy: it is usually better to have a live patient with an arterial sheath in situ; it can always be removed later when the patient has stabilized.
- Bleeding foci that are too dangerous to embolize due to inability to sacrifice downstream organ, e.g., the brain. In the presence of life-threatening hemorrhage, normal rules do not apply. If there is no surgical alternative, then it is even acceptable to sacrifice a transplant hepatic artery end, though repeat transplant might subsequently be required.
- In some cases, preservation of flow may be possible in which case stent-graft placement may be more appropriate, e.g., brachiocephalic artery injury during attempted central line placement.

Specific Complications

- Embolization following a recent operation might be disadvantageous, due to the decreased likelihood of adequate healing in the setting of post-embolization ischemia, e.g., anastomotic breakdown.
- Risk of contrast nephropathy, which may be higher in hemodynamically compromised patients.
- Access-related hemorrhagic complications including pseudoaneurym are more common if there is coagulopathy.
- "Post-embolization syndrome" following ischemia or infarction of an embolized organ, with symptoms including pain, fever, nausea, vomiting, and leukocytosis.

Anatomic Considerations

- Specific challenges in the post-operative patient are as follows:
  - Normal vascular anatomy may have been affected by the surgery. Vessels may have been ligated or there may be extra anatomic conduits especially in transplants.
  - Embolization might be difficult if the normal vasculature was sacrificed during the operation. Collaterals may have to be selected, and may prove to be much more difficult to embolize.
- The ability to embolize depends on the presence of collateral vessels and/or the ability to sacrifice downstream supply.
  - Example: embolization within the pelvis is generally possible, due to adequate collateral vasculature. However, embolization of the main renal artery may result in renal infarction due to its end-arterial supply. Do not forget better alive on dialysis than dead.
- Must assess the collateral vasculature prior to embolization. This is generally accomplished by performing a more central angiogram.

Equipment

- Catheter selection depends on the target vessel size and specific embolic agent to be employed (Section 1).
- Microcatheters allow for more distal placement and superselection of the targeted vessel, resulting in more selective embolization. This preserves adjacent tissue and collateral vessels.
- Sheaths appropriately sized.

Embolic Agents

This will depend on the exact circumstances and vessels to be occluded; the most common embolic agents are as follows:

- Coils and microcoils.
- Amplatzer device.
- Gelfoam.
- Polyvinyl alcohol particles.
- Glue.
- Stent grafts are used in large-vessel endovascular repair, such as rupture, false aneurysm, and AVFs, where preservation of distal flow is desirable.
- An occlusion balloon can be used to transiently occlude an artery and control bleeding until surgical control is achieved.

Medication

Systemic

- Supportive therapy: blood products, IV fluids, vasopressor support, sedation, and analgesia.
- Hyoscine to stop peristalsis: remember to let the aneshetist know why the patient is getting a tachycardia!
- In rare select cases, paralytic agents (succinlycholine, vecuronium) may be required in order to eliminate motion to facilitate superselective catheterization.

Transcatheter

○ Adjunctive therapy may include vasoconstrictive agents, notably when temporary control is needed in an arterial bed only (e.g., temporizing method before the patient can return to the operating room).
○ Primarily vasopressin is utilized, causing smooth muscle contraction.

Procedure

- *Access*
  ○ Preferred access is via femoral artery for simple/quick access.
  ○ Consider brachial or axillary approach if lower extremity access is not available.

Angiography and Embolization

- Required to assess vascular injury, the presence of collateral vasculature, and evaluate for variant anatomy.
- "High, hot, and a helluva lot." Bleeding vessels should be assessed by more proximal injections (high), high-injection rates (hot), and high-volume injections with prolonged imaging (a helluva lot).

Angiographic Appearance

Look for abnormalities in the following:

- In the target area.
- Adjacent to drains, surgical clips, and suture lines.
- *Extravasation*: this will be seen in unstable patients. Ill-defined blush of contrast, outside of a normal vascular territory, which enlarges and changes morphology during the angiographic run.
- *Pseudoaneursym*: focal collection of contrast, outside the confines of the normal vascular contour. Persists beyond normal arterial washout phase.
- *Arteriovenous fistula.*
- *Vascular injury following central line placement*: may visualize occlusion, luminal irregularity, intraluminal thrombus, spasm, or a dissection flap with tapering of intraluminal contrast opacification.

Clinical Scenarios

Treatment Plan and Technique

- Try to predict the likely source of the bleeding based on discussion with the surgical team, the operative note, and pre-procedure imaging.
- Consider and discuss the possible therapeutic options and balance these against the risks of doing nothing and other therapeutic alternatives.
- Discuss this with the patient/relatives if time allows, including the need to sacrifice tissues and organs
- Formulate a plan and ideally a backup plan!
- The specific embolic agent depends on the desired permanency of embolization and the ability to sacrifice downstream supply.
  - o To temporarily stop a rapidly bleeding vessel, Gelfoam pledgets or slurry are most commonly used.
  - o For permanent occlusion, where downstream flow can be safely sacrificed, coils, acrylic spheres or large particles may be used.

Unstable Patients

If the patient is unstable, or if there is rapid hemorrhage, performing the procedure in a timely fashion is essential. A temporary balloon occlusion may be beneficial either prior to a return to the operating room or while the definitive embolization procedure is being considered. Therefore, it may be better to non-selectively embolize a proximal bleeding vessel, rather than perform a lengthy selective embolization. This can only be accomplished in organs or regions with sufficient collateral flow (e.g., proximal internal iliac embolization). In this setting, distal collateral vessels prevent significant tissue necrosis.

Coagulopathic Patients

Many patients will have an underlying coagulopathy due to ongoing hemorrhage. Coagulopathies should be aggressively managed, but if the patient remains coagulopathic (e.g., disseminated intravascular coagulopathy), then the embolic agent used may have to be re-addressed.

- Coils require thrombosis; consider combining with Gelfoam to achieve the vascular occlusion "coil–Gelfoam sandwich."
- Alternatively, glue can be used as this does not require coagulation to achieve occlusion.

Active Extravasation

If temporary occlusion is desired, Gelfoam is used (slurry or pledgets). However, if permanent embolization is needed, then coils or large particles are frequently utilized.

Pseudoaneurysm

Coils are typically used due to their permanence and precise control in deployment. Several options exist for occluding a pseudoaneurysm.

- The first, and most frequently used, technique is to "trap" the pseudoaneurysm by coiling both the upstream and downstream portions of the vessel.
- Alternatively, if anatomically possible (e.g., small neck), a coil can be placed within the neck of the pseudoaneurysm.
- Some PSA may need to be treated by placing a stent graft across the neck, particularly if downstream flow cannot be sacrificed.

Iatrogenic Injury During Central Line Placement

Dissection or pseudoaneurysm formation from central line placement generally requires an operation or endovascular stenting due to the central location of the arterial injury (e.g., subclavian, carotid artery) and inability to sacrifice downstream flow.

- Avoid burning bridges—if a proximal coil is placed, it will be impossible to access distal sites later.
- The use of microcatheters may be advantageous to preserve collateral vessels, but may limit the choice of embolic materials (e.g., large particles and Gelfoam pledgets).

Post-embolization

- Routine puncture site aftercare
- Consider leaving the arterial sheath in situ if
  - o There is the possibility of further bleeding
  - o There is coagulopathy

Follow-Up

Repeat CT

- This is the key investigation.
- Remember that contrast will remain "trapped" in a thrombosed false aneurysm; this is a pitfall for the unwary and may lead to false-positive reports of continued perfusion on a contrast-enhanced scan. To prevent this, perform unenhanced scans first.
- CT may also be compromised by artifact from a large coil pack.
- If there is continued bleeding, remember to look for other potential sources.

Keypoints

- Post-operative bleeding should be urgently investigated with contrast-enhanced CT
- Knowledge of the operation is essential.
- Embolotherapy can be very challenging.
- It is essential to consider all therapeutic options with the surgical team.

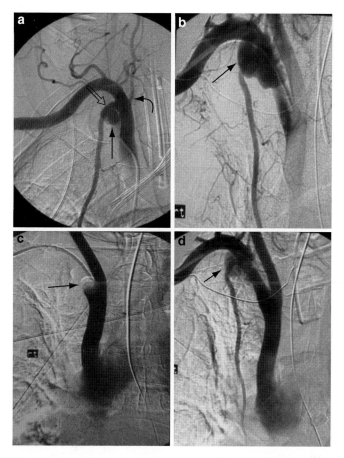

Fig. 30.1 Eighty-three-year-old man status post-attempted bedside right internal jugular central venous catheter placement. (**a**) Right subclavian angiogram performed approximately 1 week after attempted line placement demonstrates a moderate-sized pseudoaneurysm arising from the subclavian artery (*arrow*). Notice the close proximity of the internal mammary artery (*open arrow*) and vertebral artery (*curved arrow*) origins. Due to the lack of a narrow neck (precluding embolization) and the proximity of the vertebral artery origin (precluding stent-graft placement), no intervention was performed at this time. Given the patient's underlying vascular disease and age, sacrificing the vertebral artery was not considered an optimal result. The patient was placed on anticoagulation, and serial CT scans (not shown) were performed to follow the progress of the pseudoaneurysm. (**b**). Right subclavian angiogram performed 24 days after the initial angiogram demonstrates significant enlargement of the pseudoaneurysm (*arrow*). Ultrasound of the supraclavicular fossa (not shown) demonstrated a good window to access the pseudoaneurysm from a percutaneous approach. (**c**) Via a right brachial artery approach, an 11-mm occlusion balloon catheter was inflated in the suclavian artery origin (*open arrow*), central to the pesudoaneurysm but peripheral to the origin of the carotid artery. This was performed in an attempt to decrease the risk of non-target embolization of thrombin during percutaneous injection directly into the pseudoaneurysm. (**d**) Right subclavian artery angiogram following ultrasound-guided percutaneous injection of thrombin directly into the pseudoaneurysm. Angiography demonstrates decreased flow of contrast into the pseudoaneurysm (*arrow*) and patency of the cervical vessels. Continued injection of thrombin resulted in complete occlusion of the pseudoaneurysm

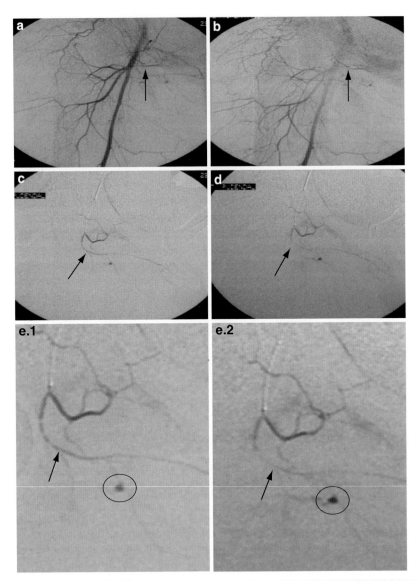

Fig. 30.2 Fifty-one-year old woman with history of intravenous drug abuse and HIV, who presented to the emergency department with signs and symptoms of pulmonary embolus. Due to the lack of venous access, a central line placement was placed in her right femoral vein, after which she was started on heparin. She developed a right groin hematoma that could not be controlled with manual compression, and her serum hematocrit dropped from 43 to 25%. (**a** and **b**) Angiography of the right common femoral artery demonstrates a small pool of contrast arising from a branch of the external pudendal artery (*arrows*). (**c** and **d**) Superselective angiography of the bleeding external pudendal artery branch redemonstrates bleeding source (*arrow*). A small amount (1 cc) of Gelfoam slurry was used to embolize the bleeding branch. Notice how the contrast pool (*circle*) enlarges and changes morphology from image to image, confirming the extravascular location of the contrast

Safety

- Embolization in the presence of sepsis should be considered a temporizing measure, as further hemorrhage is likely if there is ongoing infection.
- Embolization may lead to anastomotic dehiscence
- Remember that contrast trapped in thrombus will lead the unwary to diagnose ongoing bleeding
- Serial blood draws, to ensure the HCT remains stable. If the HCT continues to decrease, a contrast-enhanced CT or additional angiography can be pursued to assess hemorrhage.

Suggested Reading

Bauer, J.R. and Ray, C.E. (2004). Transcatheter Arterial Embolization in the Trauma Patient: A Review. *Seminars in Interventional Radiology*: 2004;21(1):11–22.

Kaufman JA. Vascular Interventions. In Kaufman, JA., Lee, MJ. (eds) *Vascular and Interventional Radiology: The Requisites*. Philadelphia: Mosby, 2003:105–113

Ray CE Jr., Waltman AC. General Principles of Embolization and Chemoembolization. In Bakal, CW., Silberzweig, J., Cynamon, J. (eds). *Vascular and Interventional Radiology: Principles and Practice*. New York: Thieme, 2002: 89–100.

Sharafuddin MJ, Sun S, Golzarian J. Embolotherapy: basic principles and applications. In Golzarian, J., Sun, S., Sharafuddin, MJ. (eds.). *Vascular Embolotherapy: A Comprehensive Approach*. Berlin Heidelberg: Springer-Verlag, 2006: 3–14.

Chapter 31
Tract Embolization

George Behrens and Nilesh H. Patel

General Concepts

- Used in various procedures and implies plugging the biopsy or drainage track using a hemostatic agent (Cowan and Traill 1998; Rosen and Rothberg 1982; Nakagawa and Nakajima 1994; Shiham and Siddiqi 2005; Allison 1988; Lyon 2006; Riddle and Bilal 2008; Androussi 2005; Schmitz-Rode and Blaum 2000 and Bourgouin and Shepard 1998).
  - Reduces risk of bleeding.
  - Reduces risk of bile leak/biloma and urine leak/urinoma.
  - Reduces risk of pneumothorax.
- Tract embolization is feasible in almost all cases.
- Reduces significantly the risk of hemorrhage in 90–95% of the cases and bile leaks in liver biopsies.
- Cases have been reported of vascular occlusion as a complication of drainage track embolization (Cowan and Traill 1998; Rosen and Rothberg 1982; Nakagawa and Nakajima 1994; Lyon 2006; Riddle and Bilal, 2008 and Androussi, 2005).

Pre-procedure Evaluation

- Careful patient evaluation is important to determinate risk factors for bleeding.
- Coagulation status, hemoglobin, and hematocrit.

Indications for Tract Embolization

- High probability of bleeding complications.
  - INR: >1.5
  - Platelets: <20,000
  - Von Willbrand's disease or other known coagulopathy.

Transcatheter Embolization and Therapy,
Techniques in Interventional Radiology, DOI 10.1007/978-1-84800-897-7_31,
© Springer-Verlag London Limited 2010

- Advanced age.
- Elevated creatinine level: creatinine >2 mg/dL (5.89 times higher bleeding risk) (Shiham and Siddiqi 2005).
- Chronic renal disease (platelet dysfunction).
- Hypertension SBP: >160; DBP: >100; MBP: >120 (3.74 times higher bleeding risk) (Shiham and Siddiqi 2005).
- Post-percutaneous hepatobiliary interventions to prevent bile leaks.
- Post-percutaneous nephroureteral interventions to prevent urinoma.
- Blood patch for co-axial core biopsy of lung lesion.

Contraindications

- No absolute contraindication.
- Fine-needle aspiration without co-axial technique.

Material Selection

Operator Preference

- *Gelfoam*
  - 20 cc and 3–6 cc syringes
  - Three-way valve stopcock
  - 0.9 normal saline
  - Scissors
  - Gelfoam
- *Metallic Coils*
  - Bentson guidewire as a coil pusher
  - Metallic coils
  - 0.018–0.035 inch depending upon the guiding needle diameter
- *N-butyl cyanoacrylate*
  - Not popular US.
  - More risk of non-target/distal embolization.
  - *N*-butyl cyanoacrilates need to be mixed with lipiodol in 1:1 ratio.
- *Autologous Blood Clot/Blood Patch*
  - Requires 10 ml of patient's blood which has been set aside for at least 15 minutes.
  - Three-way valve stopcock and second 10-cc syringe may be needed.

Procedural Steps

- The co-axial technique with introducer is required in biopsies.
- The drainage catheter needs to be exchanged for a vascular sheath or dilator/catheter.

Gelfoam

- *Gelfom slurry/suspension*
  - Cut Gelfoam sponge into square pieces which are 2–4 mm in size and place pieces into an empty 3- or 6-cc syringe.
  - In 10-cc syringe, draw up either 10 cc of saline or mixture of 7 cc of saline and 3 cc of contrast, if fluoroscopy is to be used with tract embolization.
  - Connect both syringes to the three-way valve and mix until complete suspension of the Gelfoam.
  - Inject carefully through the introducer needle/cannula slowly.
- *Gelfoam pledges*
  - A block of Gelfoam is cut into strips of 2 cm length.
  - They are tightly rolled by hand into a shape of a cigar/torpedo.
  - Load into the introducer needle/cannula or sheath.
  - Then using the sylet or introducer, push the Gelfoam pledget to desired location.

Metallic Coils

- Metallic coil is inserted into the needle/cannula/catheter and positioned at its tip (Allison 1988).
- Holding the pusher wire in place, the needle/cannula/catheter is withdrawn by 5–10 mm, allowing the coil to start forming its shape. Then push the coil out with the wire to completely deploy.
- Repeat the same procedure until the tract is embolized.

N-Butyl Cyanoacrylate

- Need to be mixed with lipiodol in a ratio of 1:1 (vial of 0.5 cc mixed with 0.5 cc of lipiodol (Lyon 2006)).
- In cases of biopsies, injected carefully through the guiding needle/cannula.
- In cases of drainage catheter, the catheter should be exchanged to a dilator over the wire.

o Always withdraw the needle/dilator tip by about 5–10 mm before beginning the injection of the mixture. Then inject the mixture slowly as you withdraw.

Autologous Clotted Blood/Blood Patch

o Need 10-ml of patient's venous blood which has been set aside for 15-minutes.
o Inject through guiding needle/cannula at a rate of approximately 1 ml per centimeter.
o If clotted blood is too thick, connect the syringe to a three-way stopcock. Connect an empty 10-cc syringe to the other end of the stopcock. Then gently agitate the clotted blood by slowly pushing it back and forth between the syringes two to three times. This should break up the clotted blood into smaller pieces that will then make it easier to inject through the guiding needle/cannula.

Post-procedure Management

• Vital signs.
• Can be performed as outpatient.
• Check for pain at site of intervention.
• US or CT if complication is suspected.

Complications

• Non-target embolization (migration of embolization material) (Riddle and Bilal 2008 and Androussi 2005).

Results

• Technical success: 98–100%.
• Complications are less than 1%.
• Decreases patient's perception of pain and decreases the amount of required analgesia (Schmitz-Rode and Blaum 2000).
• Procedural time: 15 min.

Keypoints

• Reduces risk of bile leak, urine leak, hemorrhage, and pneumothorax for relevant procedures.

- Co-axial biopsy technique or sheath required.
- Gelfoam most popular agent.
- High technical success and low complication rate (Fig. 31.1).

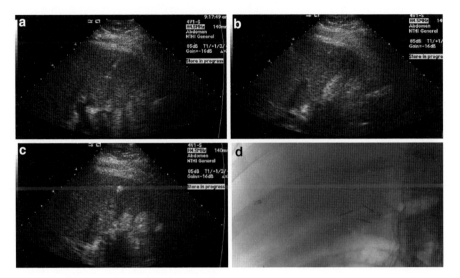

Fig. 31.1 Coil tract embolization after liver biopsy. **(a)** US image showing the tip of 17-gauge guiding needle within the peripheral aspect of the right lobe of the liver. **(b)** Shows the tip of 18-gauge automatic gun for core biopsies within the right lobe of the liver. **(c)** US image after coil deployment showing a hyperechoic structure within the biopsy tract. **(d)** Fluoroscopic image of the coil

References

1. Cowan N, Traill Z, et al. Direct percutanoeus transrenal embolization for renal artery injury following percutaneous nephrostomy. Br J Radiol 1998;71(851):1199–1201.
2. Rosen R, Rothberg M. Transhepatic embolization of hepatic artery pseudoaneurysm following biliary drainage. Radiology 1982;145:532–533.
3. Nakagawa N, Nakajima Y, et al. Immediate transbiliary embolization of a biliary–hepatic artery fistula during access for percutaneous biliary drainage. Cardiovasc Intervent Radiol 1994;17(5):295–297
4. Shiham G, Siddiqi, N, et al. Clinical risk factors associated with bleeding after native kidney biopsy. Nephrology 2005;10(3):305–310.
5. Allison, D. Percutaneous liver biopsy and track embolization with steel coils. Radiology 1988;169:261–263.
6. Lyon S, Terhaar S et al. Percutaneous embolization of transhepatic tracks for biliary intervention. Cardiovasc Intervent Radiol 2006;29:1011–1014.
7. Riddle C, Bilal A, et al. Migration of gelfoam to the gallbladder after liver biopsy. Pediatr Radiol 2008;38(7):806–809.

8. Androussi, C. Late complication following coil embolization of a biliary leak. ANZ J Surg 2005;75: 614–615.
9. Schmitz-Rode T, Blaum M, et al. Catheter tract embolization after percutaneous transhepatic biliary intervention. Rofo 2000;172(2):179–183.
10. Bourgouin PM, Shepard JA, et al. Transthoracic needle aspiration biopsy:evaluation of the blood patch technique. Radiology 1998;166(1Pt1):93–95

Chapter 32
Arterial Embolization Post-percutaneous Biopsy or Drainage

George Behrens and Nilesh H. Patel

Hemorrhage following imaging-guided biopsy and drainage procedures usually comes from a predictable site, namely the organ undergoing the biopsy or drainage procedure. Bleeding following "blind" procedures can come from almost anywhere. Imaging is necessary where there is doubt regarding the source of bleeding, or whether there is ongoing bleeding following a primary intervention. In this chapter, three common scenarios will be considered (liver, kidney, and lung), but the general principles are broadly applicable and will not be repeated.

General Considerations

Bleeding Around Drains

This scenario is usually obvious clinically, but even significant bleeding may be obscured by dressings around the drain site. Bleeding occurs due either to damage to tissue parenchyma or injury to arteries or veins en route to the drain site or within an organ. Bleeding will often stop if the tract is tamponaded by increasing the drain size, similar to the way that bleeding around a vascular sheath can be stopped by placing a larger sheath.

Drainage Catheter Upsizing

- Indicated in patients with venous bleeding and bleeding around the drain.
- The catheter is removed over-the-wire.
- A vascular sheath is placed and a contrast injection (tractogram) is performed through the sheath to look for vascular filling.
- A new catheter 1- or 2-French sizes larger than the previous catheter is placed over-the-wire.

Transcatheter Embolization and Therapy,
Techniques in Interventional Radiology, DOI 10.1007/978-1-84800-897-7_32,
© Springer-Verlag London Limited 2010

- If the catheter has no further drainage but there is concern for further bleeding from the site, the catheter should be left in situ and capped for a minimum of 4–8 hours.

Bleeding Following Biopsy

This may be occult as the bleeding may be unseen in the chest, abdomen or pelvis. Clinical suspicion is usually raised due to an increasing pulse rate and falling blood pressure. Be alert to patients who become agitated or confused, and ensure that the ward staff knows what to look for and who to call if there is concern.

Post-biopsy hemorrhage may cease spontaneously, but if there is a suggestion of ongoing bleeding or the patient is hemodynamically compromised, some form of intervention is indicated.

Risk Factors

Certain patients are at increased risk of complication and this should be noted on the aftercare instructions. Such risk factors include the following:

- Coagulopathy
- Systemic hypertension
- Related to biopsy/drainage technique
  - Central biopsies
  - Diameter of the needle/catheter
  - Numerous needle passes
- Hypervascular masses
- Cirrhosis
- Advanced age
- Steroid use
- Ascites
- Patients with known cancer have more risk of bleeding than those with diffuse diseases such as viral hepatitis

Pre-procedure Evaluation

Patient Evaluation

- *The first step in the management of post-biopsy/drainage bleeding is to resuscitate the patient!*
- Note that the patient may become hemodynamically stable during active resuscitation, if fluid replacement is keeping pace with the rate of bleeding. Such

resuscitative efforts should be considered supportive, and clinical suspicion should remain for ongoing bleeding.

Imaging

- *The second step in the management of post-biopsy/drainage bleeding is to localize the area of bleeding.*
- Hemodynamically stable patients: CT is typically performed to determine whether there is active bleeding and to attempt to determine the underlying cause (See Fig. 32.1).
- Unstable patients require emergency angiography with the intent to treat or operative intervention.

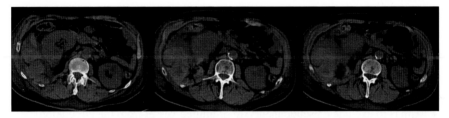

Fig. 32.1 CT examination in patient with severe hypotension after percutaneous and US-guided biopsy of the right kidney showing a large pararenal hematoma with displacement of the kidney

Laboratory

- Hemoglobin and hematocrit levels are performed serially to assess the presence of ongoing bleeding. Be aware that active resuscitation with fluids only will present with a significant decrease in hemoglobin and hematocrit levels. Additionally, brisk bleeding without resuscitation will show NO acute change in the hemoglobin or hematocrit levels and should not dissuade aggressive intervention.
- Coagulation status: the best single intervention to correct severe active bleeding post-biopsy or drainage in coagulopathic patients is to correct the coagulopathy!
- Platelet count.
- Kidney function.
- Liver function tests.

Indications for Embolization

- Unstable patients
- Hypotension or patients requiring vasopressors

- Enlarging hematoma
- Ongoing bleeding despite correction of coagulopathy or thrombocytopenia

Contraindications to Embolization

Contraindications are all relative and include the following:

- Borderline renal failure or elevated creatinine levels
- Severe contrast allergy (may use carbon dioxide)
- Inability to visualize the target vessel
- Bacteremia/sepsis
- *These contraindications should NOT preclude an intervention in a patient who needs it!*

Treatment Plan and Technique

Pseudoaneuryms and Active Bleeding

- Aim is to exclude a pseudoaneurysm or injured vessel from the circulation.
  - Exclusion methods fall into two broad categories
    - Embolization
    - Stent placement (reserved for large diameter vessels)
  - Pseudoaneurysm arising from segmental or intralobar arterial branch that does not have a collateral supply can be treated with just proximal embolization, since retrograde filling of the abnormality ("backdoor bleeding) is not possible.
  - Lesions with numerous collateral vessels need to be treated with proximal and distal coil deployment in order to exclude it from the circulation (by preventing backflow from the collateral circulation) (See Fig. 32.3 and Fig. 32.4).

Arteriovenous fistula

- Goal is to exclude the AV shunt or at least decrease the pressure enough to permit time for self-healing.
  - Superselective technique is mandatory to
    - Improve results
    - Decrease ischemic complications

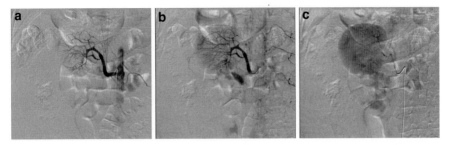

Fig. 32.2 (**a**) Selective right renal angiogram showing normal appearance of the renal artery. (**b**) There is extravasation of the contrast material from an extrarenal branch. All the intrarenal branches are intact. (**c**) Nephrogram phase showing persistent extraluminal contrast within the inferior aspect of the kidney

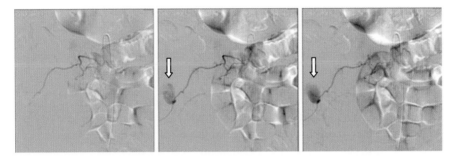

Fig. 32.3 Selective angiogram of right lumbar artery. There is a large pseudoaneurysm with active extravasation of the contrast material (*arrows*)

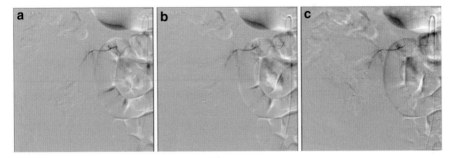

Fig. 32.4 Digital subtraction images after coil embolization of the right lumbar pseudoaneurysm using four coils. There is a complete exclusion of the sac from the circulation

- Ideally, the coils need to be deployed in the small feeding vessels, in order to reduce risk of collateral flow.
- *Particulate agents are not used in* AVF *embolization due to the risk of embolization to the venous side*!

- Stent-graft deployment should be considered in large vessels as a method to exclude the AVF while maintaining antegrade flow in the native vessel.

Materials

Catheters and Microcatheters and Guidewires

- As in other chapters for the target organ—liver, kidney, lung.

Embolization Materials

- *The best embolization agent to use may be the one with which you are most familiar!*
- *There is usually a focal bleeding point which should be targeted as precisely as possible whenever time allows.* Proximal embolizations are generally not warranted in this patient population.
- Coils and microcoils are often ideal; however, Gelfoam embolization can be performed if a temporary occlusion is desired.
- In cases where speed is of the essence or the target vessel cannot be selectively catheterized, consider proximal embolization with the following:
  - Resorbable gelatin sponge (Gelfoam)
  - Spherical polyvinyl alcohol particles (255 μ in size or larger) or tris-acryl gelatin microspheres (300 μ in size or larger)
  - *N* butyl cyanoacrylate and other glues

Medications

- Pain control: sedation and analgesia are recommended.
- Infection: prophylactic antibiotics are controversial.
- Hydration: intravenous normal saline.

Complications

- Fatal complications are rare.
- Major complications
  - Non-target embolization
  - Ischemia/tissue necrosis (usually asymptomatic)

o Intraprocedural rupture of pseudoaneurysm; embolization needs to proceed expeditiously
o Renal failure secondary to contrast-induced nephropathy
o Vascular dissection

- Minor complications
  o Post-embolization syndrome
  o Biliary stenosis due to ischemia/necrosis
  o Groin hematoma
  o Infection

Specific Organ Systems: Liver Embolization Post-percutaneous Biopsy/Drainage

General Concept and Definitions

- Severe hemorrhage in the form of hemobilia, hematoma, and/or hemoperitoneum that requires surgery or embolization is uncommon particularly when ultrasound or CT guidance is used. The mortality of liver biopsy is 0.01–0.1%
- Bleeding occurs at the puncture sites and can result in subcapsular hematomas, hemothorax, hemoperitoneum, arteriovenous fistulae, arterial–biliary or venous–biliary fistulae, and arterial pseudoaneurysm.
- Ninety-six percent of such complications appear in the first 24 h and should be suspected in any patient with falling blood pressure and rising pulse. If this is a trend, image early.
- Percutaneous transhepatic biliary drainage (PTBD) carries a 3.7-fold higher risk of arterial injury than other percutaneous transhepatic procedures.

Anatomy of the Lesion

Hematomas

- Post-biopsy/drainage hematomas and/or bleeding can arise from various locations:
  o *Intraparenchymal or subcapsular:* most common and usually self-limited
  o *Perihepatic or intraperitoneal*
  o *Intraductal (hemobilia)*
  o *Extra-abdominal (hemothorax) or at the puncture site*
- Hematomas can be complex and associated with fistulae or pseudoaneurysms.
- The location of hematoma can help to identify the vessel injured.

Arteriovenous, Arterioportal, or Arteriobiliary Fistulae

- Results from wall damage of two adjacent vascular structures or vascular structure and bile ducts, resulting in abnormal communication.
  - Arterioportal fistulae (see Chapter 16)
  - Arteriovenous fistulae (see Chapter 16)

Pseudoaneurysm

- Extrahepatic
  - Rare and potentially fatal due to severe bleeding when ruptured.
- Intrahepatic
  - Most common type resulting from hepatic biopsy/drainage
  - Strongly associated with fistulae and hematomas
  - Majority of cases are asymptomatic and resolve spontaneously

Bile Leaks

- Primary bile leak after biopsy/drainage is extremely rare.
- Small bile leaks after biopsy/drainage are treated conservatively with hydration.
- Embolization is usually not required.

Specific Indications for Liver Embolization

- Severe active hemobilia on endoscopy
- Pseudoaneurysms
  - Extrahepatic pseudoaneurysm
  - More than 10 mm in diameter
  - Enlarging pseudoaneurysm
- Enlarging perihepatic or subhepatic hematoma
- Arterioportal, arteriovenous, or arteriobiliary fistulae
  - Increased portal hypertension resulting in bleeding
  - High-flow shunt resulting in CHF, portal hypertension, or persistent GI bleed
  - Decreased liver function

Vascular Anatomy

Native Liver

- Anatomical variants are common (see Chapter 33).
- If selective hepatic artery angiography is negative, consider other arterial sources including diaphragmatic, intercostal, or inferior phrenic arteries.

Transplanted Livers

- Review of the operative note is recommended to delineate vascular anatomy.
- Post-transplant anatomy includes the following:
  - End-to-end anastomosis using a branch patch technique
  - Jump graft directly from the aorta
- Gastroduodenal artery is always absent.

Procedure/Steps

- *CT of the abdomen: obtain a CT in hemodynamically stable patients* to rule out intrathoracic or intra-abdominal bleeding.

Embolization

- Coils
  - In fistulae, the aim is to embolize the actual communication or place coils in the feeding vessel across the entire site of communication.
  - In pseudoaneurysms, the aim is to reduce the flow into the sac to permit thrombosis. Coils may be used to fill the sac or the feeding artery is embolized both proximal and distal to the site of the pseudoaneurysm. PROXIMAL EMBOLIZATION ONLY IS INSUFFICIENT, SINCE THIS CAN PERMIT RETROGRADE (BACKDOOR) BLEEDING.
- Gelfoam
  - Gelfoam slurry
  - Gelfoam pledgets
- Permanent particulate agents are usually avoided; however, they may become helpful to obtain distal control of a bleeding vessel that cannot be crossed with a microcatheter for standard distal coil embolization. Injecting large particles (>500 microns) proximal to the injured vessel will help in preventing retrograde (backdoor) bleeding.
- Percutaneous thrombin injection
  - There are some case reports of direct percutaneous thrombin injection into large pseudoaneurysm under ultrasound or CT guidance.

Results

- Technical success (blockage of bleeding vessel) rates range from 95 to 100%.
- Clinical success (cessation of bleeding) around 95%.

- Liver infarction is rare after superselective embolization, especially in a patient with normal portal circulation.
- In cases of slow rates of bleeding, especially if venous in origin, tube upsizing will tamponade and halt the bleeding.

Complications

- Biliary stenosis due to ischemia/necrosis.
- Worsening of liver function.

Renal Embolization Post-percutaneous Biopsy/Drainage

General Concept and Definitions

- The prevalence of vascular complications after renal biopsy/drainage has been reported between 3 and 5%. However, the rates of major complications are around 1–2% and usually related to bleeding, arteriovenous fistula (AVF), arteriocaliceal fistula (ACF), or pseudoaneurysm.
- Most of these complications resolve spontaneously.
- Risk of significant bleeding can be decreased with embolization of the track at the time of the procedure or simple correction of a coagulopathic state.
- Post-biopsy vascular embolization is often considered an emergency, especially in transplanted kidneys.

Anatomy of the Lesion

Hematomas

- Post-biopsy/drainage hematomas can occur in four anatomic spaces and are as follows:
  - *Collecting system:* resulting in hematuria, possible ureteral obstruction, and arteriocaliceal fistula.
  - *Intrarenal or subcapsular:* resulting in arteriovenous fistula, tamponade, and pain. In severe cases, hypertension due to subcapsular hematoma compressing the renal parenchyma ("Page kidney") can occur.
  - *Perinephric space:* hematoma formation and possibly severe hemorrhage. "Page kidney" can also occur in this space.
  - *Pararenal/extra fascial space*: resulting in large retroperitoneal or intraperitoneal hematoma.
- Location of hematoma can help to identify the vessel injured.
  - Intrarenal branch

  o Main renal artery
  o Extrarenal (e.g., lumbar artery) (see fig 32.1, 32.2 and 32.3)

Arteriovenous Fistula (see Chapter 16)

Pseudoaneurysm

- Caused by trauma to an artery, resulting in bleeding that is contained by the adventitial layer.
- Most post-biopsy/drainage pseudoaneurysms are asymptomatic and resolve spontaneously.
  o Decision to treat asymptomatic pseudoaneurysms is controversial due to the unclear and variable natural history of pseudoaneurysms. However, treatment is recommended for pseudoaneurysms larger than 10 mm or in cases of persistent hematuria.

Specific Indications for Renal Embolization

- Renal or perirenal hematoma
  o Severe bleeding
  o Symtomatic bleeding
  o Bleeding persisting for more than 72 h
- Pseudoaneurysms
  o More than 10 mm in diameter
  o Enlarging pseudoaneurysm
  o Symptomatic patients
  o Hematuria for more than 72 h
- Arteriovenous fistula
  o Persistent AVF for more than 1 month after biopsy/drainage
  o High-flow shunt resulting in CHF
  o Decreased renal function
  o Creatinine elevation
  o Decreased GFR
- The criteria for embolization in transplant recipients remain unclear.

Vascular Anatomy

Native Kidneys

- Accessory renal arteries (polar arteries) originating from the aorta and iliac arteries are common.

- If selective renal artery angiogram is negative, consider other arterial sources including lumbar, adrenal, phrenic, or mesenteric vessels.
- Ectopic kidneys and horseshoe kidneys may have very unusual arterial supplies.

Transplanted Kidneys

- Generally there is a single arterial anastomosis.
- Type of anastomosis determines angiographic approach.

Procedure/Steps

Native Kidneys

Access

- Plan according to pre-operative imaging.
- Brachial approach is recommended in patients with severe peripheral vascular disease with aortoiliac occlusion.

Angiography

- Non-selective arteriogram
  - Always recommended in order to identify other arterial sources of extravasation.
  - 15° LAO aortography can be helpful to define blood supply and anatomical variants.
- Selective arteriogram
  - Tip of the catheter within the proximal renal artery.
- Superselective angiogram

Transplant Kidneys

Access

- Plan according to the type of anastomosis.
  - *End-to-end anastomosis:* contralateral femoral approach.
  - *End-to-side anastomosis*: ipsilateral femoral approach.

Angiography

- Non-selective arteriogram is recommended to exclude other arterial sources of extravasation.
- Selective arteriogram
  - Tip of the catheter within the proximal renal artery.

- ○ 20–40° contralateral anterior oblique arteriogram with the tip of the catheter in the proximal renal artery.
- Superselective angiogram

Angiographic Appearance

- *Active bleeding:* active extravasation visualized as expanding and persistent contrast that changes morphology on delayed images.
- *Pseudoaneurysm:* persistent or stagnant contrast material in venous phase with round shape (see fig 32.3).
- *Arteriovenous fistula:* early visualization of the renal veins.

Results

- Success rates (technical and clinical) range from 80 to 100%.
- Despite superselective embolization, renal infarctions of more than 10% of the kidney volume are often noted.
- Infarctions of less than 30% are usually asymptomatic in native kidneys.
- Infarctions of more than 50% can be followed by renal failure, especially in transplanted kidneys.

Complications

Fatal Complication

- Rare.

Procedural Complication

- Major complications
  - ○ Non-target embolization: coils can dislodge and migrate. In the case of AVF, a small coil can travel through the fistulous communication to the lung.
  - ○ Ischemia/tissue necrosis: usually asymptomatic.
  - ○ Intraprocedural rupture of the pseudoaneurysm; embolization needs to proceed expeditiously.
  - ○ Renal failure secondary to contrast-induced nephropathy.
  - ○ Renal artery dissection.
- Minor complications
  - ○ Post-embolization syndrome.
  - ○ Groin hematoma.
  - ○ There is no evidence to show that the incidence of renal hypertension increases after superselective renal embolization.

Lung Embolization Post-percutaneous Biopsy/Drainage

General Concept and Definitions

- The definition of massive hemoptysis varies widely in the literature, with blood loss volumes ranging from 200 to 1000 ml per day.
- Pulmonary hemorrhage manifesting as trace hemoptysis occurs in 5–10% of cases after lung biopsies; the vast majority are self-limited.
- Massive intraparenchymal hemorrhage requiring intervention is extremely rare (0.01%), but the mortality rate can be as high as 75% if untreated. Death results from massive tracheobronchial aspiration and asphyxia rather than exanguination.
- Majority of massive bleeds arise from the bronchial circulation.
- Bleeding as a result of drainage catheter placement is classically a result of injury to intercostal arteries rather than intraparenchymal vessels.

Anatomy of the Lesion

Source of Bleeding

- Massive intraparenchymal bleeding usually arises from the bronchial circulation (90%).

Imaging Findings

- Tortuous bronchial vessel (especially in the setting of chronic pulmonary diseases)
- Neovascularity and/or hypervascularity
- Shunting to pulmonary arterial circulation
- Active extravasation of contrast material
- Bronchial artery pseudoaneurysm

Specific Indications for Lung Embolization

- Massive hemoptysis (see Chapters 35 and 36)
- Unstable patients
  - Requiring immediate ventilatory assistance
  - Requiring blood transfusions
  - Hypotensive
  - Progressive deterioration in ventilation
- Ongoing hemorrhage despite adequate resuscitation and correction of coagulopathy/thrombocytopenia

Vascular Anatomy

(see Chapters 15, 35, and 36)

Procedure/Steps

Procedure Preparation

- *The first step in the management of post-biopsy/drainage bleeding is to stabilize and secure the airway!*
- *Chest CT scans* have been reported to be superior to bronchoscopy in the evaluation of hemoptysis by
  - Localizing bleeding region/lobe.
  - Defining intraparenchymal bleed versus pleural hemorrhage.
- General anesthesia may be preferred in order to protect the airway.
- Complete patient resuscitation with correction of any coagulopathy.

Angiography

- Non-selective arteriogram
  - Always recommended to define anatomy. The tip of the flush catheter is positioned near the left subclavian artery.
- Selective and superselective arteriogram
  - Classic angiographic findings in patients with bronchial artery bleeding includes the following:

    - Bronchial artery enlargement (>3 mm).
    - Hypervascularity.
    - Parenchymal stain.
    - Bronchial to pulmonary artery shunting.
    - Frank extravasation is rarely seen and is not necessary to proceed with embolization.

- After the bronchial arteries are evaluated, the potential non-bronchial systemic collateral vessels may be interrogated.

Embolization

- Particles are the agent of choice. However, they should be used with superselective technique due to high risk of complication.
- Coils should not be used in bronchial artery embolization, because they cause proximal occlusion and preclude re-embolization.
- Contributions from collaterals from non-bronchial arteries represent an important cause of recurrent hemoptysis.

Results

- Technical success rates (occlusion of bleeding vessel) ranges from 77 to 98%.
- Technical failures are due to failure to catheterize, catheter instability precluding embolization, or high risk of non-target embolization (anterior spinal artery).

Complications

- Procedural complications are uncommon (<5%).
- Major complications
  - Spinal cord injury (<1%)
  - Non-target embolization
  - Renal failure secondary to contrast-induced nephropathy
  - Vascular dissection
- Minor complications
  - Infection

Keypoints

- Vascular complications following biopsies and drainage procedures are uncommon but may be life threatening.
- Embolization materials used are tailored to the cause of the bleeding, but typically include gelfoam, particles, or coils.
- Anatomical variants, and post-surgical changes, can delay visualization of a bleeding vessel. Evaluation of any pre-procedure cross-sectional imaging is mandatory.
- All contraindications to embolization are relative, and an embolization procedure should not be unduly delayed for such relative contraindications.

Bibliography

1. Park HS, Lee AS. Postbiopsy arterioportal fistula in HCC. AJR February 2006 186: 556–561.
2. Chavan A, Harms J, Pichlmayr Jabbour N, Reyes J, Zajko A, Nour B, Tzakis AG, Starzl TE, Van Thiel DH. Arterioportal fistula following liver biopsy. Three cases occurring in liver transplant recipients. Dig Dis Sci 1995 40:1041–1044.
3. Piccinino F, Sagnelli E, Pasquale G, Giusti G. Complications following percutaneous liver biopsy. A multicentre retrospective study on 68,276 biopsies. J Hepatol 1986 2: 165–173
4. Machicao VI, Lukens FJ, Lange SM, Scolapio JS. Arterioportal fistula causing acute pancreatitis and hemobilia after liver biopsy. J Clin Gastroenterol. Apr 2002 34(4): 481–484.

5. Fidelman N, Bloom A, Kerlan R et al. Hepatic arterial injuries after percutaneous biliary interventions in the era of laparoscopic surgery and liver transplantation: Experience with 930 patients. Radiology June 2008 247(3): 880–886.
6. Ahmed O, Balzer JO, Vogl TJ. Bleeding hepatic pseudoaneurysm complicating percutaneous liver biopsy with interventional treatment options. Eur Radiol Jan 2005 15(1):183–185.
7. Barley F, Kessel D, et al. Selective embolization of large symptomatic iatrogenic renal transplant arteriovenous fistula, Cardiovasc Interv Radiol 2006 29: 1084–1087.
8. Arata MA, Cope C. Principles used in the management of visceral aneurysms. Tech Vasc Intervent Radiol 2000 3: 124–129.
9. Dinkel HP, Danuser H, Triller J. Blunt renal trauma: minimally invasive management with microcatheter embolization experience in nine patients. Radiology 2002 223: 723–30.
10. Yoon W, Kim JK, Kim YH, Chung TW, Kang HK. Bronchial and nonbronchial systemic artery embolization for life-threatening hemoptysis: a comprehensive review. RadioGraphics 2002 22:1395–1409.
11. Do KH, Goo JM, Im JG, Kim KW, Chung JW, Park JH. Systemic arterial supply to the lungs in adults: spiral CT findings. RadioGraphics 2001 21:387–402.
12. Swanson KL, Johnson CM, Prakash UB, McKusick MA, Andrews JC, Stanson AW. Bronchial artery embolization: experience with 54 patients. Chest 2002 121: 789–795.
13. Yoon W, Kim YH, Kim JK, Kim YC, Park JG, Kang HK. Massive hemoptysis: prediction of non-bronchial systemic arterial supply with chest CT. Radiology 2003 227: 232–238.

Chapter 33
Acute Nonvariceal Upper Gastrointestinal Hemorrhage

Ian Gillespie and Hamish Ireland

Definition

Upper gastrointestinal hemorrhage (UGIH) is defined as significant bleeding from the GI tract from the lips to the ligament of Treitz (duodeno-jejunal flexure); blood loss distal to this represents lower GI bleeding and is discussed in a separate chapter.

Clinical Features

- Presentation is normally with hematemesis and/or melena. Fresh rectal bleeding ("bright red blood per rectum") may also be due to UGIH and indicates brisk bleeding.
- Hypotension implies severe life-threatening bleeding and necessitates urgent volume and red blood cell replacement. The patient should be investigated during resuscitation while they are still bleeding.
- Most cases stop spontaneously or with endoscopic therapy.
- It is essential to have a local major gastrointestinal hemorrhage management protocol in place. Endoscopists, radiologists, and surgeons must collaborate in patient management.

Causes

The underlying cause of UGIH is often unclear at presentation. Clues in the patient's history include symptoms of gastroesophageal reflux or dyspepsia, excessive alcohol consumption, consumption of nonsteroidal anti-inflammatory drugs (NSAID) or aspirin, pancreatitis, known upper gastrointestinal tumor, and history of surgery or percutaneous intervention.

The commonest causes are

- Peptic ulceration, stress ulcers, and erosions.
- *Iatrogenic*: previous surgery, endoscopy or percutaneous intervention.
- *Mallory Weiss tears*: retching/vomiting.

Transcatheter Embolization and Therapy,
Techniques in Interventional Radiology, DOI 10.1007/978-1-84800-897-7_33,
© Springer-Verlag London Limited 2010

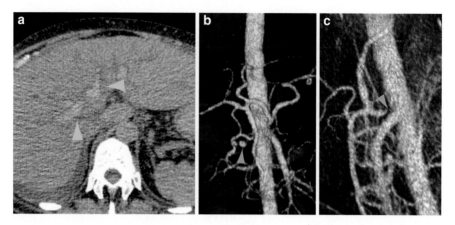

Fig. 33.1 A patient with UGIB due to bleeding from the ampulla secondary to biliary stent insertion: (**a**) Hemobilia (*yellow arrowheads*) seen on pre-contrast CT. (**b**) Shaded surface reformat showing pseudoaneurysm (*turquoise arrowhead*) of pancreaticoduodenal artery. (**c**) The celiac axis is occluded (*turquoise arrowhead*) adding difficulty to embolization

Less common causes include

- Hemobilia: most are related to biliary intervention and trauma (Fig. 33.1).
- Aortoenteric fistula – usually in a patient with a history of aortic surgery (Fig. 33.2).
- Dieulafoy's disease (enlarged submucosal artery).
- Tumors (seldom present with acute bleeding).

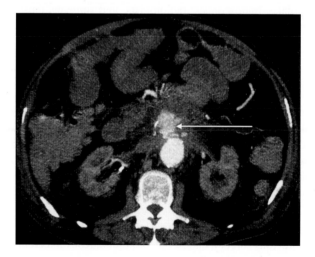

Fig. 33.2 Aortoduodenal fistula (*white arrow*). This is usually a complication of aortic surgery

Diagnostic Evaluation

Laboratory

- Check hemoglobin and coagulation status. This will often be deranged in patients with liver disease or if there has been large volume transfusion.

Endoscopy

- Endoscopy is the first-line investigation and may allow therapy including banding, sclerotherapy, adrenaline or thrombin injection, electro- or laser coagulation, and clipping. Success rates approaching 90% are reported.
- If endoscopy reveals a source, consider repeat endoscopy if bleeding recurs.
- Always ask the endoscopist to place clips at the site of bleeding to localize the lesion in patients proceeding to angiography.

Imaging

Triple-Phase Multidetector Computed Tomography Angiography (CTA)

- *Pre-contrast* to identify high-attenuation fresh thrombus, e.g., hemobilia (Fig. 33.1). Helps distinguish pseudoextravasation caused by streak artifact from bowel gas or metal.
- Arterial and venous phases
    - to identify vascular abnormalities, e.g., aneurysms, pseudoaneurysms (Fig. 33.1), arteriovenous shunting, and contrast extravasation (Fig. 33.3)
    - produce an arterial roadmap for targeting embolotherapy
- Shows features of underlying diseases that may be relevant when the bleeding has stopped.

Indications for Embolization

- Failure of endoscopy either to control the hemorrhage.

Contraindications to Embolization

These are all relative in patients with life-threatening bleeding.

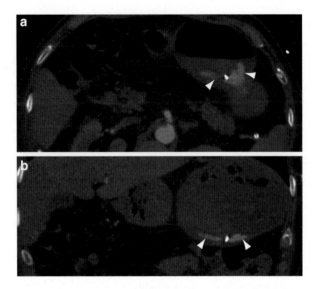

Fig. 33.3 (**a**, **b**) CTA axial slice and coronal reformat showing gastric hemorrhage (*arrowheads*)

- *Severe coagulopathy*: reduces success of embolotherapy and increases the risk of puncture site bleeding. Consider leaving the arterial sheath in situ for removal, once the coagulopathy has been corrected.
- *Portal vein occlusion*: may increase the risk of hepatic infarction following hepatic arterial embolization.
- *Very agitated patients*: may require ventilation and pharmacologic paralysis.
- *Patient has stopped bleeding*: the exception is false aneurysm, this must be treated due to the high risk of rebleeding.

Anatomy

- The upper GI tract has a rich arterial supply typically from several sources making infarction of the stomach or duodenum relatively uncommon (Table 33.1).
- Understanding the arterial anatomy is necessary to ensure successful embolization.
- Anatomical variations are common (Table 33.1).
- Failure to recognize anomalous arterial anatomy may lead to inadequate embolization or inadvertent embolization of other organs.
- Upper GI surgery may alter the anatomy. Review the notes and discuss with the surgeon to find out what was done surgically and whether there is a likely source for hemorrhage (e.g., surgical anastomoses!).

Table 33.1 Upper GI arterial anatomy

Site	Normal arterial supply	Variants
Esophagus	Bronchial, left inferior phrenic, left gastric arteries	
Stomach	Left gastric (LGA)	Complete gastroepiploic arcade in 65%,
	Splenic (via posterior/short gastric and left gastroepiploic)	incomplete in 35%
	Hepatic (via gastroduodenal/right gastroepiploic artery)	RGA 40% from CHA, 40% from L/MHA, and
	Right gastric – small and variable and may not be seen	10% RHA
Duodenum	Gastroduodenal artery (GDA)	
	Pancreaticoduodenal arcade – anterior and posterior branches (superior from GDA and inferior from SMA)	
Liver	Common hepatic artery (CHA) from celiac trunk	RHA from SMA 10–20%, accessory RHA 6%
	"Classic" anatomy in only 55% with right (RHA), middle (MHA), and left hepatic arteries (LHA) originating from common hepatic off celiac trunk. MHA arises from right or left to supply medial segment of left lobe	LHA from LGA 10–12%, accessory LHA 10% Replaced CHA from SMA 2%
Gall bladder	Cystic artery normally from right hepatic artery	From LHA or CHA
Miscellaneous	Arc of Buehler – a persistent congenital anastomosis between celiac and SMA	
	Arc of Barkow – omental arcade acts as potential collaterals among hepatic, splenic, and SMA via the anterior epiploic branches of the gastroepiploic arteries	

Equipment

- Selective catheters: cobra, sidewinder, microcatheter. May need catheters with side holes for performing angiography as well as end-hole-only catheters for embolization.
- Guide catheters or sheaths with integral valves are occasionally helpful.

Embolic Agents

- Gelfoam
- Coils – standard (0.035) and microcatheter compatible (0.018)
- Polyvinyl alcohol (PVA) particles – usually 350–500 μm
- Glue – use only with caution and experience

Medication

- Buscopan or glucagon will halt peristalsis which may otherwise lead to the mistaken identification of bowel gas movement as contrast extravasation.

Procedure

Treatment Plan

- The sole consideration is control of hemorrhage. Definitive treatment of underlying pathology comes later.
- Active resuscitation with fluid, red blood cells, and clotting factor replacement (plasma and/or platelets) is mandatory and can be carried out during angiography.
- Offer to insert central and arterial lines as this may expedite angiography.
- Assistance of anesthetic/ITU staff is essential for resuscitation, monitoring, and if necessary sedation and anesthesia.
- Establish relevance of previous surgery, surgical alternatives, and the potential impact of embolization on subsequent surgery.

Access

- Use CTA to plan the route to the bleeding site and identify collateral supply – coronal thick maximum intensity projection (MIP) images are especially helpful for displaying arterial anatomy (Fig. 33.4).
- Consider upper limb approach if catheterization is difficult.

Angiography

- Go straight to the most likely artery identified by endoscopy or CTA.
- If the bleeding point is not obvious, then review both subtracted and native images (removes bowel motion artifact).
- Celiac axis and SMA angiography are necessary for gastric or duodenal bleeding.
- Angiography of all potential feeding vessels should be repeated after embolization to ensure that anastomotic collateral supply to the bleeding site has not been overlooked.

Assessing the Lesion

Location

This should be known from endoscopy or CTA. Clips placed during endoscopy enable targeting and can considerably shorten the procedure.

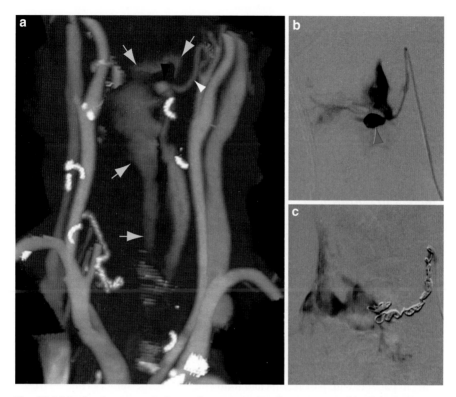

Fig. 33.4 Massive hematemesis 2 months post-esophagolaryngectomy. Bleeding from pseudoaneurysm of the lingual artery demonstrating value of CTA. (**a**) Thick MIP CTA showing lingual artery (*white arrowhead*), false aneurysm (*black arrowhead*), and extravasation (*yellow arrows*). (**b**) Selective lingual artery DSA showing false aneurysm (*red arrowhead*) with active extravasation. (**c**) Post-embolization

Angiographic Appearances

- Vascular abnormalities include aneurysms, pseudoaneurysms (Figs. 33.1, 33.2, and 33.4), arteriovenous shunting, pooling of contrast, pathological tumor circulation.
- Extravasation of contrast is the pathognomonic arteriographic feature indicating the site of hemorrhage (Figs. 33.3 and 33.4).
  - Contrast lingering after the angiographic run is completed. Extravascular contrast may mimic intravascular contrast ("pseudovein"). Prolonged filming is necessary to distinguish intraluminal contrast (from extravasation) from intravenous contrast (from an AV fistula).
  - An occluded vessel. Vascular occlusions typically represent vessels in spasm with or without superimposed thrombus. These vessels are likely to rebleed at a later time, and empiric embolization is often helpful.

Technique

- Start with cobra or sidewinder catheter shape.
- Microcatheters should be employed early in difficult or tortuous anatomy where use of standard catheters may induce spasm and lead to a failed embolization procedure.
- A guide catheter or sheath may occasionally help to stabilize access.
- Success is greater when the embolic agent is delivered as close to the point of bleeding as possible.

Gastric Bleeding

- Start with the left gastric artery (LGA).
- If LGA embolization does not control hemorrhage, then look for supply from short gastric, right gastric, gastroepiploic, and left inferior phrenic arteries.
- In erosive gastritis use gelfoam slurry to embolize each territory.

Duodenal Bleeding

- Start with gastroduodenal artery (GDA) – this is the most common site of bleeding in patients with pancreatitis and following pancreatic surgery (Fig. 33.5).
- Identify pancreaticoduodenal arteries via GDA or superior mesenteric artery (SMA).
- Coil embolization will control hemorrhage from larger accessible vessels.
- Correctly sized coils should be positioned to close both "front and back doors" (i.e., on both sides of the bleeding point). This may require catheterization from both the celiac and SMA directions (Fig. 33.6).
- If bleeding occurs from multiple tiny vessels, gelfoam or PVA particles may be useful. Deploy as selectively as possible to minimize the risk of nontarget ischemia.
- Particles (PVA or gelfoam) may be utilized in the liver to occlude branches distal to the site of hemorrhage prior to coiling the inflow artery.
- Glue may be used in place of coils but its accurate deployment is rather unpredictable and it should only be used by experienced operators.
- Extreme care must be taken to avoid nontarget territory ischemia in SMA territory.

Arterial Puncture Site

- Closure devices are especially helpful for agitated patients or those with impaired clotting.

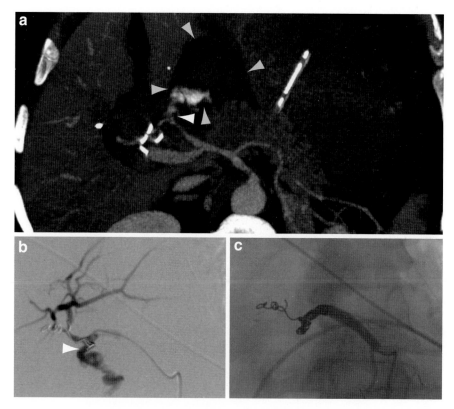

Fig. 33.5 CTA and angiographic images of upper GI hemorrhage from blown gastroduodenal artery stump post-surgery. (**a**) MIP CT reformat showing GDA stump (*white arrowhead*) and false aneurysm (*yellow arrowheads*). (**b**) During embolization, note that there is no "back door" in this circumstance. (**c**) Closure of the inflow has required occlusion of the hepatic artery. Contrast this with Chapter 29 (Fig. 33.4)

Post-embolization

- Post-embolization syndrome is uncommon with gastric and duodenal embolization.
- Bowel infarction is rare but may occur in the context of previous surgery or when PVA or liquid agents have been used.
- Duodenal stenosis secondary to ischemia is reported after pancreaticoduodenal artery embolization. The incidence of this is unknown.

Follow-up

- Patients must be carefully monitored for evidence of continued or recurrent bleeding in an ITU/HDU setting.

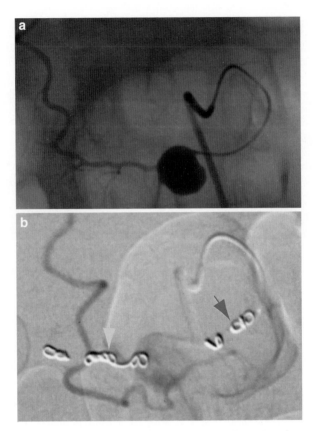

Fig. 33.6 (**a**, **b**) Angiographic images of inferior pancreaticoduodenal artery pseudoaneurysm demonstrating closure of "front" (*red arrowhead*) and "back" (*yellow arrowhead*) doors

- Further bleeding occurs in up to 20% of cases due to inadequate embolization, persistent coagulopathy, or bleeding from other sites.
- Investigation of rebleeding is the same as for the initial bleed. Artifact from metallic coils can limit the utility of CT.
- Contrast within thrombosed aneurysms can be misinterpreted as a failed embolization. Review the unenhanced scan or perform a delayed scan to confirm thrombosis.
- Repeat embolization is occasionally performed if the site of bleeding is supplied by previously unrecognized collaterals.

Alternative Therapies

- If embolotherapy is unsuccessful, then open surgery may be the only alternative.
- Historically catheter-directed vasopressin infusion has been employed in the left gastric or gastroduodenal artery territories. This technique is less successful

than embolotherapy and carries the risk of pharmacological complications (e.g., systemic ischemic effects).

Keypoints

- Endoscopy is the first choice for investigation and treatment.
- CTA is invaluable for demonstrating the bleeding site and planning the procedure.
- Knowledge of vascular anatomy is essential.
- Embolize as selectively as possible, do not hesitate to use a microcatheter.
- Do not start without the support of an anesthetist!
- Close liaison with endoscopists and surgeons is essential.

Bibliography

Lang EV. Transcatheter embolisation in management of haemorrhage from duodenal ulcer: long-term results and complications. Radiology 1992;182:703–707

Bakal CW, Silberzweig JE, Cinnamon J, Sprayregen S (Eds.)Vascular and Interventional Radiology Principles and Practice, New York-Stuttgart: Thieme 2002.

Kadir S. Atlas of normal and variant angiographic anatomy. Philadelphia, PA: WB Saunders 1991.

Kaufman JA, Lee MJ. Vascular and Interventional Radiology: The Requisites. Mosby 2004.

Millward SF. ACR Appropriateness Criteria on treatment of acute nonvariceal gastrointestinal tract bleeding. J Am Coll Radiol. 2008 Apr;5(4) 550–554.

Aina R, Oliva VL, Therasse E, Perreault P, Dufresne MP, Soulez G. Arterial embolotherapy for upper gastrointestinal haemorrhage: outcome assessment. J Vasc Interv Radiol 2001 Feb;12(2):195–200.

Schenker MP, Duszak R Jr, Soulen MC,Smith KP, Baum RA, Cope C, Freiman DB, Roberts DA, Shlansky-Goldberg RD. Upper gastrointestinal haemorrhage and transcatheter embolotherapy:clinical and technical factors impacting success and survival. J Vasc Interv Radiol. 2001 Nov;12(11):1263–1271.

Uflacker R. Atlas of Vascular Anatomy: An Angiographic Approach. 2nd Edition 2006. Lippincott Williams & Wilkins ISBN: 078176081X

Chapter 34
Acute Lower Gastrointestinal (GI) Hemorrhage

Brian Funaki

Clinical Features

- Lower GI hemorrhage is 3 times less common than upper GI hemorrhage, but more commonly seen by Interventional Radiologists due to the use of upper endoscopy as a diagnostic and therapeutic modality.
- Lower GI hemorrhage is primarily a disease of the elderly with diverticular disease, angiodysplasia, and colon cancer representing the most common etiologies of bleeding.
- Superselective embolization has proven to be a safe and effective technique for hemorrhage and has a very low risk of significant bowel ischemia.
- Diverticular hemorrhage responds best to superselective embolization.
- Patients with brisk lower GI hemorrhage may be very agitated; it is essential that an appropriate clinician is available to monitor them and supervise resuscitation.

Diagnostic Evaluation

Laboratory

Most patients have ongoing bleeding with decreasing hematocrit and hemoglobin. Adequate hydration is crucial in these cases to maintain hemodynamic stability and renal function in patients with pre-existing renal insufficiency.

Imaging: stable patients with lower GI bleeding should be screened with either Tc-99 M RBC study (Fig. 34.1) or triple-phase CTA examination (without oral contrast).

Tc-99 M RBC Study

- More sensitive than angiography.
- Imaging window prolonged which enables detection of intermittent bleeding.
- Localization of bleeding typically not used for selective surgical resection due to inaccuracy.

Transcatheter Embolization and Therapy,
Techniques in Interventional Radiology, DOI 10.1007/978-1-84800-897-7_34,
© Springer-Verlag London Limited 2010

Fig. 34.1 Tc-99 M RBC study shows bleeding from the left colon (*circle*)

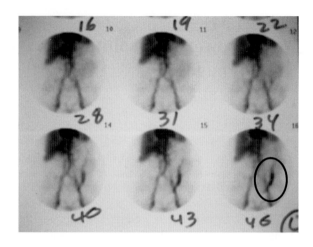

CTA

- Promising new technique that has not been widely validated to-date.
- Should be performed as unenhanced, arterially weighted, and delayed.
- Coronal reformats should be performed.
- Oral contrast should not be administered (Fig. 34.2).

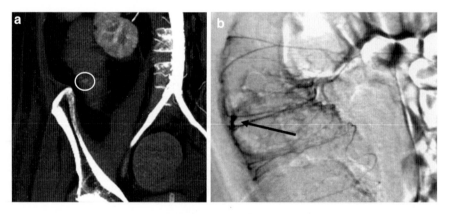

Fig. 34.2 Cecal bleeding. Computed tomographic angiogram (**a**—*circle*) and conventional digital subtraction angiogram (**b**—*arrow*) show cecal bleeding

Indications

These include the following:

- Any bleeding requiring hospitalization.

Contraindications

Contraindications are relative and include incorrectable coagulopathy.

Anatomy

The arterial anatomy to the lower GI track is highly variable and critically important for superselective embolization.

Normal Anatomy

- Right and transverse colon are supplied by superior mesenteric artery.
- Left colon and sigmoid are supplied by inferior mesenteric artery.
- Rectum is supplied by inferior mesenteric artery and hypogastric (internal iliac) arteries.

Anatomic Variation

The proximal mesenteric arcades should be scrutinized to determine collateral flow to the marginal artery (Fig. 34.3). If arcades perfuse proximal and distal portions of the marginal artery on either side of the site of bleeding, the marginal artery can be safely embolized. If not, bowel ischemia becomes a clinical concern. Also should be aware of post-surgical anatomy which can be extremely variable.

Equipment

- *Non-selective catheters:* pigtail or straight catheter if flush aortogram necessary.
- *Selective catheters:* cobra, Rosch curve 1, Rosch inferior mesenteric. Microcatheter for selective embolization.
- *Guide catheter* is helpful in rare instances of proximal mesenteric stenosis or extreme tortuosity of mesenteric arcades.

Embolic Agents

- A variety of agents have been used successfully.
- Microcoils are probably the easiest to use successfully (Fig. 34.4). They are easy to visualize, deploy accurately, and have been proven to work well.
- Polyvinyl alcohol particles (PVA) 350–500 μm have also been used and may be preferable to microcoils in tumor or angiodysplasia embolization or in refractory cases. Unlike microcoils, *PVA must be deposited directly into the vasa recta and cannot be used for marginal artery embolization.*
- Glue has been used successfully but is cost prohibitive in the United States.
- Alcohol should not be used for embolization due to high risk of bowel ischemia.

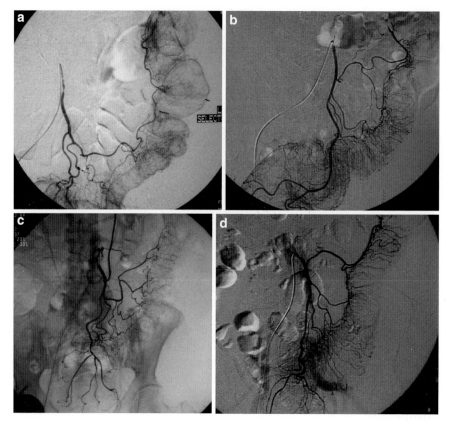

Fig. 34.3 Variable anatomy to the left colon. Multiple conventional angiograms in different patients show variability of perfusion to the left colon

Medication

- Sedation: conscious sedation with fentanyl and midazolam is helpful in most cases.
- Glucagon: glucagon 1 mg IV or hyoscine 20–40 mg can be given to prevent bowel peristalsis which can interfere with image interpretation.

Procedure

Access

- Vast majority of procedures performed from a femoral artery access.
- 4–5Fr vasculary sheath inserted in most cases.

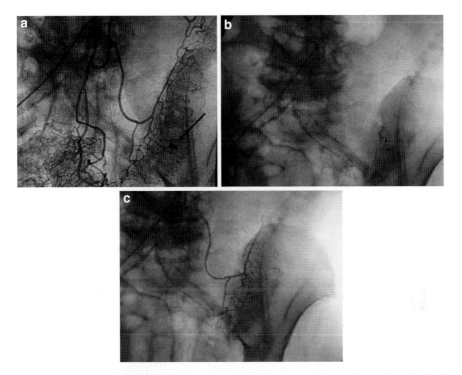

Fig. 34.4 Embolization of diverticular bleeding. (**a**) Inferior mesenteric angiogram showing focal bleeding at the junction of the sigmoid colon and left colon. (**b**) Fluoroscopic image shows micro-coils deployed in sigmoid colon. (**c**) Post-embolization angiogram showing cessation of bleeding (*arrows*)

Angiography

Lateral flush aortography can be helpful in patients to define proximal mesenteric vessel origins.

- If pre-procedure imaging has been performed, the artery supplying the bleeding site should be catheterized first. If initial angiography is unrevealing, the other mesenteric vessels should also be interrogated.
- If all three (or four, if the hypogastric arteries are imaged) angiograms fail to show bleeding, then the initial artery may be recatheterized for repeat angiography. Lower GI bleeding is frequently intermittent; the artery bleeds, becomes vasospastic, and stops bleeding, then rebleeds.
- If the bleeding site is very accurately localized on pre-procedural imaging, then subselective angiography can be performed.
- Carbon dioxide can be used in patients with renal failure and is thought to be more sensitive to bleeding than liquid contrast media by some investigators.

Angiographic Appearance

- *Active hemorrhage* is recognized by extravasation of contrast into the bowel which persists through the venous phase of angiography.
- The hallmark of *angiodysplasia* is an early draining vein. These lesions are more common in the right colon.
- Should also recognize tumor vascularity—chaotic neovascularization replacing the typical branching pattern.

Treatment Plan and Technique

Any site of active bleeding should be embolized. A microcatheter is advanced to the most distal accessible vessel which is usually either the vasa recta or marginal artery.

Embolization

- Goal is to reduce perfusion pressure to site of hemorrhage and devascularize smallest segment of bowel possible.
- Embolic agent is deposited as selectively as possible.
  - Microcoils can be deposited in marginal artery (if proximal arcades maintain flow proximal and distal to site of bleeding) or vasa recta. If the marginal artery is embolized, typically a 3–4 cm segment is occluded with 3–4 mm diameter microcoils.
  - PVA must be deposited into vasa recta.

Follow-Up

Elective colonoscopy should be performed to exclude malignancy as a source of bleeding and to assess for evidence of ischemia.

Alternative Therapies

Colonoscopy for diverticular hemorrhage is most successful after a 6–8 h bowel preparation ("bowel purge"). It is usually best applied to patients with slow or intermittent bleeding and is not indicated in patients with severe active bleeding.

Specific Complications

Renal failure can be managed by a nephrologist.

Bowel ischemia is rare if superselective embolization is performed but more common with proximal embolization or when a large segment of bowel is devascularized.

Keypoints

- Lower gastrointestinal hemorrhage tends to be intermittent; thus screening studies such as Tc-99M RBC scan or CTA may be helpful prior to angiography.
- Microcoils are the author's preferred embolic agent. Polyvinyl alcohol particles may also be used successfully.
- All patients should have follow-up colonoscopy after embolization to exclude malignancy as a source of bleeding.
- The risk of ischemia with superselective embolization is minimal.

Suggested Reading

Darcy M. Treatment of lower gastrointestinal bleeding: vasopressin infusion versus embolization. J Vasc Interv Radiol 2003; 14: 535–543

Funaki B. Microcatheter embolization of lower gastrointestinal hemorrhage: an old idea whose time has come. Cardiovasc Intervent Radiol 2004; 27: 591–599

Chapter 35
Bronchial Artery Embolization

Simon McPherson

Clinical Features

- Major hemoptysis with respiratory compromise is an emergency. Bronchoscopic airway management ± unilateral lung ventilation can be lifesaving.
- Hemoptysis kills by drowning the patient in their own blood. Death is by asphyxiation from major airway obstruction, *not* by exsanguination.
- Systemic arterial supply accounts for >95% of major hemoptyses.
- Neo-angiogenesis is caused by the underlying condition. Bleeding is from systemically pressurized abnormal pulmonary parenchyma.
- Bronchial artery embolization (BAE) stops bleeding by reducing this pressure.

The commonest causes are as follows:

- Chronic lung disease
  - Cystic fibrosis
  - Bronchiectasis from other causes
- Infection
  - Tuberculosis
  - Aspergillosis
  - Abscess
  - Chronic pneumonia
- Malignancy
  - Bronchogenic cancer
  - Metastases—rarely
- Congenital heart disease
- Leaking thoracic aortic anuerysm/penetrating ulcer

Pulmonary arterial and venous bleeding (Chapter 36) are rare. Consider in patients with a history/risk of the following:

- Trauma, including iatrogenic (e.g., recent Swan–Ganz catheter)
- Tuberculosis (Rasmussen's aneurysm)

Transcatheter Embolization and Therapy,
Techniques in Interventional Radiology, DOI 10.1007/978-1-84800-897-7_35,
© Springer-Verlag London Limited 2010

- Right-sided endocarditis or infected DVT (especially IV drug abusers)
- Hereditary hemorrhagic telangectasia

Diagnostic Evaluation

- Assessment of the degree of respiratory compromise and skilled airway management are essential.
- Medical management may need to be supplemented by bronchoscopic pulmonary clearance.
- Use history, imaging, and bronchoscopy to try to lateralize the site of bleeding and to demonstrate the underlying cause. Overspill often results in blood in both lungs.

Laboratory

- Arterial blood gas and oxygen saturation.
- Full blood count. Anemia is rare; anemia and thrombocytopenia should be corrected.
- Any clotting abnormalities must be corrected.
- Assess for renal impairment and ensure adequate hydration.

Imaging

CXR

- Unilateral changes are uncommon but can lateralize the bleeding site and allow targeted embolization.
- Compare with previous films if available. New changes indicate the side to be assessed first.

CT

- Non-contrast-enhanced CT may show the likely side of bleeding.
- Contrast enhancement is unnecessary (except where a pulmonary artery cause is suspected). Identification of the bronchial artery origins on CT does not significantly aid BAE.
- If a pulmonary arterial cause is suspected, then contrast enhancement may show a pseudoaneurysm. This is often more evident on multiplanar reformats.

Indications

Life-Threatening Hemoptysis

- The conventional definition uses the volume of blood expectorated.
- This is variable (200–500 ml/24 h) and difficult to accurately quantify.
- A more useful definition is any hemoptysis that causes significant airway compromise.

BAE Should Also Be Considered in

- Sudden onset of hemoptysis with increasing volumes. Such smaller "herald" bleeds often precede a catastrophic hemorrhage.
- Patients with chronic lung disease, such as cystic fibrosis, when minor recurrent hemoptysis precludes effective airway clearance maneuvers or adversely affects the quality of life.

Adjunctive and Alternative Therapies

- Supportive measures (oxygen, bronchodilators, hydration, etc).
- With major hemoptysis, nurse the patient with the affected lung dependent to decrease overspill into the non-bleeding lung.
- Bronchoscopic airway management and, if necessary, single-lung ventilation.
- Treat any infection; infection often precipitates hemoptysis.
- Tranexamic acid can occasionally be helpful in minor recurrent hemoptysis.
- Open surgical options should be discussed. They are usually the second-line intervention except for those with potentially surgically curable malignancy.
- CT-guided antifungal instillation into aspergillomas has been advocated as a supplementary treatment to BAE.

Contraindications

- No absolute contraindication exists. In those with severe iodinated contrast reactions, consider using gadolinium. CO_2 *must not be used* above the diaphragm.
- All other contraindications are relative and the risk of not treating massive hemoptysis generally outweighs any risks.

Specific Complications

- Neurological deficits are the most important
  - Spinal (paraplegia – partial or complete). Due to embolization of anterior spinal artery collaterals.

o Cerebrovascular – very rare. Due to non-target embolization during subclavian branch or aortic arch BAE.
- Odontophagia/difficulty swallowing—transient (3%). Esophageal necrosis has been reported.
- Chest-wall pain – transient.
- Angina/myocardial infarction (coronary artery connections).
- Airway necrosis has been reported.

All Complications Are Minimized by

- Meticulous angiographic technique
- Avoiding liquid agents (glue), and by using particles larger than 300 µm
- Selective use of coils for vessels that cannot be occluded with particles

Anatomy

Normal Bronchial Artery Anatomy

Bronchial arteries supply trachea, bronchi, esophagus, posterior mediastinum, and act as vasa vasorum for pulmonary arteries.

- Most bronchial arteries arise at the level of the left main bronchus (90% T5–6).
- Multiple arteries (including broncho-intercostal trunks) and conjoined origins are common.
- Broncho-intercostal trunk more common on the right.
- Multiple arteries are more common on the left.
- Bronchial artery origins arise from the anterior aorta.
- Broncho-intercostal arteries arise from the posterior aorta.
- Normal bronchial arteries are limited to medial 1/3 or 1/2 of lung field.

Key Points in Bronchial Arteriography

- Bronchial arteries follow a meandering course toward pulmonary hilum along the line of the bronchi.
- Intercostals follow undersurface of ribs and pass laterally.
- Bronchial–intercostal trunks have a slightly angulated cranial course; the bronchial branch descends sharply caudally toward pulmonary hilum (Fig. 35.1).
- Spinal branches
  o Anterior medullary arteries: initially course sharply cranially. A tight hairpin (180°) bend is followed by the straight midline anterior spinal artery (Fig. 35.2).

Fig. 35.1 Combined
bronchial–intercostal trunk
(*white arrow*) arterial phase
showing bronchial arteries
(*black arrowheads*) and
intercostal arteries (*white
arrowheads*). Note early
filling of pulmonary vein
(*black arrowhead*)

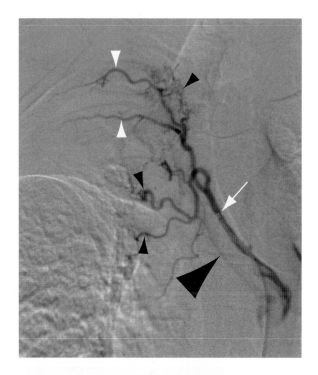

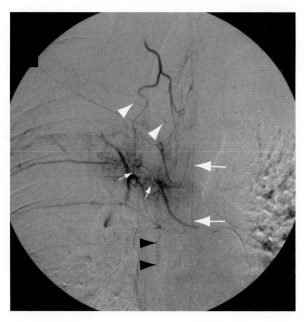

Fig. 35.2 Angiography in a patient with recurrent hemoptysis following embolization. Previously
deployed coils in bronchial arteries (*white arrowheads* and *small white arrows*) and internal mammary
artery (*black arrowheads*). Note filling of the anterior spinal artery (*large white arrows*)

o Dorsal and ventral radicular arteries – smaller vessels from segmental spinal arteries – course medially with a vertical, off-midline, not perfectly straight course. Unintentional radicular artery embolization rarely has clinical sequelae.

Aberrant/Variant Anatomy

- Bronchial arteries arising outside of T5/6 are considered anomalous.
- Arteries that can supply the bronchial circulation include the following:
- Intercostals
- Internal mammary (Fig. 35.3a)
- Inferior thyroid
- Costo-cervical
- Superior intercostal
- Inferior phrenic
- Subclavian (Fig. 35.4)
- Brachiocephalic

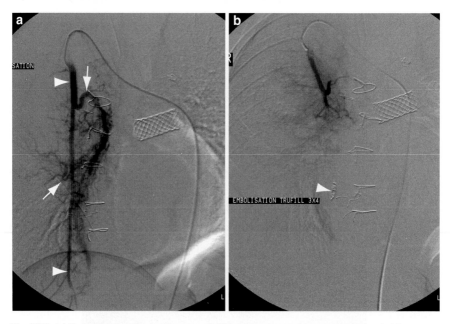

Fig. 35.3 (**a**) Bronchial arteries (*white arrows*) filling from internal mammary artery (*white arrowhead*) (**b**) following embolization with coils and polyvinyl alcohol particles. Note coils (*white arrowhead*) have been deployed beyond the lower bronchial supply to protect distal internal mammary circulation

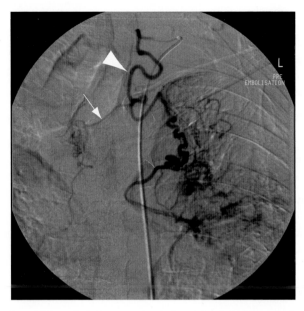

Fig. 35.4 Large bronchial supply (*white arrowhead*) from left subclavian artery. Supply to left (*red arrowheads*) and right lungs (*white arrow*)

Important common anastomoses exist between the bronchial arteries and the following:

- Anterior spinal artery
  - arise from central segments
  - more common on the right
- Pulmonary artery
- Mediastinal (including esophageal)
- Coronary arteries

These all have the potential to

- Cause significant non-target embolization
- Result in incomplete embolization or recurrent bleeding

Equipment

Catheters

Non-selective Catheters

- Pigtail flush catheter.

Selective Catheters

- Reversed curve catheters such as
  - Amplatz left coronary 1
  - Mikaelson
  - Simmons (sidewinder)

allow a more stable ostial position than forward/upward facing catheters (e.g., Cobra).

- Microcatheters are required in the majority.

Sheaths and Guide Catheters

- Long sheaths or guiding catheters can be helpful to provide support or alter the approach to a bronchial artery.

Embolic Agents

- Particles are the agent of choice. The aim is to permanently occlude the abnormal circulation distally but not at a level that will cause tissue necrosis. PVA 350–500 μm is most commonly used. Embolization is terminated when forward flow is almost terminated.
- Larger particles may be used when large pulmonary arterial or venous shunts are present. Gelfoam slurry or coils are occasionally used to occlude very large shunts. Gelfoam slurry can be injected via a microcatheter, if a dilute slurry is injected with an angioplasty indeflator. A distal position must be obtained to minimize the risk of Gelfoam reflux.
- Coils (steel conventional or platinum micro coils) may also be used to
  - Protect the distal circulation (Fig. 35.3b).
  - Occlude abnormal vessels with spinal, esophageal or coronary supply – usually this would be done distally and then proximally to the branch. The distal embolization prevents retrograde passage of particles and non-target embolization when other pathological vessels are embolized.
  - Coils should *not* be used to occlude proximal bronchial arteries, especially when embolizing patients with chronic diseases. This proximal embolization will lead to formation of significant collateral vessels, which are often much more difficult to catheterize in the setting of recurrent hemoptysis.

Medication

- High-quality angiography is the key to safe BAE. This requires a co-operative patient, and BAE may take 2 hours or more. If there is any doubt about the patient's ability to cope, then enlist the help of an anesthetist.

- Patients who are in extremis may be managed with selective intubation to protect the non-bleeding lung during BAE.
- Catheter-induced vasospasm can be treated with vasodilators. Vasospasm may result in vessel recanalization and failed BAE.

Infection Control

o Patients with current infection should be on antibiotic treatment. Prophylactic antibiotics are not required.

Hydration

o Adequate hydration aids airway clearance and reduces the risk of contrast nephrotoxicity.

Angiography

Access and Angiography

- Common femoral 4Fr or 5Fr access is sufficient in the overwhelming majority.
- A flush aortic run, with a frame rate of 3–4 frames per second in shallow left anterior oblique, may be useful to demonstrate the origins of the bronchial arteries. The absence of abnormal circulation on this run does not exclude pathological bronchial circulation.
- Selective catheterization is necessary to detect pathological circulation.
- Occasionally, arm access is required for aberrant vessels from the subclavian or the inner curve of the aortic arch.

Angiographic Appearance

First look for pathological bronchial circulation. One or more of the following will be seen.

- Enlarged main bronchial artery (<3 mm)
- Hypertrophied bronchial radicles (visualization of normal bronchial arteries limited to medial 1/3 or 1/2 of lung field)
- Dense parenchymal blush
- Pulmonary arterial or venous shunting (Fig. 35.5)
- Pseudoaneurysms (rare) (Fig. 36.6)
- Active extravasation (very rare and NOT a prerequisite for embolization)

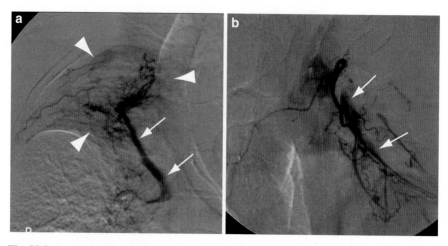

Fig. 35.5 Communications with pulmonary vein and artery. (**a**) Late arterial phase. Parenchymal stain (*white arrowheads*) and shunting into pulmonary vein (*white arrows*) (same patient as in Fig. 35.1). (**b**) Filling of pulmonary artery (*white arrows*) during arterial phase of bronchial angiography

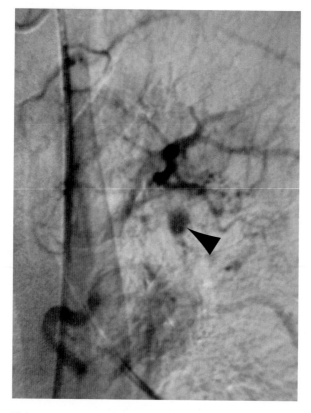

Fig. 35.6 Bronchial artery false aneurysm (*black arrowhead*)

Next, Identify Any Spinal Supply That

- Arises from proximal bronchial or intercostal arteries (medial to pedicle).
- Passes sharply cranially and then has a tight hairpin (180°) bend before supplying the straight midline anterior spinal artery (Fig. 35.2)

Embolization

- When embolizing –
  - o Inject embolic agent slowly to avoid reflux and non-target embolization.
  - o Continuous high-quality screening during embolization is mandatory, and repeat angiograms should be performed frequently. Spinal and other important collaterals may open up as the target vessel is being occluded. Intermittent-check angiographic runs are recommended.
  - o Do not inject intercostals at the vessel origin as this increases the chance of radiculomedullary branch embolization. Advance the catheter a few centimeters into the vessel (at least beyond the pedicle) to avoid particle reflux.

Clinical Scenarios

- BAE starts with airway management. Make sure that you have adequate clinical support for this. Intubation and ventilation may be much safer for the patient and will also improve angiographic quality.
- If possible, lateralize the source of hemorrhage before starting. This will simplify and shorten the procedure.
- Patients may feel a unilateral gurgling sensation or discomfort when bleeding occurs. This is a reliable lateralizing symptom.
- Where clinical or imaging lateralization is not possible, bilateral BAE is required (the underlying disease commonly causes bilateral pathological changes and the culprit lesion cannot be identified).

Treatment Plan and Technique

- Start with the side most likely to be bleeding, When lateralization of the cause has not been possible, treat any abnormal circulation on both sides.
- In massive hemoptysis, ALL POTENTIAL NON-BRONCHIAL SYSTEMIC COLLATERALS SHOULD BE ASSESSED, after treatment of all identifiable bronchial arteries. Embolizing bronchial arteries alone is a common cause of embolization failure.
- In less severe hemoptysis, it may be appropriate to assess the response to BAE alone (the risk of persistent hemoptysis being weighed against the risk of complication(s) from more extensive embolization).

Aftercare

- Observe for signs/evidence of neurological deficit.
- If spinal cord damage occurs, it is likely due to focal infarction (transverse myelitis) caused by hypoperfusion from more proximal occlusion of spinal branches.
- Supplemental oxygen, IV fluids, and blood pressure maintenance (mean arterial pressure above 80 mmHg) are recommended.
- A spinal drain should be inserted, if spinal cord infarction cannot be immediately confirmed.

Arterial Puncture Site

- A closure device may be useful. It allows patients with respiratory compromise to immediately achieve a more comfortable sitting position.

Post-embolization

- Chest-wall pain and pain/difficulty swallowing are common and transient.
- If significant hemoptysis persists or recurs, repeat angiography is performed.
  - Check that the embolized vessels remain occluded.
  - Look for accessory bronchial arteries and collateral bronchial supply, particularly from the intercostal, internal mammary, inferior phrenic and subclavian arteries (including thyrocervical, costo-cervical, and lateral thoracic branches of the subclavian).
  - Consider pulmonary angiography, if no bronchial arterial abnormality is detected.

Follow-Up

Most patients have chronic pathology. Many will require repeated embolization every 2–3 years, as new collateral vessels open up. Patients, and their physicians, should be made aware that recurrence of hemoptysis is to be anticipated and that BAE is repeatable. However, these embolizations become increasingly challenging as more collaterals develop.

Keypoints

- Knowledge of normal, aberrant, and collateral bronchial arterial circulation is a prerequisite. Multiple supplying vessels are the norm.

- BAE involves the identification and then catheterization of multiple small vessels. Diligent angiographic technique is required. Even microcatheters may be difficult to advance.
- Preserve the main arterial trunk to allow future access/prevent particulate reflux.
- Coils and other proximal occlusion techniques are rarely indicated, as they block the access vessel without occluding the abnormal parenchymal circulation.

Safety

- Have a low threshold for asking for anesthetic support.
- Identify any spinal arterial supply.
  - Requires high-quality magnified screening and check angiographic acquisitions.
  - Modify the embolization technique if identified – this is often an indication for coil embolization distal and proximal to the spinal branch.

Suggested Reading

[1] Uflacker R, Kaemmerer A, Picon P et al. Bronchial artery embolization in the management of haemoptysis: technical aspects and long-term results. Radiology 1985; 157: 637–644
[2] Yoon W, Kim JK, Kim YH et al. Bronchial and nonbronchial systemic artery embolization for life threatening haemoptysis: a comprehensive review. Radiographics 2002; 22:1395–1409
[3] Mauro, Murphy, Thomson, Venbrux and Zollikofer. Bronchial artery embolization. In: Image guided interventions (Vol II). Eds Irani Z and Keller FS (2008) pp. 931–938 Elsevier ISBN 978-1-4-4160-29649

Chapter 36
Pulmonary Hemorrhage (Non-bronchial)

Hamed Aryafar and Thomas Kinney

Clinical features are as listed in Chapter 35.

The most useful definition of massive hemoptysis is a volume sufficient to cause life-threatening condition. In the literature, this ranges from 100 to 1000 cc per day.

- Emergency surgery performed for hemorrhage has a 17–40% mortality.

Etiology

- 90% of massive hemoptysis derives from bronchial or systemic arteries, 5% from the pulmonary arteries, and 5% from other systemic arteries or from miscellaneous causes such as aorto-bronchial fistula.
- Pulmonary artery abnormalities co-exist with systemic abnormalities in up to 10% of patients.

Causes of Pulmonary Arterial Hemorrhage

- Pulmonary artery aneurysm/pseudoaneurysm (Rassmusen's aneurysm: see Fig. 36.1)
- Pulmonary AVM (Chapter 15)
- Pulmonary artery iatrogenic injury from Swan-Ganz catheter placement
- Pulmonary embolus
- Pulmonary hypertension
- Mitral stenosis
- Trauma

Transcatheter Embolization and Therapy,
Techniques in Interventional Radiology, DOI 10.1007/978-1-84800-897-7_36,
© Springer-Verlag London Limited 2010

Fig. 36.1 A male patient with TB who had massive hemoptysis unresponsive to conservative treatment. He had a negative bronchial angiogram, and a pulmonary arteriogram was performed. This showed extensive cavitary change to the left upper lobe with a Rasmussen's aneurysm along the inferior margin of the cavity; this was successfully embolized with coils

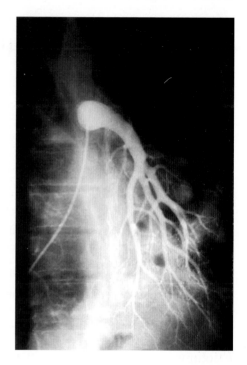

Diagnostic Evaluation

- Clinical assessment and airway management are crucial.
- Must exclude other source of bleeding such as nose, mouth, pharynx, and hematemesis.

Laboratory

- Arterial blood gas and oxygen saturation.
- Any clotting abnormalities must be corrected.

Imaging

- Plain radiographs are often normal and seldom establish the source.
- Bronchoscopy (not always performed, but may give more information regarding etiology and side of bleeding for planned embolotherapy).
- Contrast-enhanced computed tomography scan (CECT) (Chapter 9).
  - o Useful for evaluation of anatomy and possible direct diagnosis of source of hemorrhage. Some advocate CT scan prior to bronchoscopy. The primary goal

is to identify which lung the hemoptysis arises from and possibly pinpoint the specific pulmonary segment.

o A secondary goal is to determine if the bleeding arises from the pulmonary artery or intercostals or systemic collaterals.

o Lastly, if the supply arises from the pulmonary arterial supply, it is important to determine if the anatomy is simple (one feeding artery) or complex (multiple feeding arteries).

Pulmonary angiography: The logistical requirements for treating acute or chronic recurrent hemoptysis include the following:

o Availability of high-quality digital angiographic equipment
o On-call interventional radiologist and radiologic technologist and nurse
o Embolization material and a variety of different catheters (including stent grafts)
o Availability of an intensive care unit and advanced airway management. Patients may require intubation (including selective endobronchial balloon occlusion) prior to the procedure

Indications

Pulmonary arteriography is indicated

- In patients with hemoptysis suspected to be arising from the pulmonary circulation.
- When conservative medical therapy fails.
- In operative candidates when surgery cannot be performed.
- Recurrent hemoptysis in patients with bilateral widespread disease.
- To control bleeding as a temporary measure before definitive surgery is planned.

Contraindications

- *All contraindications are relative!*
- Severe pulmonary arterial hypertension is a contraindication to pump angiography.
- Inability to find exact source of bleeding via diagnostic pathway or clinical instability would preclude treatment.
- Due to the contrast load, renal insufficiency is a relative contraindication.
- A recent electrocardiogram is necessary to exclude a left bundle branch block. Right heart block induced by attempted catheterization of the pulmonary arteries may result in complete heart block. If the patient has right heart block, then a temporary pacemaker (transvenous or transcutaneous) is required before angiography.

Equipment

Catheters

- Pulmonary artery catheterization for diagnosis (Fig. 36.2)
  - 5 Fr Omniflush catheter
  - 7 Fr Grollman Catheter
  - 6–7 Fr Pigtail catheter with tip-deflecting wire technique
  - Balloon flotation catheter
- Selective catheterization for transcatheter therapy
  - 5 Fr Kumpe, headhunter, or cobra for conventional-sized coils
  - 7–8 Fr White Lumax Catheters
  - 3 Fr microcatheters for situations requiring subselective embolization with microcoils
  - 4–7 Fr sheath or 5–9 Fr guide catheter (for Amplatzer Vascular Plug II)

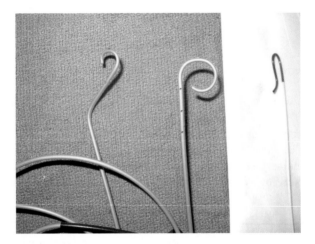

Fig. 36.2 Catheters to use for pulmonary artery catheterization. From left to right, these include the Grollman, Pigtail catheter (used with tip-deflecting wire technique), and the Ominflush catheter

Embolic Agents

- Amplatzer vascular plug
- Embolization coils (stainless steel, platinum (Nestor), detachable (GDC or other))

Exclusion

- Covered stent graft.

Medications

- Consider moderate sedation for patient.
- Atropine 0.5 mg IV for prophylaxis against bradycardia.
- Antibiotic prophylaxis (e.g., 1 gm cefazolin).
- Some patients may require endotracheal intubation to protect aspiration into the unaffected lung.

Procedure

Access: femoral (more common), brachial, or jugular vein.

Pulmonary Artery Catheterization

Always monitor for ectopic ventricular beats, particularly for ventricular tachycardia.

- Omniflush technique: the 5 Fr catheter is advanced to the right atrium. At that level, a stiff hydrophilic guidewire is inserted, which opens the curve of the catheter directing the guidewire superiorly toward the right ventricular outflow tract and pulmonary artery.
- Grollman catheter technique: the pre-shaped catheter is positioned with the Pigtail in the right atrium. Twisting the catheter directs the catheter tip through the tricuspid valve and further catheter twisting and advancement selects the right ventricular outflow and main pulmonary artery.
- Pigtail and deflecting wire technique: the Pigtail is advanced to the right atrium. The tip deflecting wire is inserted into the catheter near the catheter tip and the wire deflected towards the right ventricle. The catheter is fed forward off the wire into the right ventricle. The deflection of the wire is released, straightening the catheter which is advanced through the right ventricular outflow tract and into the main pulmonary artery.
- Balloon flotation catheter: analogous to Swan-Ganz catheter insertion. The balloon catheter is inserted to the right atrium; the balloon is inflated with air and carefully advanced under fluoroscopy into the pulmonary circulation.
- In the setting where a right-to-left shunt is suspected, careful attention must be paid to decreasing the risk of small clot or air bubble injection. Even a small thrombus or air embolus in the setting of such a shunt could prove to be devastating to the patient, particularly if the embolus travels to the heart or brain.

Pulmonary Arterial Pressures

o Pulmonary arterial pressures are typically determined. Elevated pressures may
  alter the diagnostic and therapeutic techniques (e.g., decreasing rate and volume
  during angiography).

Pulmonary Angiography

o Pulmonary artery injection (15–20 cc/s for total of 30–40 cc) with rapid digital
  subtraction imaging (>15 frames/second) on side causing suspected hemoptysis.
o If possible, respirations are suspended.
o Multiple views, including obliques and cranially–caudally angulated views, may
  be helpful for subselective catheterization and defining the pathologic lesion
  (aneurysm neck, number of supplying arteries, sizes and lengths of arteries for
  coil selection or stent-graft implantation).

Assess Bleeding

• Prior imaging (CT) will be helpful in determination of source.
• The most common finding is an aneurysm, pseudoaneurysm, or arteriovenous
  fistula.
• Demonstration of contrast extravasation is highly unusual, and the lack of definite
  contrast extravasation should not preclude embolization if a bleeding source is
  noted.

Embolization

• In cases where embolization is considered, the coils should exclude the aneurysm
  completely (Fig. 36.3). The coils should be appropriately sized for diameter
  and length to achieve adequate coverage without excluding normal pulmonary
  segments. Situations with communication to the pulmonary veins warrant extra
  consideration, as air or coil embolism may result in significant complications.
  Proper sizing of coils, detachable coils, and the Amplatzer plugs are useful in
  these situations. If a particular case involves stent grafting, appropriate sheaths,
  stent graft diameters, and lengths are crucial.

Follow-up angiography: if hemoptysis persists despite transcatheter pulmonary
artery therapies, consider a systemic source (Chapter 35).

Alternative approach: conventional surgery or rarely direct percutaneous
embolization of diseased vessel(s).

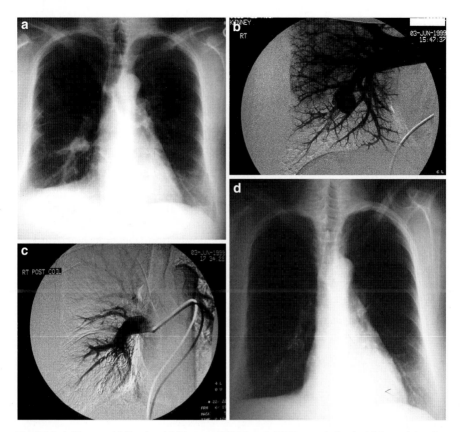

Fig. 36.3 A 37-year-old female with history of IVDA and AIDS was admitted with bacterial endocarditis (staph aureus). After antibiotic therapy she improved but had a persistent right-lung opacity (**a**). She developed massive hemoptysis and was evaluated by cardiothoracic surgery but was denied surgery. She underwent pulmonary arteriography, which showed a pseudoaneurysm arising from a right lower lobe subsegmental pulmonary artery branch (**b**). This was embolized with coils distal to the aneurysm, within the aneurysmal sac, and proximal to the aneurysm (**c**). The patient was evaluated at 1 year follow-up, which showed no evidence for recurrent aneurysm by CT and chest radiograph (**d**)

Complications/Follow-Up

o Rebleeding (early/late) can occur. This is usually due to a failure to recognize the involvement of other pulmonary/bronchial arteries or of non-bronchial systemic vessels that were not identified and occluded during the first procedure.

o Late rebleeding is generally due to disease progression, but may result from recanalization of embolization coils.

o Lung parenchyma ischemia with pleuritis (usually from large segment embolization therapy).

o Non-target embolization to other pulmonary segments. Systemic embolization of coils, thrombus, or air if communication to the pulmonary vein is present.
o Dysrhythmias.
o Hemoptysis.
o Contrast allergies.
o Contrast-induced renal failure.

Keypoints

1. Pre-procedure imaging and/or bronchoscopy may be helpful in determining the site of bleeding.
2. The majority of massive hemoptysis arises from the bronchial artery (discussed in another chapter of this book).
3. Care must be taken in the setting of a right-to-left shunt, in order to prevent paradoxical embolization.
4. Large permanent agents, such as coils and Amplatzer plugs, are typically used for pulmonary artery hemorrhage.
5. If bleeding persists after pulmonary embolization, consider systemic arterial sources.

Suggested Reading

1. Andersen PE Imaging and Interventional Radiological Treatment of Hemoptysis, Acta Radiologica 2006; 47(8): 780–792
2. Yoon W, Kim JK, Kim YH, Chung TW, Kang HK. Bronchial and nonbronchial systemic artery embolization for life-threatening hemoptysis: a comprehensive review. Radiographics 2002; 22: 1395–1409.
3. Pulmonary and Bronchial arteries. In Valji K (ed). Vascular and Interventional Radiology. Philadelphia, Saunders Elsevier, 2006; 347: 259–282.

Chapter 37
Endoleaks Following EVAR

Stephen Johnson, Jennifer Fraser, and Rajan Gupta

Clinical Features

- Continued perfusion of an abdominal aortic aneurysm (AAA) after endovascular stent-graft deployment has been termed an "endoleak."
- There are five types of endoleaks:
  - Type I: inadequate seal at the proximal or distal attachment sites.
  - Type II: continued blood flow through a patent inferior mesenteric artery (IMA), lumbar artery or hypogastric artery. Requires an inflow and outflow artery. (Most common type of endoleak.)
  - Type III: midgraft leak from fabric holes or an inadequate seal between graft components.
  - Type IV: transgraft flow from porosity of the graft (usually takes place immediately after placement).
  - Type V: also known as endotension; aneurysm enlargement without an identifiable leak.

- Endoleaks contributing to continued perfusion of the aneurysmal sac can lead to enlargement and possibly rupture of the sac.
- Treatment involves interrupting vessel flow and includes the use of coils, onyx (ethylene–vinyl alcohol) and thrombin ± gelfoam.
- Embolization can be performed either at the time of EVAR or during a subsequent procedure.

Diagnostic Evaluation

Laboratory

Prior to the procedure, patients should have labs drawn for CBC, BUN/Cr, and PT/INR.

Transcatheter Embolization and Therapy,
Techniques in Interventional Radiology, DOI 10.1007/978-1-84800-897-7_37,
© Springer-Verlag London Limited 2010

Imaging

Patients undergoing EVAR should have CT imaging prior to EVAR to evaluate vascular anatomy.

Direct fluoroscopic imaging is used at the time of EVAR to identify endoleaks and proper graft placement.

Patients should undergo subsequent CT evaluation at 1 month, 6 months, and yearly for evidence of aneurysmal growth (i.e., endoleak).

Indications

Presence of an endoleak, aneurysmal growth.

Alternative Therapies

Open surgical repair, ligation of feeding arteries.

Watchful waiting—follow endoleak with CT for continued aneurysmal growth.

Contraindications

Inability to access aneurysm sac, patient unable to tolerate second procedure.

Specific Complications

Common: failure of embolization with continued perfusion of aneurysmal sac, enlargement of aneurysm.

Uncommon: bowel or spinal ischemia.

Anatomy

Since EVAR is performed to repair an abdominal aneurysm, the related vasculature anatomy can be very diseased and difficult to access. Therefore, imaging prior to the procedure is essential. Additionally, the anatomy of contributing arteries varies greatly and must be visualized with either angiography or direct fluoroscopy with contrast.

Normal Anatomy

Patent bilateral femoral arteries, iliac arteries, and abdominal aorta.

Aberrant Anatomy

Tortuous vasculature, stenotic, or atherosclerotic arteries.

Equipment

Catheters

- *Non-selective catheters:* 4 Fr kumpke
- *Selective catheters:* microcatheters
- *Guide catheter*

Embolic Agents

- Multiple approaches to embolization have been used and they vary depending on the type and severity of the endoleak. Embolization should continue until there is no further pulsatile blood return. Confirmation is obtained with contrast injection during direct fluoroscopy.
- *Coils*
  - ○ Embolic coils can be used for selective embolization of vessels feeding the endoleak, as well as to embolize the aneurysmal sac itself.
  - ○ Stainless steel coils vs. platinum coils

    - • Stainless steel coils are more difficult to see under fluoroscopy than platinum coils.
    - • However, stainless steel coils are preferred because they cause fewer artifacts on follow-up imaging.

  - ○ Coils can also be particularly effective for the treatment of retrograde endoleaks.
- *Onyx*
  - ○ Onyx embolizes by filling the aneurysm sac with an elastic polymer which conforms closely to the wall of the sac, occluding flow.
- *Thrombin*
  - ○ Can be used with or without Gelfoam.
  - ○ As a liquid mixture, thrombin ± Gelfoam can be injected directly into the aneurysmal sac to induce embolization.
  - ○ Must be used cautiously to avoid non-selective embolization.

Medication

- *Pain control*: conscious sedation using PRN Fentanyl and Versed if not using general anesthesia.
- *Infection control:* prophylactic antibiotics (e.g., Cephazolin).
- *Sickness control:* PRN antiemetics.
- *Hydration*: IV fluids.

Angiography

Access

- Femoral artery access via one or both femoral arteries at the time of EVAR.
- Translumbar access into aneurysm sac.

Angiography

Direct fluoroscopic angiography is obtained either at the time of EVAR or during a subsequent procedure to identify the source(s) of the endoleak.

- Selective catheterization with contrast injection of feeding arteries, such as the IMA or lumbar arteries, can be done to identify source of endoleak.

Assessing the Lesion

- Assessment of the lesion can be done at the time of EVAR or during follow-up evaluation.
- At the time of EVAR, a catheter placed in the excluded sac can signify the presence of an endoleak with the return of pulsatile blood flow (type II endoleak).
- Types I and III can be detected at the time of graft deployment with fluoroscopic imaging.
- Endoleaks can also be assessed using follow-up CT. The aneurysmal sac can be measured and analyzed for interval growth.

Angiographic Appearance

- The endoleak is identified angiographically by the extravasation of contrast from within the graft lumen into the aneurysm sac (type I and III endoleaks).
- Type II endoleaks can be identified during angiography by the presence of contrast traveling from a peripherally catheterized vessel into the excluded aneurysm sac.

Treatment Plan and Technique

There are several different approaches to endoleak treatment, and treatment varies with the type of endoleak present.

- Type I: identified at the time of graft placement and can be corrected by securing the graft attachment sites with angioplasty balloons, stents, or stent-graft extensions.

- Type II: currently, type II endoleaks are treated either at the time of EVAR through a transarterial approach or during a secondary procedure via direct translumbar endoleak puncture. Different types of embolization materials are outlined above.
- Type III: Type III endoleaks can be corrected by covering the defect with a stent-graft extension.
- Type IV: This type of endoleak is not associated with aneurysmal growth and rupture; therefore, treatment generally involves monitoring of the aneurysmal sac with subsequent CT scans.
- Type V: the etiology of graft-related endotension is unknown, and therefore treatment has not yet been established.

Aftercare

Arterial puncture site: monitor for hematoma, extravasation.

Post-embolization

Patients should be monitored for signs of embolization-related bowel or spinal ischemia and continued endoleak with aneurysm sac growth.

Follow-Up

Follow-up CT angiogram at 1 month, 6 months, and yearly for aneurysmal growth (Fig. 37.1)

Keypoints

- Endoleaks are a common complication of endovascular AAA repair (EVAR) and can lead to aneurysm growth and rupture.
- There are five different types of endoleaks.
- Endoleaks may be identified at the time of EVAR or upon follow-up imaging.
- Treatment of endoleaks depends on the type of endoleak present.
- Treatment of type I and III endoleaks may involve graft extensions, ballooning or stents.
- Treatment of type II endoleaks involves the use of embolic coils, onyx, or thrombin, and can be done at the time of EVAR or during a secondary procedure through a translumbar sac puncture.

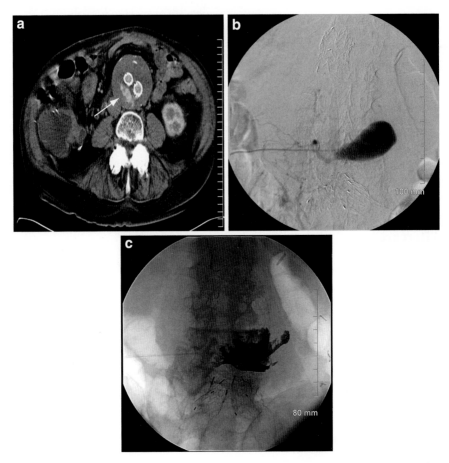

Fig. 37.1 (**a**) Contrast-enhanced CT scan, venous phase, in a patient undergoing routine imaging follow-up after bifurcated endograft placement. Notice the contrast accumulation in the aneurysm sac (*arrow*). On review of the non-contrast-enhanced CT (not shown), the finding was not visualized. (**b**) Contrast injection following direct puncture of the aneurysm sac under fluoroscopic guidance demonstrating retrograde filling of a lumbar arterial branch. (**c**) Fluoroscopic image following injection of onyx

Suggested Readings

Golzarian J, Maes ED, Sun S. Endoleak: treatment options. Tach Vasc Interv Radiol 2005;8(1): 41–49

Stavropoulos SW, Baum RA. Catheter-based treatments of endoleaks. Semin Vasc Surg 2004;17(4):279–283

Chapter 38
Internal Iliac Artery—Isolated Aneurysm and Pre-EVAR Embolization

David O. Kessel

Clinical Features

This is a relatively uncommon indication for internal iliac artery territory embolization compared with embolization for uterine fibroids, pelvic trauma, and hemorrhage. Prophylactic embolization to prevent type II endoleak pre-endovascular aneurysm repair (EVAR) is much more common than embolization for isolated internal iliac artery aneurysm (IIAA).

- Most internal IIAAs are asymptomatic and occur in the context of aortoiliac aneurysm. Isolated IIAA are rare.
- Symptomatic aneurysms may present with rupture or compression of adjacent structures.
- IIAAs are challenging to repair surgically, and endovascular treatment is the preferred option.
- In male patients, pre-procedure history must document erectile function and presence or absence of buttock claudication.

Diagnostic Evaluation

Most IIAA will be detected as incidental findings on ultrasound, CT, or MRI. Evaluation is similar to that for endovascular aneurysm repair. If aneurysms are symptomatic or greater than 4 cm in diameter, then CT angiography with reconstruction is the investigation of choice.

Laboratory

Beware of renal impairment and ensure adequate hydration. Consult renal physicians if necessary.

Transcatheter Embolization and Therapy,
Techniques in Interventional Radiology, DOI 10.1007/978-1-84800-897-7_38,
© Springer-Verlag London Limited 2010

Imaging

Use contrast-enhanced CT/MRI (Fig. 38.1) to

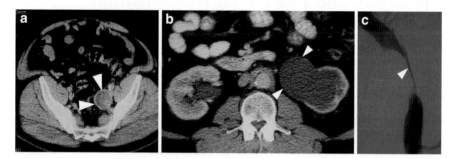

Fig. 38.1 (**a**) 5 cm IIAA (*arrowheads*) presenting with deep vein thrombosis, (**b**) associated left hydronephrosis (*arrowheads*), and (**c**) external iliac vein compression (*arrowheads*)

- Demonstrate patency of the contralateral internal iliac artery
- The length and size of the internal iliac artery
- Verify the size of the aneurysm
- Demonstrate the extent of involvement of the aortoiliac segments
- Demonstrate whether other structures are affected
- Assess factors that will influence the approach (e.g., iliac artery tortuosity and configuration of the aortic bifurcation)

Indications

- Symptomatic, large, or ruptured IIAA
- Need to occlude internal iliac artery (± IIAA) in association with aortoiliac aneurysm pre-EVAR

Alternative Therapies

- Branched stent grafts for some aortoiliac aneurysms
- Aorto-uniiliac stent graft with femorofemoral crossover, and contralateral external iliac to IIA stent graft
- Aneurysm resection or primary repair

Contraindications

- Contraindications are relative and relate to the indication and severity of the underlying disease, and thus there is little that will prevent emergency embolization for hemorrhage.

Specific Complications

- Buttock claudication
- Erectile dysfunction
- Descending colon/sigmoid colon/rectal ischemia
- Bladder ischemia

Complications are most common if the entire internal iliac circulation is embolized (i.e., bilateral embolization or embolization of the only IIA) or if embolization involves the branches of the IIA.

Anatomy

Normal Anatomy

- The vast majority of patients have conventional aortoiliac arterial anatomy.
- The common iliac artery bifurcates to form internal and external iliac arteries.
- The internal iliac artery bifurcates into anterior and posterior divisions, which supply pelvic organs as well as the gluteal muscles.
- Occlusion of the internal iliac artery proximal to its bifurcation is less likely to result in ischemia.
- Principal consideration will be anatomical factors influencing the approach for emoblization.

Aberrant anatomy: very uncommon, but there are also iatrogenic (post-operative) variations in pelvic vasculature.

- Persistent sciatic artery supplying the leg. Embolization might be needed in this context as the persistent sciatic artery is prone to aneurysm developing. In this case, embolization needs to be combined with revascularization of the leg.
- Renal transplant anastomosed to internal iliac artery.
- Iliofemoral crossover graft.

Equipment

Catheters

- *Non-selective catheters:* Pigtail or straight catheter if flush aortogram necessary.
- *Selective catheters:* cobra, renal double curve, sidewinder to catheterize the IIA or cross the aortic bifurcation. Microcatheter occasionally needed for selective embolization.
- *Guide catheter with detachable hemostatic valve* if using Amplatzer vascular plugs (AVP) or working over the aortic bifurcation.

Embolic Agents

- *Pre-EVAR*: AVP, coils to proximal IIA.
- *Selective IIAA*: AVP, coils to occlude distal circulation; AVP, coils, or CIA-EIA stent graft to occlude inflow.

Medication

- *Antiperistaltic*: Hyoscine (Buscopan) will improve angiography.
- *Infection control:* Pre-procedural broad-spectrum antibiotics.

Angiography

Access

- Plan according to the pre-procedure imaging.
- >90% from the femoral artery.
- Contralateral approach may give a more stable catheter position and may be useful in tortuous vessels.
- Brachial artery may be used in difficult cases, but ensure that you have sufficiently long catheters (>100 cm) and exchange length guidewires.

Angiography

- AP and iliac oblique projections may be necessary.
- Craniocaudal tilt is sometimes required in IIAA to clarify distal anatomy.

Assessing the Iliac Artery

Key features are as follows:
- Patency of contralateral internal iliac artery in terms of risk of developing ischemic sequalae.
- Diameter and length for choosing appropriate coils/plugs.
- Extent of any aneurysm.

Angiographic Appearance

- The iliac arteries are frequently tortuous in the presence of abdominal aortic aneurysms.

Clinical Scenarios

Pre-EVAR Embolization

- The goal is prevention of type II endoleak.

- Permanent occlusion of the internal iliac artery proximal to its bifurcation.
- Ensure that there is complete occlusion before proceeding to EVAR, as any leak will be much more difficult to treat subsequently.
- Coils may be packed against an AVP to complete embolization.
- If both IIA are to be occluded, consider interval therapy to allow collateral development.

Embolization in Patients with IIAA

- The goal is to treat the IIAA by exclusion from the circulation.
- Either proximal or distal isolation needed to prevent retrograde filling of aneurysms via pelvic arterial collaterals (Fig. 38.2) or distal embolization and stent graft from CIA to EIA to occlude the inflow.

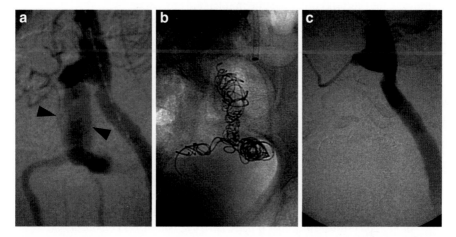

Fig. 38.2 Same patient as in Fig. 38.1. (**a**) The IIAA (*black arrowheads*) extends down to the bifurcation of the IIA. (**b**) Coils placed into the anterior and posterior divisions of the IIA and packing of the aneurysm. (**c**) Completion angiogram showing exclusion of the IIAA. The iliac vein was subsequently stented, the patient has been asymptomatic and 5 years regular duplex surveillance has shown the aneurysm to be thrombosed and the iliac vein to be patent

Aftercare

Arterial Puncture Site
- Routine care.
- Try to avoid closure device if the patient is about to undergo EVAR, as inflammatory change can complicate surgery.

Post-embolization

- Check for ischemic complications.

- Buttock claudication typically improves over several weeks, even with bilateral embolization.

Follow-Up

- CT or ultrasound to confirm exclusion of aneurysm or absence of type II endoleak.

Keypoints

Review the pre-procedural imaging to plan the procedure.
Ensure you understand the rationale for treating each patient, as this will ensure.

- Use coils or AVP ± stent graft.
- Correct endpoints.
- Document that the patient recognizes the risks of pelvic ischemia.

Safety

Never start embolization until you have personally reviewed the imaging.
Stick to the indications for the procedure, use appropriate agents, and remember that the endpoints depend on the indication.
Stop if uncertain, especially if there is risk of non-target embolization!

Suggested Reading

Parry DJ, Kessel D, Scott DJA. Simplifying the internal iliac artery aneurysm. Ann R Coll Surg Engl 2001; 83: 302–308

Chapter 39
Embolization of Visceral Arterial Aneurysms

A.N. Keeling

Clinical Features

- This chapter covers aneurysms of the abdominal visceral arteries excluding renal artery aneurysms which are covered in Chapter 40.
- Visceral arterial aneurysms (VAA) may be true aneurysms or pseudoaneurysms; they are defined as a localized dilatation >1.5 times the expected arterial diameter. A prevalence of 0.1–2% up to 10% with reported in autopsy series.
- Etiology is variable and depends on the site. Most patients with VAA are in their sixties. Pregnancy is a recognized risk factor for rupture.
- Recent increase in diagnosis of visceral aneurysms is most likely due to the incidental finding of asymptomatic VAA with contemporary imaging and imaging reformats (Fig. 39.2a, 39.2c).
- One-third VAA are associated with non-visceral aneurysms, one-third are multiple.

Natural History

- Little is known about the natural history; some have been observed to remain stable or be slow growing on serial imaging.

Clinical Presentation

Many asymptomatic VAA are diagnosed incidentally on imaging; symptomatic aneurysms present with rupture or distal complications.

Rupture

- Rupture risk is up to 22% and rupture has a high reported mortality said to be as high as 90% for celiac axis, 50% for hepatic artery, and 36% for splenic artery. Mortality is likely to be highest in patients with significant co-morbidity, e.g., pancreatitis (Chapter 29) and in the post-operative period especially in patients with sepsis.

Transcatheter Embolization and Therapy,
Techniques in Interventional Radiology, DOI 10.1007/978-1-84800-897-7_39,
© Springer-Verlag London Limited 2010

- *Non-fatal rupture*: this has variable clinical manifestation depending on the site and severity of bleeding.
- Site of bleeding: hematemesis, hemobilia, hematochezia, bleeding from surgical drain.
- Severity of bleeding: hemodynamic compromise with abdominal pain indicates massive rupture.
- Herald bleeding: a small warning bleed is not uncommon; this can presage massive bleeding and is an indication for urgent intervention.
- Rupture into the portal vein results in arterio-portal fistula and severe portal hypertension.
- *End-organ complications*
- Ischemia (upper GIT ischemia, pancreatitis).
- Infarction secondary to distal embolization of thrombus.
- Abscess formation secondary to super infection of end-organ infarct.

Specific Sites

Splenic Artery

- Incidence of 0.78%
- Females > males in a 4:1 ratio
- 20% of patients have multiple aneurysms
- 70% are true aneurysms
- Etiology:

  1. Portal hypertension
  2. Inflammatory process – 10% of chronic pancreatitis
  3. Trauma
  4. Mycotic
  5. Other risk factors: essential hypertension, polyarteritis nodosa, fibrodysplasia, systemic lupus erythematosis, Ehlers–Danlos syndrome and neurofibromatosis
  6. Repeated pregnancies

Hepatic Artery

- Male > females in a 2:1 ratio
- Similar etiology to splenic arterial aneurysms, with >20% secondary to *trauma* or *iatrogenic* (surgery, percutaneous biopsy, liver transplant) causes
- 80% extra-hepatic location
- >50% false aneurysms
- Presentation: asymptomatic or non-specific pain
  Rupture – *Hepatobiliary tract*: hemobilia, jaundice, GI bleed
  Peritoneal cavity: abdominal pain, hypotension, abdominal distension

- Mortality rate of rupture >35%, which exceeds the mortality rate associated with splenic artery rupture

Celiac Artery

- Males = females
- Etiology: arteriosclerosis and medial degeneration, trauma, dissection, Takayasu's arteritis, syphilitic aneurysms (now uncommon)
- Lifetime risk of rupture of about 6%

Superior Mesenteric Artery

- Males = females
- Etiology: septic emboli in about one-third

Other causes: arteriosclerosis, dissection, polyarteritis nodosa, pancreatitis, biliary tract disease, neurofibromatosis, trauma

- Some SMA aneurysms are termed high-flow aneurysms and result from compromise of the celiac artery. In these situations, treating the underlying cause (the celiac axis stenosis) will usually cause the aneurysm to regress.
- Clinical manifestations: >90% are symptomatic, most commonly pain and gastrointestinal bleeding. Acute mesenteric ischemia may result from thromboembolism.
- Intervention is recommended for all patients.

Diagnostic Evaluation

Clinical

- Asymptomatic vs symptomatic
- Double-rupture phenomenon
- Risk factor for rupture – pregnancy
- Abdominal bruit on auscultation

Laboratory

- Anemia if ruptured, abnormal LFTs if biliary tract obstruction is secondary to hemobilia, raised amylase/white cell count/inflammatory markers if associated with pancreatitis.

Imaging

- *Plain film*: aneurysmal sac calcification can be identified within the right or left upper quadrant.
- *Ultrasound (US)*: echopoor fluid-like sac structure can be identified. Can be echogenic if the wall is calcified or isoechoic if there is thrombus within the sac. Associated conditions can be diagnosed (e.g., pancreatitis, abscess).
- *Color Doppler*: flow within the sac can be identified. Ying-Yang sign can be elicited in a pseudoaneurysm. Feeding and draining vessels can sometimes be identified.
- *MDCT and MDCTA*: better spatial resoultion has enabled accurate diagnosis of aneurysm location and morphology, the parent artery anatomy, potential etiology, and associated end-organ complications.
- *MRI and MRA*: aneurysm location and morphology can be determined; the parent artery anatomy, potential etiology, and associated end-organ complications can also be determined. Spatial resolution is not as good as CT.
- *DSA*: remains the gold standard. Enables treatment planning because afferent and efferent vessels can be identified, any vessels arising from the sac can be seen, and allows intervention at the same session.

Indications for Treatment

- Presentation: rupture is an emergency asymptomatic, incidentally diagnosed may need to be treated if criteria below are met.
- Size >2 cm is usually treated.
- Etiology: all pseudoaneurysms should be treated due to rupture risk; some true aneurysms have an indolent course and can be managed expectantly.
- Morphology: calcified wall does not confer protection from rupture.
- Location: will determine type of treatment undertaken.
- Number: increased number is associated with an increased rupture risk.
- Presence of end-organ complications: infarcts, ischemia, abscess formation, associated inflammation.
- Presence of high flow states:
- *Pregnancy* increases blood flow through the aneurysm and estrogens affect the elastic lamina of the wall, both increasing the risk of sac growth and rupture. Maternal death with rupture = 75%, fetal death = 95%.
- *Cirrhosis with portal hypertension*: associated with splenic arterial aneurysms, increasing the risk of rupture and death.
- *Liver transplantation*: risk of rupture 40–80%.

Contraindications to Treatment

- Size: <2 cm in asymptomatic, single, true aneurysm without associated high flow state/end-organ complications/inflammation is a relative contraindication for treatment. However, the decision regarding treatment should be made on an individual patient basis.

Relevant Anatomy

Normal Anatomy (≈ 50%)

- Celiac artery: arises from the anterior aspect of the abdominal aorta at T11/12, divides into splenic artery, common hepatic artery, and left gastric artery. Common hepatic bifurcates into the gastroduodenal artery and hepatic artery proper.
- Superior mesenteric artery: arises from the anterior aspect of the abdominal aorta at T12/L1.

Aberrant Anatomy (≈ 44% with One Arterial Variant, ≈ 6% with Two Arterial Variants)

- Celiac artery: replaced left hepatic artery arising from the left gastric artery; can have common origin with SMA; arises higher/lower from the aorta; hepatic and splenic arteries can arise directly from the abdominal aorta.
- Superior mesenteric artery: can have replaced/accessory right/left/common hepatic artery/gastroduodenal artery arising from the SMA.

Equipment

- *Catheters*: Non-selective: Pigtail, Omniflush; selective: Cobra, SosOmni, Sidewinder/Simmonds, Rim, Microcatheters.
- *Wires*: glidewire, hydrophilic, various microwires (0.014).
- *Coils*: detachable preferred (can be retrieved if operator not satisfied with resting position), pushable fibered coils. Microcoils may be needed.
- *Liquid embolics*: glue, Onyx.
- *Stent-grafts*: self expandable (Viabahn, Fluency, Atrium, Wallstent (stiffer, less flexible)); balloon expandable: more precise deployment (Jostent (coronary stent-graft, smaller sizes), Advanti, Iscat).

Medication

- Sedation and analgesia: intraprocedural intravenous sedation if required. May need analgesia and anti-emetic post-procedure to manage post-embolization syndrome. General anesthesia may be useful if using Onyx, which can be extremely painful.

- Anticoagulation: only necessary if using a stent-graft. Recommend aspirin for life and clopidegrol for 6 weeks – 3 months post-stenting (if stenting performed electively, can give anti-platelet agents pre-stenting).

Procedure

- *Access:* >90% from the common femoral artery. Remember the brachial approach if difficulty with celiac/SMA angulation.
- *Angiography:* flush aortogram, lateral position to determine origin of celiac/SMA or aberrant anatomy. Selective angiogram of parent artery to identify afferent/efferent/additional arteries feeding the aneurysmal sac.
- *Assessing the aneurysm:* location and size of the aneurysm are usually known from non-invasive angiographic imaging. Determine if the aneurysm occurs at a parent vessel origin/branch point. Angiographic appearance: saccular/fusiform, size of neck if saccular, parent vessel caliber/tortuosity/calcification.
- *Forming an embolization treatment plan:* goal is to completely exclude the aneurysm from the arterial circulation.
  - *Pack the sac*: with true, saccular, or narrow-necked aneurysms selective embolization of the sac with coils or glue until fully occluded. (Figure 39.2)
  - *Sandwich technique*: with true/pseudoaneurysm, saccular/fusiform aneurysm, exclude the aneurysm by coiling the afferent and efferent arteries (i.e., coil the "front and back door"). (Figure 39.1)
  - *Stent-graft*: with true/pseudoaneurysm, saccular/fusiform aneurysm, exclude the aneurysm with a covered stent. Ensure the parent vessel is of good caliber and non-tortorous, with an adequate proximal and distal artery for landing zones/guidewires/sheath/guidecath. Stent grafts are generally oversized by ≈20%.
  - *Combination*: use both the "pack the sac" and "sandwich" techniques, if feeding vessels supplying the sac/very large sac/failed coiling or if loss of access of efferent artery. (Figure 39.2)
  - *Balloon remodeling*: used to pack the sac with wider neck to prevent coil/glue protrusion. Microcatheter is placed into aneurysm and occlusion balloon inflated across the neck of the aneurysm. Aneurysm can be packed with coils to exclude parent artery or Onyx can be used to form a cast of the aneurysm. (Be careful to use a microcatheter compatible with Onyx as non-compatible microcatheters can disintegrate.)
  - *Balloon occlusion*: inflate balloon proximally to reduce flow in order to prevent distal coil migration during sandwich embolization.
- *Immediate post-procedure care:* vital signs and clinical observation for recurrent bleeding from the aneurysm. Arterial access site observation, analgesia, antiemetics, IV fluids for post-embolization syndrome. Image before discharge to detect sac re-perfusion – modality depends on site.
- *Long-term follow-up:* clinical evaluation, imaging if re-perfusion suspected, repeat embolization if rupture.

Results

- There are a number of reasonably sized series in the literature reporting outcome for endovascular therapy of visceral aneurysms.
- Technical success varies from 93 to 98%.
- Agents used are mainly coils (detachable and pushable), glue and more latterly, Onyx.
- Post-embolization syndrome occurred in 6–30%.
- Sac reperfusion occurred in 6–7% requiring reintervention.
- 8% periprocedural mortality reported in one series (from aneurysm rupture).

Alternative Therapies

- *Percutaneous thrombin injection*: if suitable anatomy (i.e., narrow neck, suitable location, clear and safe access route). Thrombin injection may be useful in splenic artery aneurysms associated with pancreatitis.

  After failed or partial endovascular embolization result
  > May deploy coils via percutaneous needle approach if thrombin alone fails.
  > Use US/CT/endoscopic US as image guidance methods
  > Potential complications: distal embolization via aneurysmal neck if wide.
  > Sac reperfusion via parent vessel or side branch feeders.

- *Surgery:* bypass with vein graft or prosthetic graft (prosthetic grafts have lower risk of occlusion than saphenous vein grafts).
  Direct aortic reimplantation of celiac or superior mesenteric artery for proximal aneurysms.
- *Conservative:* watchful waiting if small size (<2 cm), no possibility of pregnancy, true aneurysm, no end-organ complications, and no history of portal hypertension.

Specific Complications: Methods to Reduce Complications

- Rupture of aneurysm during embolization: avoid packing the sac of a pseudoaneurysm.
- End-organ infarction: try to preserve some end-organ blood supply.
- Abscess formation within infarcted tissue: prophylactic antibiotics.
- Post-embolization syndrome: antiemetics, analgesia, in fluids.
- Recurrence/reperfusion of sac: follow-up imaging to detect, embolize to complete stasis during first procedure.
- Stent-graft migration/kinking/occlusion/thrombosis: routine anticoagulation.
- Distal coil embolization: use long coil initially to form a nest.

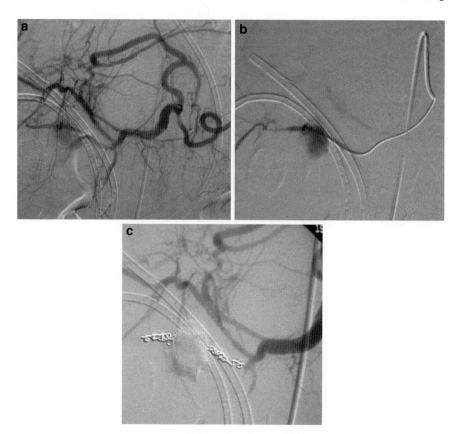

Fig. 39.1 A 71-year-old with painless obstructive jaundice secondary to a Klatskin tumor. Biliary drainage was performed. Hemobilia from the biliary drain necessitated blood transfusion. A DSA of the celiac artery demonstrated a large pseudoaneurysm arising from a right hepatic arterial branch. As the vessel was in a non-critical vascular territory, it was elected to embolize both the entry and exit arteries with coils, i.e., the sandwich technique, using a microcatheter. A repeat DSA demonstrated no contrast filling of the feeder artery or the pseudoaneurysm (Keeling, A.N., McGrath, F.P., Lee, M.J., Interventional Radiology in the Diagnosis, Management, and Follow-Up of Pseudoaneurysms, *Cardiovascular and Interventional Radiology* 2009; 32: 10)

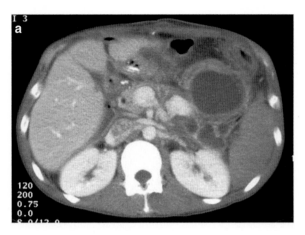

Fig. 39.2a A 42-year-old alcoholic with acute pancreatitis became septic and thus had a contrast-enhanced CT abdomen to identify any abscess formation. Of note there was a large abscess in the left upper quadrant. This was drained at the time of the CT examination. However, there was also a large splenic arterial pseudoaneurysm and an arterio-venous fistula between the splenic artery and vein. (Keeling, A.N., McGrath, F.P., Lee, M.J., Interventional Radiology in the Diagnosis, Management, and Follow-Up of Pseudoaneurysms, *Cardiovascular and Interventional Radiology* 2009; 32: 7)

Fig. 39.2b A DSA following coiling (coiling was performed after treatment of the local sepsis) of the pseudoaneurysm demonstrates no contrast filling of the pseudoaneurysm. Note also the drainage catheter within the large abscess cavity. (Keeling, A.N., McGrath, F.P., Lee, M.J., Interventional Radiology in the Diagnosis, Management, and Follow-Up of Pseudoaneurysms, *Cardiovascular and Interventional Radiology* 2009; 32: 7)

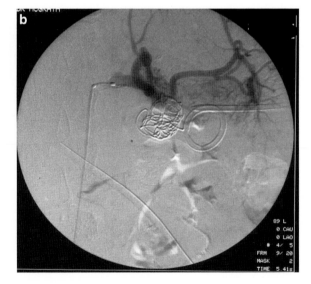

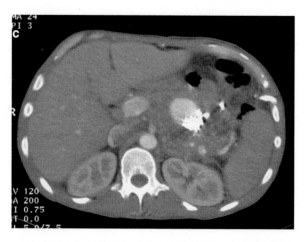

Fig. 39.2c A repeat contrast-enhanced CT abdomen 1 week later to check the abscess showed the coils within the pseudoaneurysm sac. However, there is an enlargement of the sac with marked contrast enhancement within it, indicating reperfusion (Keeling, A.N., McGrath, F.P., Lee, M.J., Interventional Radiology in the Diagnosis, Management, and Follow-Up of Pseudoaneurysms, *Cardiovascular and Interventional Radiology* 2009; 32: 7)

Fig. 39.2d A repeat DSA confirms the CT findings and demonstrates the sac filling with contrast material. (Keeling, A.N., McGrath, F.P., Lee, M.J., Interventional Radiology in the Diagnosis, Management, and Follow-Up of Pseudoaneurysms, *Cardiovascular and Interventional Radiology* 2009; 32: 7)

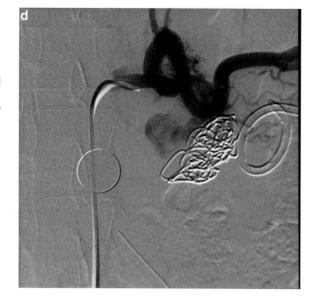

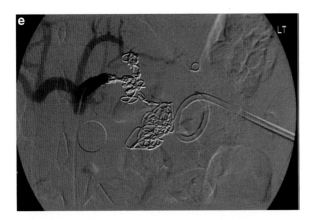

Fig. 39.2e The splenic artery proximal and distal to the neck of the psuedoaneurysm was coiled to exclude the pseudoaneurysm. A repeat DSA confirms no filling of the sac with contrast. The pseudoaneurysm did not recur on follow-up CT. (Keeling, A.N., McGrath, F.P., Lee, M.J., Interventional Radiology in the Diagnosis, Management, and Follow-Up of Pseudoaneurysms, *Cardiovascular and Interventional Radiology* 2009; 32: 7)

Keypoints

- High mortality from visceral arterial aneurysm rupture.
- Embolization is a valuable life-saving procedure.
- Non-invasive imaging is useful for treatment planning.
- Treat ruptures, pseudoaneurysms, true aneurysms >2 cm, high-risk patients – pregnancy, high flow states, transplants.
- Be aware of the different embolization techniques; consider combination techniques.
- Stent-grafts are quick to deploy – consider if ruptured.

Suggested Reading

Tulsyan N, Kashyap VS, Greenbery RK, Sarac TP, Clair DG, Pierce G, Ouriel K. The endovascular management of visceral artery aneurysms and pseudoaneurysms. J Vasc Surg 2007;45:276–283.

Sachdev U, Baril DT, Ellozy SH et al. Management of aneurysms involving branches of the celiac and superior mesenteric arteries: a comparison of surgical and endovascular therapy. J Vasc Surg 2006;44:718–724.

Saltzberg SS, Maldonado TS, Lamparello PJ et al. Is endovascular therapy the preferred treatment for all visceral artery aneurysms? Ann Vasc Surg 2005;19:507–515.

Carr SC, Pearce WH, Vogelzang RL, McCarthy WJ, Nemcek AA Jr, Yao JS. Current management of visceral artery aneurysms. Surgery 1996;120:627–633.

Chapter 40
Renal Artery Aneurysms

M.J. Lee

Clinical Features

- Renal artery aneurysms (RAA) are rare, accounting for 0.1% of visceral aneurysms.
- Sixty percent of patients are female, with the right kidney more often affected than the left.
- Sixty percent of RAA occur at the division of the renal artery; only 10% are intraparenchymal.
- 80% are saccular and 20% are fusiform.
- Causes include: fibro-muscular dysplasia, atherosclerosis, Ehler Danlos, Marfans, trauma/iatrogenic.
- Other causes of smaller aneurysms include: polyarteritis nodosa and amphetamine abuse.
- Aneurysms may also occur as part of angiomyolipoma.
- RAA is usually found incidentally and is often associated with hypertension.
- Rupture is the most feared complication. There is an increased risk of rupture in pregnancy with a greater than 70% maternal mortality and almost 100% fetal mortality.

Diagnostic Evaluation

Clinical

- Hypertension is commonly associated with RAA. Occasionally a bruit may be auscultated over the kidney.

Laboratory

- Renal function should be measured.

Transcatheter Embolization and Therapy,
Techniques in Interventional Radiology, DOI 10.1007/978-1-84800-897-7_40,
© Springer-Verlag London Limited 2010

Imaging

- Renal scintigraphy should be performed to document renal function as a base line.
- CT angiography is the best test to elucidate the location of the aneurysm and renal artery anatomy.
- If endovascular intervention is considered, angiography is useful to confirm CTA findings and determine the best obliquity to display the aneurysm in profile.

Treatment Indications

- Size greater than 2 cm in males or post-menopausal women.
- Local complications, such as dissection, distal embolization or rupture.
- Urological symptoms such as hematuria or pain.

All women of childbearing age with RAA irrespective of size. Some investigators recommend treatment of RAA in this population only if the size is greater than 1 cm

Contraindications

- These are relative as most RAA can be treated endovascularly, with novel embolic techniques.

Equipment

- Equipment will vary depending on the method of treatment, but may include some or all of the following:
  - 5Fr cobra catheter or sidewinder
  - 6Fr guiding catheter
  - Microcatheters and microwires
  - Detachable coils
  - Amplatzer vascular plugs
  - Detachable balloons
  - Onyx
  - Stents and stent grafts

Procedure

Access

- Access is usually through the groin, but occasionally may be from the arm.

Angiography

- A flush aortogram is only needed if CT has not delineated the number and location of the renal arteries.
- Selective angiography is then performed, with oblique or craniocaudad angulation as required to fully display the aneurysm in profile. This is one circumstance when rotational angiography can be helpful.
- Note: it is always worthwhile to perform angiography at a different session to plan for treatment or to treat in a staged fashion for complex lesions.

Assessing Lesions

- The location of the aneurysm with regard to the main renal artery, branch vessels, neck size (narrow or wide neck), and whether the lesion is intraparenchymal.
- For truly intraparenchymal lesions, it may be possible to sacrifice the portion of the kidney supplied by the artery containing in the aneurysm. This, however, is a rare occurrence.

Forming a Treatment Plan

- Numerous options are available depending on the location of the aneurysm, and whether it has a narrow neck or wide neck. Not all RAAs are suitable for endovascular treatment. If function is paramount and there are multiple branches arising from the aneurysm, surgical alternatives such as bench dissection should be considered.

Covered Stent

- Covered stents can be used if the RAA is arising from the main renal artery and there is a proximal and distal landing zone.
- Remember most aneurysms are at the bifurcation of the main renal artery and therefore use of a covered stent will involve sacrifice of renal tissue.

Balloon Remodeling

- This requires two vascular access points or use of a sheath/guide catheter able to accommodate two separate catheter systems.
- Balloon remodeling can be used if the RAA has a wide neck, which increases the risk of coil extrusion.
- A microcatheter is first placed into the RAA and a separate angioplasty balloon inflated across the neck of the RAA.

- Using the balloon as a buttress the RAA can be coiled, preferable with detachable coils until completely occluded. The balloon is then deflated and the balloon and microcatheter removed.
- More than one modelling balloon may be necessary to protect the renal circulation in complex aneurysms or when using polymers such as Onyx.

Bare Stent Assisted

- Stent-assisted coiling involves placement of a stent across an aneurysm neck, and subsequent coil embolization through a microcatheter that is placed through the interstices of the stent. The stent then keeps the coils from migrating back into the feeding artery.
- Stent-assisted coiling can be used for bifurcation aneurysms, where there is a risk of non-target embolization of adjacent branch arteries.
- Stents for neurointervention are preferred as they are quite flexible and have a loosely woven mesh.
- Stents include the Neuroform stent (Boston Scientific), the Leo Stent (Pyramed), the Enterprise Stent (Cordis), and the Solitaire Stent (EV3).
- Note: the Solitaire Stent is the only stent that is detachable, which means that it can be either left permanently in situ or removed at the end of the coiling procedure.

Primary Coiling

- Primary coiling is suitable for many RAA.
- Generally, if the neck of the aneurysm is less than 50% of the maximum diameter of the aneurysm, primary coiling is often feasible.
- Detachable coils are preferred for control.
- A large framing coil is first inserted, with placement of additional coils until the aneurysm is packed completely. The coil sizes can be reduced as the RAA fills with coils.
- Consider using a hydrogel coil for the neck of the aneurysm (Hydrogel coils swell to three to four times their normal size and are useful for occluding the neck of the aneurysms.).

Performing the Embolization

- Remember that RAAs are often complex aneurysms, and decisions should be made by a multidisciplinary team that includes experienced Transplant Urology, Nephrology, and IR services.

- Individual decisions are required for each patient because of the differing sizes and locations of RAA.
- Once decided on a treatment plan, take your time and carry it out with care.
- Do not be afraid to call for help, if needed.

Embolization Endpoint

- The embolization procedure is complete when the entire aneurysm is excluded including the neck. If the neck is not adequately embolized, there is a significant risk of recanalization of the aneurysm.

Immediate Post-procedure Care

- Care is similar to all angioplasty procedures.
- Serum creatine is obtained after 24 h.

Long-Term Follow-Up

- Follow-up imaging can be difficult depending on the embolic agent used.
- If coils are used, they will often cause an acoustic shadow on ultrasound, making it difficult to accurately visualize flow within the aneurysm.
- Similarly for MRA, coils can cause artifact making aneurysm assessment difficult.
- Angiography is the most useful modality to exclude any reperfusion of the RAA. Follow-up angiography is typically performed at 6-months. If the aneurysm remains excluded on angiography at 6 months, follow-up with ultrasound, CTA, or MRA can be performed at yearly intervals for up to 5 years.

Results

- Published results for endovascular aneurysm repair are limited as this is a rare aneurysm.
- More and more small series using novel embolization techniques are appearing in the literature.

Alternative Therapies

- Imaging follow-up is used for aneurysms that are under 2 cm in size in males or post-menopausal women.
- A number of surgical options are available including the following.

In Vivo Aneurysmectomy

- This implies operating on the kidney in situ, with resection of the aneurysm and either primary closure, patch angioplasty, or RAA resection with the placement of a graft.

Ex Vivo Resection and Autotransplant

- Ex vivo resection implies removing the kidney and performing bench surgery to remove the aneurysm and autotransplanting the kidney to the iliac artery.

Nephrectomy

- Either partial or total nephrectomies can be performed.
- The largest surgical series of 252 RAA in 168 patients had a total nephrectomy rate of 28% (25 planned nephrectomies and 8 unplanned nephrectomies).
  - During a mean follow-up over 91 months, there were two graft failures and a 60% significant decrease in blood pressure.
- Endovascular treatments are usually preferable where renal tissue can be sacrificed.

Complications

- Complications mainly relate to non-target embolization.
- These can be avoided by meticulous attention to detail and careful treatment planning.
- Considerable experience is necessary for treating complex RAA.

Keypoints

- The management plan should be made in consultation with the patient. All relevant clinical staff should be involved in the decision-making process (interventional radiologists, vascular surgeons, nephrologists, physicians, and sometimes obstetricians) usually in the context of a multidisciplinary team meeting.
- High-quality pre-procedural imaging is important for embolization planning.

- Angiography separate to the embolization procedure may be necessary for complex aneurysms.
- Choose a treatment plan appropriate to the aneurysm.
- Do not forget to totally exclude the neck of the aneurysm.
- Call for help or refer if uncomfortable (Figs. 40.1, 40.2, 40.3, and 40.4)

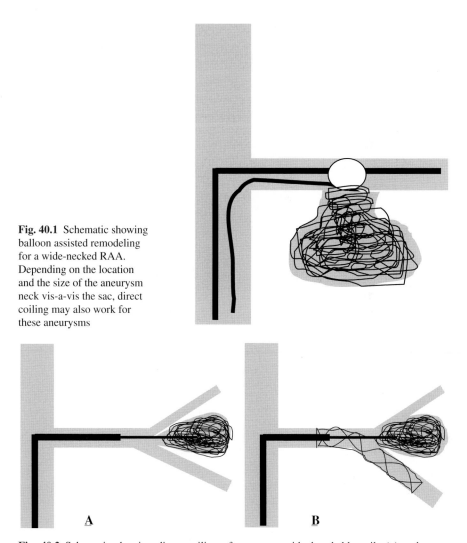

Fig. 40.1 Schematic showing balloon assisted remodeling for a wide-necked RAA. Depending on the location and the size of the aneurysm neck vis-a-vis the sac, direct coiling may also work for these aneurysms

A

B

Fig. 40.2 Schematic showing direct coiling of aneurysm with detachable coils (**a**) and stent-assisted coiling (**b**)

Fig. 40.3 Sixty-four-year-old female with incidentally discovered 2.7-cm RAA on a background of FMD (**a**). Proximal and distal landing zones were adequate for a covered stent. (**b**) A Gore Viabahn-covered stent (6 mm tapering to 4 mm distally) was placed to exclude the RAA

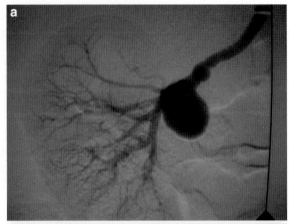

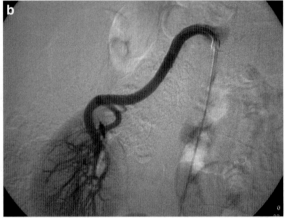

Fig. 40.4 Forty-four-year-old
female with FMD and
incidentally discovered RAA.
The RAA measured 3.2 cm
and the neck 1.3 cm. Note
that it also is arising at a
trifurcation. (**a**) Coiling using
a microcatheter was
performed and the aneurysm
packed and excluded with
detachable coils; (**b**) 6-month
follow-up angiogram was
stable

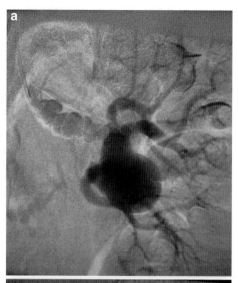

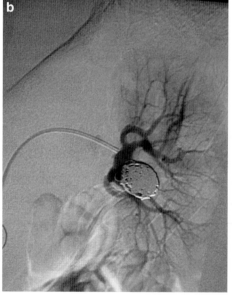

Suggested Reading

Abath C, Andrade G, Cavalcanti D, Brito N, Marques R. Complex renal artery aneurysms: Liquids or coils? Tech Vasc Intervent Radiol 2007;10:299–307.

Bastounis E, Pikoulis E, Georgopoulos S, Alexion D, Leppaniemi A, Boulafendis D. Surgery for renal artery aneurysms: A combined series of two large centers. Eur Urol 1998;33:22–27.

Garg N, Pipinos II, Longo M, Thorell WE, Lynch TG, Johanning JM. Detachaable coils for repair of extraparenchymal renal artery aneurysms: An alternative to surgical therapy. Ann Vasc Surg 2007;21:97–110.

Hislop SJ, Patel SA, Abt PL, Singh MJ, Illig KA. Therapy of renal artery aneurysms in New York State: Outcomes of patients undergoing open and endovascular repair. Ann Vasc Surg 2009;23:194–200.

Manninen HI, Berg M, Vanninen RL. Stent-assisted coil embolisation of wide-necked renal artery bifurcation aneurysms. J Vasc Radiol 2008;19:487–492.

Nosher JL, Chung J, Brevetti LS, Graham AM, Siegel RL. Visceral and renal artery aneurysms: A pictorial essay on endovascular therapy. Radiographics 2006;26:1687–1704.

Chapter 41
Pre-operative Portal Vein Embolization

Trevor Cleveland

Pre-operative Portal Vein Embolization

Clinical Features

- The most common indications for the procedure are localized metastatic liver invasion or primary liver tumor.
- Portal vein embolization is performed in patients undergoing liver resection in whom the residual liver volume will not provide sufficient function (Fig. 41.1).
- This may be because the remaining (usually the left) lobe of the liver is small or because the resection needs to be extensive (extended hepatectomy).
- The intention of embolization is to divert portal venous blood flow from the liver to be resected into the segment that will remain following resection.
- This increased perfusion carries growth factors and hormones, stimulating the residual liver to hypertrophy.
- The lobe containing the cancer will be the one embolized.
- The procedure is performed 4 to 6 weeks prior to the definitive liver resection to allow hypertrophy.

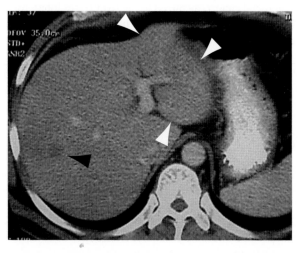

Fig. 41.1 CT showing tumor in right lobe of liver (*black arrowhead*) and small left lobe of the liver (*white arrowheads*)

Transcatheter Embolization and Therapy,
Techniques in Interventional Radiology, DOI 10.1007/978-1-84800-897-7_41,
© Springer-Verlag London Limited 2010

Diagnostic Evaluation

Laboratory

- The procedure is performed transhepatically; hence, all patients should have their clotting status checked and corrected prior to embolization.
- Renal function with conventional renoprotection if indicated.

Imaging

Use contrast-enhanced CT and or MRI to

- Identify the location of the diseased segment/s
- Assess the size and location of the liver that will remain following the planned surgery
- Demonstrate patency of the portal venous system
- Plan the likely approach for percutaneous access
- Assess for ascites
- Identify any evidence of other distant metastatic disease. This is essential as new disease is common in this group of patients, and may preclude the surgery making portal vein embolization contraindicated.

Indications

- Metastatic colorectal cancer, localized to the liver (right lobe), for which surgical resection is planned. This procedure is indicated if the remaining segment/s of the liver are judged to be insufficient in size to be compatible with survival in the post-operative period.
- Primary liver tumor, for which resection is planned, when the remaining liver is considered to be inadequate.

Contraindications

- Metastatic disease outside the liver – this is a contraindication to resection.
- Sufficient healthy liver to sustain function following the planned resection.
- Ascites: as with any transhepatic procedure, this is not an absolute contraindication; the ascites can be drained. The etiology must be considered as
  - Embolization will exacerbate portal hypertension
  - Portal vein occlusion is a contraindication to surgery
  - Malignant ascites is a contraindication to surgery

- Severely deranged clotting: this indicates that there is already insufficient synthetic hepatic function.

Specific Complications

Embolic material should not be introduced into segments that are to be retained. This may become difficult as the flow to the lobe for embolization becomes slow as embolization progresses. If glue or particles are injected into the incorrect lobe, there is little that can be done to reverse this. Coils can be retrieved using a snare.

Anatomy

- The segmental anatomy of the liver and portal vein variations should be understood.
- The confines of the planned resection should be discussed with the referring surgeon.
- The pre-procedural imaging should be used to plan the extent of the portal venous system for embolization.
- The portal venous system will be accessed percutaneously. The position and size of the hepatic lobes, the portal veins, and the diseased liver should all be ascertained from the pre-procedural imaging.
- Metastases are almost always situated in the right lobe of the liver, and the left lobe will be small (otherwise pre-operative portal vein embolization will not be necessary). The relationship of the liver, the rib cage, and the pleura should be considered, from the perspective of percutaneous access.

Equipment

- Ultrasound of sufficient quality to visualize the portal vein and needle.
- A micro-puncture set.

Catheters

- 4–5F vascular sheath with radiopaque tip. The sheath must be long enough to reach and be stable in the portal branch (Fig. 41.2).
- Selective catheters with and without side holes for portal venography and portal vein catheterization and embolization.
  o Contralateral lobe puncture: Berenstein, Cobra, Headhunter, multi-purpose
  o Ipsilateral lobe access: Sidewinder/Simmonds, SosOmni (Fig. 41.3)
- If using glue, ensure that the catheter hub is not polycarbonate.

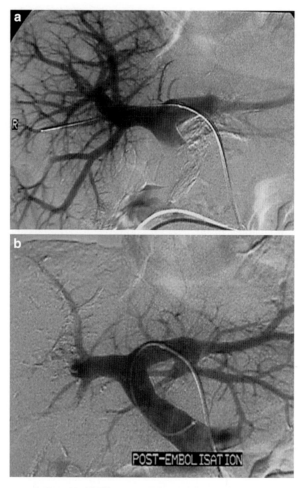

Fig. 41.2 (**a**) Portal venogram obtained via sheath inserted into left portal vein. The majority of flow enters the larger right lobe. Left portal vein puncture allows ready access to all right liver segments. (**b**) Completion venogram post-embolization shows blood flow directed into the left lobe of the liver with no flow into the periphery of the right lobe

Embolic Agents

The intention of the embolization is to completely stop flow in the portal vein to the segments that are to be removed. This diverts blood flow (containing growth factors and hormones) to the remaining liver, stimulating it to hypertrophy.

- *Cyanoacrylate glue*: it is the preferred agent. Portal vein embolization is a relatively safe procedure and is a good opportunity to learn how to use glue.

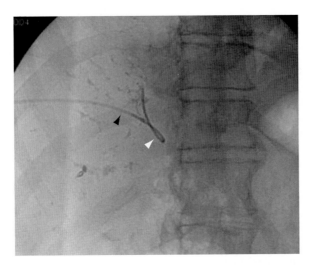

Fig. 41.3 Coil embolization of the access segment (*white arrowhead*) as the catheter (*black arrowhead*) is withdrawn

- o Glue is effective, efficient, and low cost in Europe (although expensive in the United States) (Fig. 41.4).
- o Cyanoacrylate glue should be mixed with Lipiodol (proportions 1:2.5).
- o 5% Dextrose solution is needed to flush catheters and to prevent pre-mature setting of the glue.

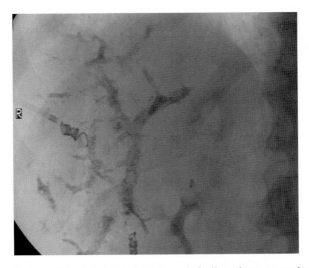

Fig. 41.4 Embolization of the right lobe of the liver via ipsilateral puncture using a sidewinder catheter

Alternatives Include

- *Particulate materials*: Gelfoam and PVA may be used for embolization. The volume to be embolized is large, so large particles should be used. Remember that Gelfoam is a temporary agent and must be combined with coils.
- *Coils:* these are often combined with Gelfoam to ensure permanent occlusion.
- *Amplatzer vascular plugs:* these are relatively expensive, and may require a fairly large-diameter delivery device.

Medications

- *Sedation and systemic analgesia:* access for this procedure may be painful, and a benzodiazepine (such as midazolam) and opiate should be administered. There is usually little pain following the procedure.
- *Local anaesthesia* is used for the percutaneous access.

Angiography

Access

The access point is chosen according to the segments to be embolized based on the planned resection and pre-procedural imaging.

- The patient is positioned in an angiographic suite, with their right arm above their head.
- Use ultrasound to image the target portal access site and target the percutaneous puncture.
- The puncture may be made either in the lobe to be preserved or in the lobe to be resected.
- The vascular sheath is positioned in the portal venous branch. Once this has been achieved, it is often helpful to suture the sheath in place.

Angiography

- A portal venogram should be performed by passing a catheter with side holes into the main portal vein, followed by a hand injection of contrast (Fig. 41.2).
- It is essential to identify the portal venous anatomy with certainty.
- AP and oblique projections may be necessary.
- Comparison with multi-planar reformats of CT/MR images may help with orientation.

Clinical Scenarios

Treatment Plan and Technique

The most common scenario is embolization of the right portal vein.

- If possible, a route is selected to access the portal vein in the left lobe of the liver. This has the advantage of embolization being in the direction of flow in the portal vein.
- Left-lobe puncture may be impossible, if the lobe is small.
- The right lobe of the liver may be used. Some surgeons prefer that the lobe being preserved *not* be used for the embolization. If the right lobe is accessed, then
  - o Embolization of the punctured vein will be "against the flow". Care must be taken not to glue the catheter/sheath in the liver.
  - o Care should be paid to avoiding access through a diseased area to avoid the risk of tumor seeding.
- Percutaneous access is performed under ultrasound control using a micro-access set.
- The vascular sheath is positioned with the radiopaque tip visible in the portal venous branch. Once this has been achieved, it is often helpful to suture the sheath in place.
- Portal venography is performed (Fig. 41.2).
- A simple curved catheter without side holes can be used for selective catheterization and embolization of the target right-lobe portal vein branches.
- If glue is being used, when in position in the target branch:
  - o The catheters and syringes should all be flushed with 5% dextrose solution.
  - o Inject small aliquots of the glue mixture (0.25–0.5 ml or less) under fluoroscopic guidance until near stasis is achieved.
  - o Remember that the catheter contains a "reservoir" of glue which should either be aspirated or carefully flushed through with the dextrose solution.
  - o Repeat this procedure for each branch to be embolized.
  - o Perform check-venography to demonstrate satisfactory (complete) occlusion.
- The access track should be embolized (using a Gelfoam pledget or a coil) when the access sheath is removed (Fig. 41.3).

Additional Considerations

- If the same lobe has been accessed as for embolization, then more complex-shaped catheters (Fig. 41.4) will probably be needed for selective segmental catheterization (e.g., Sidewinder/Simmonds, SosOmni).
- If the segment used for access requires embolization, then great care should be taken with glue, to avoid gluing the access sheath into the liver. It may be more suitable to use particles and/or coils for this final segment (Fig. 41.3).

Aftercare

- As with any transhepatic procedure, pulse and blood pressure should be recorded for 24 h in case of bleeding.
- Pain after the procedure is completed is usually minimal, as the embolized liver segments retain their hepatic arterial supply, and so cellular ischemia/necrosis does not occur.

Follow-Up

CT/MRI should be performed 4–5 weeks after the embolization. This can be used for the following:
- Assess the success of the embolization (by comparison with the pre-procedural images).
- Assess the increase in liver volume. This will influence the timing of the definitive hepatic resection (Fig. 41.5).
- Look for development of new disease in the hypertrophied lobe and outside the liver.

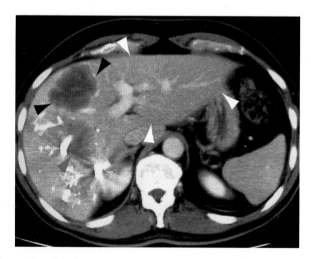

Fig. 41.5 CT scan 5 weeks after embolization with glue (same patient as in Fig. 41.1). The left lobe of the liver has enlarged (*white arrowheads*). Glue and Lipiodol are seen in the right lobe (*yellow arrows*), the original lesion has enlarged (*red arrowhead* – compare with Fig. 41.1) and a new metastatic deposit (*black arrowheads*) is seen

Keypoints

- Portal vein embolization is performed on one hepatic lobe to stimulate hypertrophy of the other.
- Portal vein embolization does not cause hepatocellular death.
- Pre-operative imaging with CT or MRI is vital to planning.
- Small left hepatic lobes may be difficult to access percutaneously.
- Glue is a cheap (in Europe) and effective agent for embolization.
- Post-operative imaging should be performed 4–5 weeks after embolization to plan the timing of liver resection.

Suggested Reading

1. Lochan R. Pre Operative Portal Vein Embolisation for Primary and Secondary Liver Tumours. Cochrane Review 2008.
2. Abulkahir A; Limongelli P; Healey A; Damrah O; Tait P; Jackson J; Habib N; Jiao L. Preoperative Portal Vein Embolization for Major Liver Resection: A Meta-Analysis. Ann surg. 2008; 247(1): 49–57
3. Hemming A, Reed I, Howard R, Fujita S, Hochwald S, Caridi J, Hawkins I, Vauthey J-N. Preoperative Portal Vein Embolization for Extended Hepatectomy. Ann Surg. 2003; 237(5): 686–693
4. Di Stefano D, de Baere T, Denys A, Hakime A, Gorin G, Gillet M, Saric J, Trillaud H, Petit P, Bartoli J-M, Elias D, Delpero J-M. Preoperative Percutaneous Portal Vein Embolization: Evaluation of Adverse Events in 188 Patients. Radiology 2005; 234: 625–630
5. Gallego C, Velasco M, Marcuello P, Tejedor D, De Campo L, Friera A. Congenital and Acquired Anomalies of the Portal Venous System RadioGraphics 2002; 22: 141–159.
6. Madoff DC, Hicks ME, Vauthey J-N, Charnsangavej C, Morello FA, Ahrar K, Wallace MJ, Gupta S. Transhepatic Portal Vein Embolization: Anatomy, Indications, and Technical Considerations. RadioGraphics 2002; 22: 1063–1076

Chapter 42
Epistaxis

Anthie M. Papadopoulou and Andrew Platts

Definition: epistaxis is defined as acute hemorrhage from the nostril, nasal cavity, or nasopharynx.

Clinical Features

- Most epistaxis is self-limiting; patients tend to present if bleeding is prolonged, heavy, or repeated.
- Severe epistaxis can be life threatening due to airway compromise and blood loss.
- Spontaneous idiopathic epistaxis accounts for approximately 80% of cases.
- Risk factors include smoking, hypertension, atherosclerotic disease, coagulopathy/thrombocytopenia, and oral anticoagulant/antiplatelet agent use.
- Unusual causes of epistaxis include hereditary hemorrhagic telangiectasia, internal carotid artery aneurysm, vascular malformations, trauma, and post-surgical complications, tumors such as juvenile nasal angiofibroma, solitary fibrous tumor of the nasopharynx, and carcinoma of the nose and throat.
- Less than 10% of patients require treatment, and the vast majority of these will be successfully treated by an emergency physician.
- Epistaxis is classified according to anatomic location—anterior and posterior.
  - Anterior hemorrhage is most common; posterior hemorrhage tends to be more severe.

Diagnostic Evaluation

Nasal Endoscopy

- This is performed to define the location of bleeding as well as to rule out predisposing factors such as telangiectasias or neoplasm.

Transcatheter Embolization and Therapy,
Techniques in Interventional Radiology, DOI 10.1007/978-1-84800-897-7_42,
© Springer-Verlag London Limited 2010

Imaging

- Radiologic assessment is not routinely required and should be tailored to the clinical situation.
- Cross-sectional imaging with CT and MR is usually reserved for cases where a neoplasm, trauma, or post-surgery is the suspected cause of bleeding.
- Angiography is usually only performed in the context of intervention.

Laboratory

This should not delay treatment of massive epistaxis. Some laboratory investigations will have been performed as part of the diagnostic pathway to determine the cause and severity of the epistaxis.

- *Coagulation profile.* If there is life-threatening hemorrhage, then coagulation status and platelet count must be closely monitored to evaluate for disseminated intravascular coagulopathy. Coagulation disorders may be the underlying cause, and abnormalities will be exacerbated by fluid replacement and blood transfusion. Appropriate measures should be aggressively instituted to correct coagulopathy.

Management of Epistaxis

The severity and location of the bleeding as well as any predisposing and underlying factors determine the subsequent treatment approach.

Initial Therapy

- Airway management and resuscitation.
- Nasal packing and chemical or electrocautery are usually successful if the source of bleeding is from the anterior septal area. Packing is first-line therapy for posterior epistaxis; the use of an epistaxis balloon as an alternative form of tamponade is also widely advocated.
- Transantral surgical ligation of the internal maxillary artery (IMA).
- Transnasal endoscopic sphenopalatine artery ligation (TESPAL).

Indications for Embolization

- Definitive therapy for severe intractable epistaxis refractory to chemical/electrocautery, and anterior and posterior packing/balloon tamponade.
- Definitive therapy for post-traumatic pseudoaneurysms resulting in epistaxis.
- Pre-operative embolization of juvenile nasal angiofibroma and other tumors (Fig. 42.1) can improve visualization of the surgical field and result in a more complete and uncomplicated resection. Recent advances in transnasal endoscopic resection techniques rely on pre-operative embotherapy to reduce intraoperative blood loss.

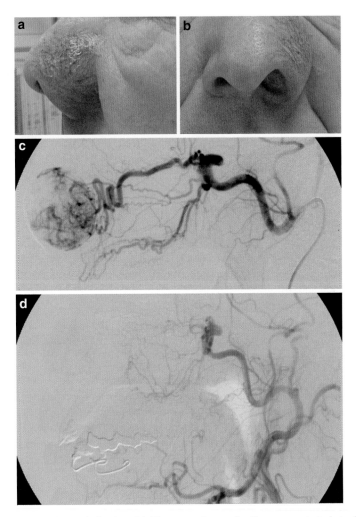

Fig. 42.1 Pre-operative embolization. (**a**) Hypervascular renal cell cancer metastasis to the lateral nasal wall. (**b**) Selective catheterization of the internal maxillary artery showing tumor supply (**c**) following superselective embolization of multiple feeding branched with 300–500 μ PVA, the tumor circulation is obliterated. The patient subsequently underwent resection without blood loss. (Courtesy Dr David O. Kessel and Dr Jai Patel)

Contraindications

These are relative in massive life-threatening epistaxis.

- True allergy to iodinated contrast is a relative contraindication to angiography. Gadolinium chelates may be considered as an alternative.
- Other contraindications (such as renal insufficiency) are relative.

Specific Complications

The patient must be aware of and consented for the following:

- Significant rates of recurrence (up to 25%).
- Frequent post-procedure complications include facial pain and numbness, which are often self-limiting. Skin sloughing and hard palate necrosis have also been reported as an uncommon complication.
- Major complications include stroke and blindness.

Anatomy

Normal Anatomy

- The arterial supply to the nasal fossa is complex, involving branches from both the internal and external carotid arteries. Multiple anastomoses are also present (Fig. 42.2a and b).
- External carotid artery (ECA) supply
  - Sphenopalatine and greater palatine arteries from the IMA.
  - Septal branch of the superior labial artery, arising from the facial artery.
- Internal carotid artery (ICA) supply
  - Anterior and posterior ethmoidal branches of the ophthalmic artery.
- *Knowledge of the potentially dangerous anastomoses around the skull base is mandatory.* These may allow embolic material to pass from the extracranial circulation to the intracranial circulation during embolization resulting in stroke or blindness. These anastomoses involve the inferolateral trunk, ethmoidal collaterals, meningo-hypophyseal arteries, and occipital-vertebral arteries.

Aberrant Anatomy

- The commonest anomalous origin of the ophthalmic artery is from the middle meningeal artery, which occurs in about 1% of cases.
- The infraorbital artery, a branch of the pterygopalatine segment of the internal maxillary artery, has been shown to contribute to the nasal mucosal supply.

Equipment

Catheters

- *Non-selective catheters:* a pigtail catheter is sometimes needed for arch aortography.

Fig. 42.2 Arterial supply of
(**a**) the lateral and (**b**) the
medial nasal walls (courtesy
of Dr J M Harris)

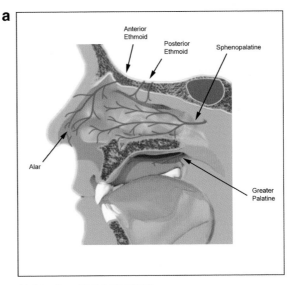

Arterial anatomy of the lateral nasal wall

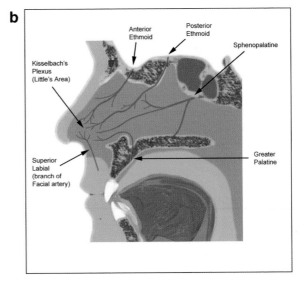

Arterial anatomy of the medial nasal wall

- *Selective catheters:* Vertebral, sidewinder II, microcatheter with a 30–45° curve, guidewire with 30–45° curve.
- *Guide catheter:* 6Fr with a 0.067″ lumen. This allows guiding contrast injections as well as continuous flushing with heparinized saline from a pressurized bag to prevent clot formation.
- *C-arm angiographic equipment with road map capability.*

Embolic Agents

The choice of agent depends on the clinical context and angiographic findings.

- Polyvinyl alcohol (PVA) particles (250–300 μm).
- Gelfoam slurry/pledgets.
- Coils can be used successfully in cases when the bleeding source correlates with a focal arterial anomaly on diagnostic angiography, and superselective single vessel embolization is possible (e.g., trauma resulting in epistaxis). Coils are not recommended for proximal embolization in spontaneous epistaxis because they make the distal vessel inaccessible in cases of recurrent bleeding.
- Liquid embolic agents (cyanoacrylate or Onyx^{TM}) may be used, but there is increased risk of non-target embolization.

Medication

- *General anaesthesia:* is necessary in cases of airway compromise, and in children and poorly compliant patients.
- *Analgesia:* intravenous opiates in combination with sedatives such as benzodiazepines are usually administered peri- and intraprocedurally. Anti-inflammatory analgesics are often necessary after the procedure, as patients often report temporofacial pain.
- *Antibiotics:* penicillin/cephalosporin if nasal packing is present.
- *Heparin:* this sounds paradoxical during an embolization procedure but is necessary to prevent pericatheter thrombus formation with the risk of cerebral embolization and stroke. The patient is given a 5000 IU bolus, with 1000 IU per hour thereafter during the embolization procedure. If available, an activated clotting time (ACT) should be used to control heparinization—the objective being to achieve and maintain a doubling of the baseline reading.

Angiography

Access

- Common femoral artery.

Angiography

- Complete ECA angiography is imperative because bleeding can originate from unsuspected sites such as the accessory meningeal artery or the infraorbital artery, intracranial, and ophthalmic artery anastomoses are also identified.
- The most useful angiographic view of the ECA is the lateral view, which profiles nearly all vessels. However, distal portions of the IMA are best demonstrated on a frontal view.

- Selective views of ECA branches are also mandatory before embolotherapy.
- ICA angiography is imperative. Although rare, aneurysms of the ICA can present with epistaxis. In addition, demonstration of ICA anatomy prior to embolization is important because of the presence of ECA-to-ICA anastomoses and demonstration of the supply to the ophthalmic artery. Remember that these anastomoses may enlarge in the presence of ICA occlusion.

Angiographic Appearance

- Diffuse, bilateral mucosal hypervascularity with early venous opacification is the most common finding in patients with intractable epistaxis. The actual bleeding site is rarely visualized, particularly in patients who have packing in place.
- Juvenile nasal angiofibroma is demonstrated as a hypervascular mass. The blood supply initially originates from the ipsilateral IMA, but as the tumor grows, supply is recruited from other arteries including the contralateral IMA, the ascending pharyngeal, and ICA branches, as well as other sites such as spinal and occipital arteries.
- Pseudoaneurysms of the ICA and vascular malformations resulting in epistaxis can be demonstrated.
- In epistaxis following trauma, direct vessel injury is usually demonstrated and may consist of vessel laceration/transection or vessel irregularity. Pseudoaneurysms, contrast extravasation, or arteriovenous fistula formation are also possible findings on angiography.

Clinical Scenarios

The treatment plan and embolic agent used depend on the indication, the cause, and location of bleeding, as well as the angiographic findings.

Treatment Plan and Technique

- Nasal packing with radiopaque materials such as bismuth iodophore paste (BIPP)-drenched swabs should be replaced with non-opaque material prior to angiography.

Spontaneous Epistaxis

- The nose should be packed with radiolucent material during the procedure and unpacked at the end.
- The purpose of the procedure is not to achieve complete devascularization but to decrease arterial inflow pressure to allow clotting and epithelial repair.

- Most commonly, the precise site of bleeding is not known. Bilateral IMA embolization with particles is necessary in such cases because of the side-to-side anastomoses that can be recruited to the bleeding nasal mucosa. The microcatheter should be advanced distal to branches with high potential for dangerous anastomosis collaterals such as the middle meningeal, accessory meningeal, and superficial temporal arteries to avoid non-target embolization.
- For patients with an anterior source of bleeding, particle embolization of the nasal branches of the facial artery should also be performed carefully so that the distal supply of the terminal alar artery, which supplies the skin of the nasal ala, is preserved.
- Catheter-induced vasospasm is a common occurrence with superselective catheterization of ECA branches. This significantly alters flow distally, even to the point of stasis. Gentle microcatheter manipulation and minimal guidewire manipulation can minimize vasospasm. Glycerine trinitrate (GTN 50–500 µg) can be administered to treat vasospasm after the catheter has been retracted proximal to the point of vasospasm.
- Liquid embolic agents (NBCA, Onyx^{TM}) are not recommended for use routinely because of the risk of non-target embolization or tissue necrosis. Their use has been advocated in rare cases where a focal angiographic abnormality or extravasation is demonstrated but the feeding vessel cannot be catheterized.

Juvenile Nasal Angiofibroma

- PVA particles are the agent of choice in the pre-operative embolization of juvenile nasal angiofibroma.
- The goal is to obliterate the capillary bed while preserving normal tissue.

Hereditary Hemorrhagic Telangiectasia

- Approach similar to that for spontaneous epistaxis with bilateral IMA embolization.
- There is a higher recurrence rate and need for re-intervention.

Trauma Including Traumatic Pseudoaneurysms

- Coils or covered stents may be used in the case of pseudoaneurysms.

Aftercare

Arterial Puncture Site

- A closure device is useful when the patient has been anti-coagulated during the procedure.

Post-embolization

- No specific care is needed.
- Do not forget the following:
  - o To continue resuscitation/transfusion as necessary
  - o To manage risk factors
  - o That rebleeding is common

Follow-Up

No routine follow-up needed.

Keypoints

- Epistaxis can result from a multitude of causes, the commonest being the spontaneous or idiopathic form.
- Embolotherapy in the management of spontaneous epistaxis is reserved for cases refractory to topical or conservative measures.
- Embolotherapy is essential prior to some endoscopic tumor resection procedures.

Safety

- Knowledge of the arterial anatomy, the angiographic and embolization technique, and potential complications and how to avoid these are imperative for ensuring a good outcome.

Bibliography

Gifford TO, Capt MC, Orlandi, RR. Epistaxis. Otolaryngol Clin N Am 2008; 41: 525–536.
Mahadevia AA, Murphy KJ, Obray R, Gailloud P. Embolization for intractable epistaxis. Tech Vasc Interventional Rad 2005; 8:134–138.
Nguyen QA. Epistaxis eMedicine http://www.emedicine.com/ent/TOPIC701.HTM
Smith T. Embolization in the external carotid artery. J Vasc Interv Radiol 2006; 17:1897–1913.

Chapter 43
Meningiomas and Paragangliomas

H.L.D. Makalanda and Andrew Platts

Clinical Features

- Meningiomas are extra-axial brain tumors derived from arachnoid cells of neural crest origin. They comprise 20% of primary intra-cranial tumors and are more common in older patients and women (M:F = 2:1). They also have some syndromal associations.
- Paragangliomas (glomus tumors) arise from neural crest cells and typically arise at four locations and are as follows:
  - Carotid body (caroticum)
  - Jugular foramen of the temporal bone (jugulare)
  - Tympanic plexus (tympanicum)
  - Vagal nerve (vagale)
    - They are slow growing and most frequently found in women of the fifth and sixth decade.
    - May be multifocal in as many as 22% of patients.
- The optimal treatment for these tumors is complete resection where possible. Pre-operative embolization reduces operative time and intra-operative blood loss when resecting these vascular tumors. It provides a particularly useful adjunct when the tumors exhibit hypervascularity or when they encase vital structures.

Diagnostic Evaluation

Laboratory

As for any angiographic examination (e.g., clotting and renal profiles).

Transcatheter Embolization and Therapy,
Techniques in Interventional Radiology, DOI 10.1007/978-1-84800-897-7_43,
© Springer-Verlag London Limited 2010

Imaging

- Never start embolization until you have formally reviewed the pre-procedure imaging.
- Use contrast-enhanced CT/MRI with multi-planar reformats to
  o Establish diagnosis (differential diagnosis: hemangiopericytoma, angiosarcoma).
  o Demonstrate location and tumor extent.
  o Assess operability.
  o Assess tumor vascularity.
  o Delineate tumor extension to
    o Major arteries
    o Major veins
    o Cranial nerves
    o Dural venous sinuses
    o Calvarium

  Use angiography to

- Plan embolization by identifying feeding vessels (dural and pial) and assess feasibility and safety of embolization.
- Detect arterio-arterial anastamoses, abnormal branches, or trans-osseous supply.
- Assess the collateral circulation to the brain.
- Assess the intensity of tumor staining and flow characteristics.
- Acquire information about the venous drainage, any cortical venous changes, and patency of adjacent major dural venous sinuses.

Indications

- Pre-operative embolization: making the tumors smaller, softer, and less bloody allowing easier manipulation and removal at surgery. Embolization of the ECA branches controls deep hemorrhagic sites. Pial bleeding is usually easy to control surgically.
- Stand-alone embolotherapy of tumors has been reported in a small series, but is rarely performed.

Contraindications

- Renal insufficiency and coagulopathy are relative contraindications, and should ideally be corrected before this semi-elective procedure is performed.

- Gadolinium may be used in patients with a true allergic reaction to iodinated contrast.

Alternative Therapies

Direct injection of liquid embolic agents into hypervascular paragangliomas has been proven safe and efficacious in some studies. Both NBCA and Onyx^{TM} have been used.

Specific Complications

These include non-target embolization causing the following:

- Stroke
- Blindness
- Cranial nerve palsy

Anatomy

Assess the vascular supply on the pre-procedural imaging. Multiple vessels supplying the tumor indicate that the case will take longer to perform. The anatomy is markedly variable depending upon tumor location.

Normal Anatomy

- Commonly supplied by the dural arteries. These include the following:
  - External carotid artery branches

    - Middle meningeal (MMA)
    - Accessory meningeal
    - Ascending pharyngeal—of particular importance in paragangliomas
    - Occipital transmastoid
  - Internal carotid artery (ICA) branches

    - Tentorial
    - Inferolateral trunk
  - Vertebral artery branches

    - Posterior meningeal
- All these branches need to be assessed to exclude aberrant anatomy. However, the feeding arteries can often be deduced from the tumor location (Tables 43.1 and 43.2).

Table 43.1 Meningioma location and supply

Meningioma location	Supply
Falx/parasagittal/convexity	MMA—usually ECA occasionally from ICA—ophthalmic
	Anterior falx artery—usually from ICA –ophthalmic
	Superficial temporal artery –ECA
	Anterior ethmoidal branches—usually from ICA –ophthalmic
	Direct supply from pial branches of ICA
Sphenoid wing	MMA—usually ECA occasionally from ICA—ophthalmic
	Meningo-hypophyseal artery—from cavernous ICA
	Middle cranial fossa meningeal branches from ophthalmic
Olfactory groove/planum sphenoidale	Usually from ICA—ophthalmic, anterior, and posterior ethmoidal branches.
	MMA—usually ECA occasionally from ICA –ophthalmic
Parasellar/pertroclinoid/ petrous apex	MMA—usually ECA occasionally from ICA –ophthalmic
	Dorsal meningeal from VA
	Occipital artery from ECA
	Ascending pharyngeal from ECA
Tentorium	Tentorial artery—ICA branch
	MMA—usually ECA occasionally from ICA –ophthalmic
	Occipital artery from ECA
Infratentorial	Tentorial artery—ICA branch
	MMA—usually ECA occasionally from ICA—ophthalmic
	Occipital artery from ECA
	Ascending pharyngeal from ECA
	Dorsal meningeal from VA
	Cerebellar branches from vertebral and basilar arteries

Abbreviations: MMA—middle meningeal artery; ECA—external carotid artery; ICA—internal carotid artery; VA—vertebral artery

Table 43.2 Paraganglioma location and supply

Glomus caroticuum	ICA and ECA supply
Glomus vagale	ICA and ECA supply particularly ascending pharyngeal
Glomus jugulare	VA branches
	ECA branches occipital, post-auricular, MMA, posterior division of ascending pharyngeal
Glomus tympanicum	VA branches
	ECA branches occipital, post-auricular, MMA, posterior division of ascending pharyngeal

Aberrant Anatomy

Secondary supply may be derived from pial branches and are as follows:

- Anterior cerebral artery (ACA)
- Middle cerebral artery (MCA)
- Posterior cerebral artery (PCA)

Strategy

- The goal is to reduce the tumor vascularity, thereby reducing surgical blood loss and dissection time.
- The most important vessels to devascularize are those that feed the tumor deep to the surgical approach. There is little point in embolizing the middle meningeal or superficial temporal supply to a convexity meningioma when the surgical exposure will result in these branches being clipped early during the surgical approach.
- Pial branches from the ICA are not normally embolized, since the risk of non-target embolization and stroke is unacceptably high.

Equipment

- *Roadmap capability*
- *Non-selective catheters:* none required.
- *Selective catheters:* vertebral, Sidewinder 2. Microcatheter for selective embolization.
- *Guide catheter:* 6Fr with 0.067 lumen allowing guiding contrast injections, as well as constant flush by attaching to a pressurized heparinized saline bag via a rotating hemostatic valve. This ensures that the dead space around the microcatheter is flushed and clot accumulation is prevented.

Embolic Agents

- *Polyvinyl alcohol (PVA) particles*—300–500 μm, unless shunting or very large vascular tumor are present in which case larger particles should be used.
- *Acrylic polymer microspheres* (Embospheres)—300–500 μm unless shunting or very large vascular tumor when larger particles may be used.
- *Coils* – may be placed within the MMA proximal to the tumor bed, allowing easier surgical transection of the artery.

Medication

- *General anesthesia:* addresses both patient compliance and analgesic requirement during the procedure. If provocative testing is to be employed, the procedure must be performed under local anesthetic with mild sedation.
- *Heparin:* 5000 IU bolus with 1000 IU per hour thereafter during the embolization procedure.

- *Lidocaine:* can be used as a provocative test to ensure safe catheter placement prior to embolization. Inject 1 ml of 1% plain lidocaine and check that the patient does not develop a cranial nerve palsy or facial sensory change.
- *Pain control*: analgesia should be prescribed for the recovery period.
- *Sickness control*: anti-emetics should also be prescribed to control symptoms of post-embolization syndrome.

Procedure

Access

- Plan according to the pre-operative imaging.
- Almost always approached from the common femoral artery

Angiography

- Selective six-vessel angiography (both ICA, ECA, and vertebrals) can be helpful in patients with large tumors when the blood supply may not derive exclusively from a single branch, and when the exact supply is unclear from the pre-procedure imaging.
- The following must be identified and examined to avoid potentially disastrous complications.

  - The distal internal maxillary artery (potential communication with the ICA).
  - The neuromeningeal trunk of the ascending pharyngeal artery (supply to 9th, 10th, and 11th cranial nerves).
  - The odontoid branch of the ascending pharyngeal artery (potential vertebral artery anastamosis).
  - Meningolacrimal branch of the MMA (potential retinal supply).

- Pre-embolization testing by injection of a small-dose of lidocaine (1 ml 1% plain lidocaine without epinephrine or buffer) may be used to identify that the blood supply to cranial nerves is not jeopardized.

  - Temporary cranial nerve deficit increases the risk of embolization.
  - After the microcatheter has been properly and safely positioned, embolic material is injected under constant, real-time digital-subtraction fluoroscopy (road map). This optimizes visualization of tumor staining and filling of non-target vessels to allow penetration of the material into the tumor bed thereby producing devascularization and subsequent necrosis.[/11]

- The pial supply is generally not embolized pre-operatively (due to the risk of CVA).

Assessing the Lesion

Location

- The location of the tumor should be known from the pre-operative imaging.

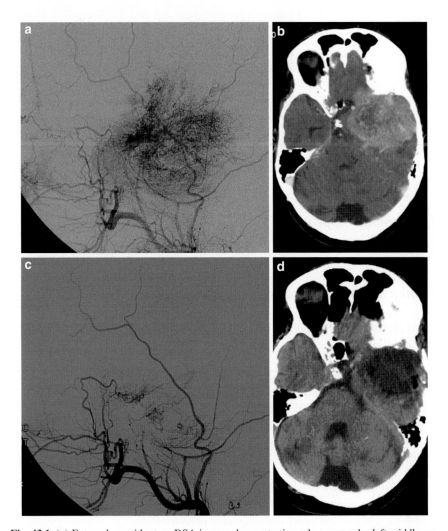

Fig. 43.1 (**a**) External carotid artery DSA images demonstrating a hypervascular left middle cranial fossa meningioma supplied by enlarged posterior ethmoidal and middle meningeal arteries. Note the typical DSA sunburst tumor blush pre-embolization. (**b**) Corresponding CT image. (**c**) Post-embolization. Tumor vascularity is markedly reduced post-embolization. (**d**) CT illustrates the tumor necrosis post-embolization and prior to surgery

Fig. 43.2 DSA images of
right common carotid artery
angiograms demonstrating a
right glomus jugulare tumor
(*white arrowheads*) (**a**) pre-
(**b**) post (*right*) embolization.
Note the pruning of
peripheral vessels
post-embolization

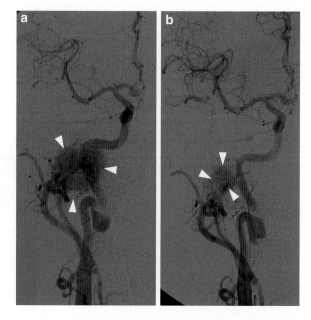

Angiographic Appearance

- A typical starburst blush pattern identifies the tumor (Figs. 43.1 and 43.2).

Treatment Plan and Technique

The treatment plan and embolic agent depends on the tumor anatomy and operator experience.

- The goal is to obliterate the tumor capillary bed to produce devascularization of the tumor while preserving normal tissue. Occluding the feeding artery confers little benefit over surgical ligation of these vessels intra-operatively.
- When the flow of embolic particle begins to slow, embolization is halted to prevent reflux of particles into non-target territories.
- Always try and embolize as selectively as possible using microcatheters to navigate into each feeding vessel. PVA particles or acrylic microspheres are used to embolize as distally as possible.
- The catheter must not be wedged. Flow around the microcatheter delivers the embolic agent to the target without undue pressurization.
- Embolization is complete when the majority of tumor flow has been obliterated—remember that the goal is to try to make the surgery simpler by reducing blood supply from branches of the ECA. Benefit vs. risk of embolizing a particular vessel should always be considered.

- A coil may be placed at the end of the procedure to aid surgical ligation intraoperatively; this is not usually required.
- Care should be used to ensure the dead space within the catheter is cleared to avoid non-target embolization.
- Leave any tumor supply arising from the pial vessels. These are easier to tackle during surgical resection. You will cause more harm than good. Provocative testing with lidocaine has been used in some centers to ensure safe embolization.
- Inform the surgeon what you have done, especially if significant supply persists.

Arterial Puncture Site

- Use a closure device unless there is provision for adequate recovery time postprocedure and for the effects of heparin to resolve.

Post-embolization Syndrome

- Ensure that the patient is prepared for this and knows that pain and sickness can be treated effectively.
- Treatment is supportive.
- Ensure that the ward staff knows what to look for and do.

Follow-Up

- Patients may require follow-up imaging. Some advocate this to assess timing of subsequent resection.
- Timing of subsequent resection debated. Some say timing of embolization has no effect on ease of tumor resection and should therefore be performed within 24 h. Others advocate 7–10 day delay following embolization for maximal tumoral necrosis to occur.

Keypoints

- Review the pre-procedural imaging to plan the procedure.
- Consider and treat the possible collateral supply.
- Aim for targeted selective capillary bed embolization.

Safety

- Never start embolization until you have personally reviewed the imaging.
- *Stop if uncertain, especially if there is risk of non-target embolization.*

Suggested Reading

Byrne J. Interventional Neuroradiology: Theory and Practice. Chapter 11: 213–234. Cary, NC: Oxford Press, 2002.

Dowd CF, Halbach VV, Higashida RT. Meningiomas: the role of preoperative angiography and embolization. Neurosurg Focus 2003; 15(1):E10.

Smith T. Embolization in the external carotid artery. J Vasc Interv Radiol 2006; 17:1897–1913.

Chapter 44
Gonadal Vein Reflux: Varicocele and Pelvic Congestion

Lindsay Machan

Clinical Features

Due to the gender differences, the consequences of gonadal vein reflux are different in males and females. There is, however, considerable overlap in the techniques used to manage symptomatic reflux. Throughout this chapter, gender-specific differences will be referred to separately.

- Gonadal vein reflux is common in males and females, although it is usually asymptomatic.
- Spermatic vein reflux is associated with abnormal sperm production, groin pain, and testicular atrophy (particularly in adolescents).
- Ovarian vein reflux can result in chronic pelvic pain and can complicate the treatment of labial or leg varicosities.
- Chronic pelvic pain has many causes and there is considerable overlap of symptoms.
- Pelvic congestion syndrome remains controversial and is normally only diagnosed when no other cause of symptoms can be found on clinical and imaging assessment.
- Pelvic venous ectasia can be a normal consequence of pregnancy; however flow remains antegrade. In pelvic congestion syndrome, patients have retrograde ovarian vein flow.
- Gonadal vein embolization is an elective procedure usually performed in otherwise healthy patients. Appropriate indications for emergency treatment are exquisitely rare.

Diagnostic Evaluation

- Detailed clinical assessment by a gynecologist is required for women with chronic pelvic pain, in order to exclude other causes of symptoms.
- In men, a consultation with urologist or infertility specialist is necessary.

Transcatheter Embolization and Therapy,
Techniques in Interventional Radiology, DOI 10.1007/978-1-84800-897-7_44,
© Springer-Verlag London Limited 2010

Imaging/Investigation

Females with Pelvic Pain

- The purpose of imaging is to exclude alternative causes of chronic pelvic pain.
- Pelvic varicosities are frequent incidental findings on computed tomography and magnetic resonance imaging in asymptomatic patients investigated for other problems. They are often not demonstrated on studies such as pelvic ultrasound.
- Patients seldom require other specific imaging prior to venography.

Males with Varicocele

- Scrotal ultrasound is the mainstay of investigation.
- Assess pampiniform plexuses, and look for evidence of reflux during Valsava maneuver.
- In older patient with left-sided varicocele, remember to assess the left kidney and renal vein.
- Exclude factors that may prevent improvement of semen quality, e.g., severe dystrophic changes in the testicle, congenital absence of vas deferens.
- Transrectal ultrasound if low semen volume.

Indications

Females

- Chronic pelvic pain that cannot be explained by another diagnosis.
- Pelvic varicosities seen at laparoscopic or open surgery in a patient with appropriate symptoms.
- Severe labial/perineal varicosities.
- Lower extremity varicose veins recurrent after adequate surgical/endovascular treatment.
- Symptomatic lower extremity varicose veins not secondary to typical truncal or perforator vein reflux.
- Prior to endovenous ablation of lower extremity varicose veins in patients with pelvic congestive symptoms.

Males

- Infertility and appropriate semen abnormalities
- Groin pain
- Adolescent varicocele
- Testicular atrophy
- Recurrence post-surgery

Alternative Therapies

Ovarian Vein Reflux

- *Surgery*: hysterectomy and salpingoophorectomy, oophorectomy, ovarian vein ligation.
- *Medical*: medroxyprogesterone acetate, ergots, psychotherapy.

Male Varicocele

- *Surgery*: open surgical, laparoscopic, or microsurgical ligation $\pm$ antegrade sclerosis.
- *Medical*: assisted fertility techniques (e.g., IVF, ICSI).

Contraindications

General

- Severe anaphylactoid reactions to radiographic contrast media
- Uncorrectable coagulopathy
- Severe renal insufficiency
- Phobia to medical implants

Specific

- Female: other cause of chronic pelvic pain that has not been adequately treated.
- Male: primary disorder of sperm production (e.g., generation of spermatazoa without heads)
- Anatomy
  - When the gonadal vein is the route of venous return from lower extremities (e.g., chronic pelvic venous occlusion or congenital abnormality).
  - When there is no absolute assurance of the embolic agent remaining within the gonadal vein once it has been deployed.

Complications

- *Vasovagal episodes* during the procedure are common, particularly in men.
- *Post-embolization syndrome (PES)*: 80–90% of females treated for pelvic congestion suffer from a degree of PES. There is considerable variation in severity and duration.
- *Back or scrotal pain*: approximately 10% of males develop testicular phlebitis; *in 1% this is debilitating*.

- Treatment for pain and PES is at least 5 days of continuous anti-inflammatory agents and reduced activity until symptoms resolve.

Anatomy

- Assessed by venography during embolization procedure.
- Pre-procedure non-invasive imaging to define anatomy is not essential.

Normal Anatomy

- Left gonadal vein almost always drains into the left renal vein.
- Right gonadal vein usually drains directly into the vena cava.

Female

- The entire pelvic venous network is virtually devoid of valves and interconnects by venous plexuses surrounding rectum, bladder, vagina, uterus, and ovaries.
- Uterine and vaginal plexuses drain mainly into internal iliac veins, but there are extensive communications with the ovarian venous plexus.

Male

- A varicocele is varicose dilation of the pampiniform plexus that drains the testicle and epididymis. The pampiniform plexus drains into the internal spermatic vein.
- Additional small veins drain into saphenous, external iliac, and internal iliac systems.

Aberrant Anatomy

- Variations and duplications of the gonadal and renal veins are common.
- Insertion of right gonadal vein into IVC is variable; it may be anterior or even to left of midline.
- Right gonadal vein drains into the right renal vein in 8%.
- Intact valves at orifice, with reflux more distally, can occur.
- In retroaortic or circumaortic left renal vein, gonadal vein usually arises from lower limb of renal vein and is more easily cannulated from femoral approach.
- "Nutcracker phenomenon" compression of left renal vein by superior mesenteric artery) is described in up to 83% of patients with varices.
- Collateral communications with portal or systemic veins are common but usually of no significance.

Equipment

Catheters

- *Selective catheters:*
- For jugular approach—6 Fr or 7 Fr multipurpose (MPA) catheter
- For femoral approach—

  - 5 Fr Cobra catheter for left gonadal vein
  - 5 Fr Sos or Simmons type-II catheter for right gonadal vein

- *Guide catheter*—some use 180° curve guide catheter (e.g., Hopkins curve)
- *Microcatheters* are occasionally needed

Embolic Agents

- Coils/microcoils
- 3% tetradecyl sulfate or equivalent sclerosant
- Cyanoacrylate adhesive

Medication

- *Pain control*: intraprocedural analgesics as needed. Post-procedure for PES, non-steroidal anti-inflammatory drugs are the mainstay of treatment.
- *Infection control:* standard aseptic precautions. No prophylactic antibiotics needed.
- *Sickness control:* as necessary.
- *Hydration*: avoid dehydration.

Venography

Access

- Right internal jugular (>90%) or right femoral vein.
- Femoral approach usually necessary if retroaortic LRV.

Venography

Jugular route: multipurpose shape catheter

- Left renal venogram performed with the patient performing a Valsalva maneuver to identify the origin of the left gonadal vein and any important collateral vessels.

- If gonadal vein reflux and varicosities are seen, then the catheter is advanced into the upper left gonadal vein. Further venography is performed to identify the anatomy and all collateral channels.
- Same multipurpose shape catheter is then directed into right gonadal vein. Venography and embolization, if needed, are performed in the same fashion as described for the left.
- If ovarian venograms are negative, then bilateral internal iliac venograms are performed. Pudendal vein reflux can cause symptomatic pelvic varicosities. Some interventionists routinely study the internal iliac vein.

Transfemoral Route

- *Left*: Cobra catheter or 180° guide catheter directed into the peripheral left renal vein. Selective gonadal venography and embolization are performed using the same diagnostic criteria and methods as for transjugular route.
- *Right*: Simmons II catheter or equivalent and right gonadal venogram performed.

Angiographic Appearance

Ovarian Vein

- There are multiple published criteria for positive venogram including ovarian vein reflux, dilated ovarian veins, and delay in clearance of contrast medium.
- The author's opinion is
  - Retrograde flow within the ovarian vein (white arrows) AND visualization of paraovarian varicosities (black arrows) constitutes a positive study.
  - Reflux of contrast down to the ovary without opacification of varicosities is a negative venogram, *regardless* of the diameter of the ovarian vein.
- Opacification of entire pelvic venous system after ovarian vein injection is normal.

Spermatic Vein

- Positive study—reflux into pampiniform plexus of 1–2 cc of gently injected contrast from catheter in non-wedged position in upper spermatic vein or above.

Clinical Scenarios

- Chronic pelvic pain does not respond to embolization in all patients (70–80% symptom improvement in women, 85–90% in men).
- As with other chronic pain syndromes, symptoms may take up to 6 months to respond.

- Delay of 3–6 months after ovarian vein embolization before treatment of labial or lower extremity varicosities is recommended.

Treatment Plan and Technique

Ovarian Vein

- Catheter should be directed selectively into the origin of each of the two or three caudal branches of the main ovarian vein.
- Tetradecyl sulfate 3% (2 cc mixed with 0.5 cc of contrast) or equivalent sclerosant injected with the patient performing Valsalva maneuver until static sclerosant is seen at the catheter tip.
- Trickle in more sclerosant as the catheter is slowly withdrawn to just above the iliac crest.
- Coil (usually 30-8-10) is laid in an elongated configuration to within 2 cm of the ovarian vein origin.
- Perform gentle venogram to confirm occlusion and exclusion of all parallel channels.
- If rapid retrograde flow in ovarian vein persists, overlap a second elongated coil with the first in the configuration of a double helix.

Spermatic Vein

- All branches large enough for selective catheterization should be occluded with coils or glue at internal inguinal ring (level of roof of acetabulum).
- If coils are used, sclerosant, e.g., tetradecyl sulfate 3% (2 cc mixed with 0.5 cc of contrast), injected as catheter withdrawn to immediately above the iliac crest.
- Prevention of reflux of liquid into the pampiniform plexus by external compression at the level of the inguinal ring is mandatory or the patient will develop pampiniform phlebitis.
- After sclerosant is injected, it is critical not to inject contrast vigorously or the sclerosant will be displaced.
- Coil (usually 30-8-10) is laid in an elongated configuration to within 2 cm of the spermatic vein origin.
- Gentle post-embolization venogram performed to confirm occlusion and exclude parallel channels. If rapid retrograde flow persists in the spermatic vein, overlap a second elongated coil with the first in the configuration of a double helix.

Aftercare

- Bedrest for 1 h post-procedure.

Venous Puncture Site

- Manual compression and dressing.

Post-embolization

- Mild pelvic cramping is common and treated with over-the-counter anti-inflammatory agents as needed.
- Patient to avoid any activity involving Valsalva maneuver, such as lifting or sports, for three full days beginning day after the procedure.
- If persistent discomfort at the end of 3 days, continue these instructions until symptoms resolve.
- The first period after ovarian vein embolization is often unusually heavy.

Follow-Up

- Clinical assessment and ultrasound 3 months post-procedure.
- Post-treatment ultrasound will normally reveal persistent dilated veins, but normal or no accentuation of flow with Valsalva manoeuvre maneuver.
- If varicocele treatment for infertility, sperm count and urologic assessment at 3 months.

Keypoints

- Other causes of chronic pelvic pain must be excluded before ovarian vein embolization is performed.
- In ovarian embolization, similar clinical results are achieved regardless of embolic agent, whether liquids are used, or if internal iliac veins are also occluded.
- In spermatic vein occlusion, a liquid (sclerosant if coils used or glue alone) results in higher technical success and lower recanalization rates than coils alone.

Safety

Never start embolization until you have personally reviewed the indications.

Stick to the indications for the procedure, use appropriate agents, and remember that the patient does not have a life-threatening illness.

Suggested Readings

Check JH. Treatment of male infertility. Clin Exp Obstet Gynecol. 2007;34(4):201–206

Ganeshan A, Upponi S, Hon LQ, Uthappa MC, Warakaulle DR, Uberoi R. Chronic pelvic pain due to pelvic congestion syndrome: the role of diagnostic and interventional radiology. Cardiovasc Intervent Radiol. 2007;30(6):1105–1111.

Liddle AD, Davies AH. Pelvic congestion syndrome: chronic pelvic pain caused by ovarian and internal iliac varices. Phlebology 2007;22(3):100–104.

Stones RW. Pelvic vascular congestion—half a century later. Clinical Obst Gyn 2003;46:831–856.

Sze DY, Kao JS, Frisoli JK, McCallum SW, Kennedy WA 2nd, Razavi MK. Persistent and recurrent postsurgical varicoceles: venographic anatomy and treatment with N-butyl cyanoacrylate embolization. J Vasc Interv Radiol. 2008;19(4):539–545

Chapter 45
Varicose Veins

David West

Definition

Varicose veins are abnormal dilated veins secondary to abnormal flow due to venous insufficiency. Varicose veins can occur at many sites; this chapter will focus on varicose veins in the lower limb.

Clinical Features

- Varicose veins are very common affecting up to 40% of the population.
- Classically affect medial aspect of the limb (great saphenous vein territory) (Fig. 45.1) or posterior calf (small saphenous vein territory) but many variations exist.
- Patients complain frequently of aching, itching, restless legs, aching and tiredness which are worst when standing.
- May lead to severe skin discoloration due to the deposition of hemosiderin.
- Some patients may present with skin ulceration.
- Occasionally mild trauma will cause severe hemorrhage.

Causes of Venous Insufficiency

- Valve failure (genetic and by far the most common)
- Muscle pump failure
- Deep venous obstruction, e.g., secondary to deep vein thrombosis (DVT) or proximal venous obstruction, e.g., May-Thurner syndrome.

All these are normally permanent but can occasionally be temporary (e.g., pregnancy-induced).

Transcatheter Embolization and Therapy,
Techniques in Interventional Radiology, DOI 10.1007/978-1-84800-897-7_45,
© Springer-Verlag London Limited 2010

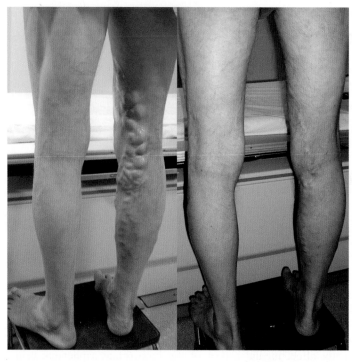

Fig. 45.1 (**a**) Gross great saphenous varicose veins pre-treatment. (**b**) Same patient after EVLA ablation of great saphenous vein

Natural History of Varicose Veins

- Varicose veins do not spontaneously disappear except sometimes following pregnancy.
- Progression is highly variable. Some progress rapidly over weeks whereas others remain static for many years.
- Serious skin changes (e.g., ulceration 0.5–1.5%) which cannot be predicted.

Diagnostic Evaluation

If involved in the treatment of varicose veins, it is important to be able to assess the patient clinically.

History: to elicit the following:

- How seriously the problem is affecting patient's life.
- Past medical history of DVT, congenital venous problems.
- Details of previous treatment for varicose veins. Veins that have not undergone previous therapy are the simplest to manage.

Physical examination

- Patient standing position with bare legs.
- Visual inspection to detect and record
  - Ulceration and other skin changes.
  - Appearance and distribution of varicosities.
  - Scars from previous surgery.
  - Birth marks.
- Palpation to detect defects in fascia which may indicate incompetent perforators.
- Measure the circumference of both legs.
- Do not attempt to detect presence of reflux by physical examination.

Imaging

- The aim of imaging varicose veins is to establish and document the following:
  - Patency of deep veins
  - Anatomy and size of the superficial and deep venous systems
  - Distribution of varicosities
  - Presence, degree, and sites of reflux
- Color duplex scanning with the patient standing is the gold standard.
  - Concentrate on the sapheno-femoral vein junction (SFJ) and sapheno-popliteal vein (SPJ) junction in primary varicose veins.
  - Use adjunctive compression and Valsalva maneuvers.
  - Look for sustained reflux.
- In complex cases exquisite images can be obtained using CT and MR venography but these do not demonstrate abnormal flow.
- Direct venography is occasionally necessary and usually only performed at the time of therapy.
- Consider deep venous stenosis as a contributory cause. This should be treated by angioplasty or stenting before treating the reflux symptoms.

Indications for Treatment

Varicose veins are benign and treatment is aimed at symptom relief (e.g., cosmetic, pain relief etc.)

- Varicose veins associated with ulceration or impending ulceration should be actively treated.
- Other symptoms should be treated according to patient preference and local expertize.

Alternative Therapies

Surgery

The gold-standard surgical technique is to tie-off all superficial branches at the SFJ or SPJ, strip the refluxing saphenous vein, and avulse the varicosities.

Occlusion techniques: these are established as alternatives to surgery.

- There are two principal mechanisms and are as follows:
  - o Heating (laser and radiofrequency)
  - o Chemical (sclerotherapy)
- Catheter-based techniques may be used in primary varicose veins or recurrent varicosities.
- Unlike surgery, the refluxing venous source is left in situ but the lumen is permanently occluded.
- Subsequent therapy may be needed to deal with troublesome residual varicosities.
- Normally only two truncal veins can be treated at one session.

Contraindications

- *Occluded deep vein.* This leaves the superficial veins as the sole route of venous return and is an absolute contraindication. Note that in the presence of deep venous reflux the condition of the leg can be dramatically improved by treating the superficial reflux.
- *Procoagulant conditions* (e.g., oral contraceptive pill) are a relative contraindication to foam sclerotherapy.

Special situations that may increase difficulty: although with experience most patients can be treated by endovascular means, some cases present special challenges.

- Young fit women who exercise regularly have veins which are prone to spasm.
- Very tortuous and very superficial veins.
- Short wide communications with the deep veins (e.g., in the popliteal fossa) can still be treated using either laser or RF SEPS (Fig. 45.2) but require special attention to prevent damage to deep veins. The use of foam sclerotherapy blocked by an occlusion balloon catheter can also be useful in this situation.
- Thermal treatment of a duplicated truncal vein can cause the second vein to go into spasm. To prevent this, catheterize both before heating either.

General Complications of Venous Ablation Therapy

- Superficial thrombophlebitis
- Deep vein thrombosis

Fig. 45.2 RF SEPS needle in position in perforator

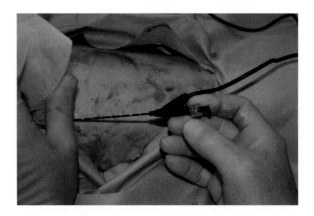

Specific Complications of Thermal ablation

- Burns, nerve injuries
- Aching and bruising (worse after laser)

Specific Complications of Foam Sclerotherapy

- Transient visual loss.
- Skin discoloration is common although usually lasts less than 1 year.
- Ulceration and allergy are rare.

Anatomy and Physiology

Normal Venous Anatomy

- Contain bicuspid valves allowing flow only from superficial to deep and toe to heart.
- Deep veins anatomically follow the arterial supply. Deep veins lie between the muscles of the legs. The deep system comprises calf veins, popliteal vein, femoral vein, external and common iliac veins.
- Superficial veins. Lie between two layers of fascia.
  - o Great saphenous vein drains into common femoral vein at the SFJ in the groin.
  - o Small saphenous vein drains into popliteal vein in popliteal fossa (SPJ).
  - o Anterolateral thigh vein coursing across the thigh from lateral to medial and joining the great saphenous vein at or near the SFJ.
- Perforating veins.
  - o Communicate between superficial and deep systems at several points on the lateral and medial sides of the leg.

Aberrant anatomy: Many variants exist including the following.

- Parallel duplicate channels of the femoral vein are very common.
- Giacomini vein—extension of small saphenous vein to join the great saphenous vein.

Awareness of this variable anatomy is essential to the proper management of varicose veins.

Normal Lower Limb Venous Physiology

- Calf muscle contraction compresses the deep veins.
- In presence of competent valves, blood is forced toward the heart.
- Calf muscles relaxation reduces pressure in the deep veins, blood passes from superficial to the deep veins.
- Cycle repeats enabling blood to pass against gravity from foot to heart.

Equipment

Imaging

- Color duplex ultrasound scanner 7.5–12 MHz linear probe.
- Access to fluoroscopy if possible.

Needles

19G for initial venous puncture.

Micropuncture sets for small veins or those prone to spasm, e.g., young fit women, tortuous, and superficial branches.

Guidewires

- 0.035″ double-ended J/straight standard wire.
- 0.035″ hydrophilic wire for tortuous veins and those in spasm.
- 0.025″ or 0.018″ for use with VNUSclosureFast® system.

Catheters/Introducer Sheaths

- 7F 9 cm sheath for VNUSclosureFast®.
- 4–6F 45–80 cm sheath for introduction of laser fibers. These should have visible markings at least every centimeter to judge pullback rate (Fig. 45.3).
- Diagnostic angiographic catheters as necessary.

Fig. 45.3 Laser fiber in position in calibrated sheath

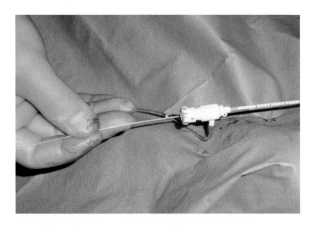

Miscellaneous

- Luer-lock syringes and three-way taps for sclerosant foam production.
- Avulsion hooks (for stab phlebectomy).
- Occlusion balloon catheters.
- Tilting couch.
- Class-2 compression hosiery/compression bandaging.

Medication

Pain control: Diclofenac 500 mg SR OD as required (post-procedure).
Local anesthetic.
Initial cannulation: 5 ml 1% lidocaine without adrenaline.
Tumescent analgesia: 20 ml 2% lidocaine with adrenaline diluted with saline to 100 ml (0.4%) and 400 ml (0.1%).

Treatment Plan and Technique

Treatment principles: regardless which technique is used, there are three elements to consider and are as follows:

1. To abolish all sources of reflux starting with the most proximal (cranial): gonadal vein, iliac vein, SFJ, SPJ, perforating vein.
2. To occlude the main incompetent vein.
3. To treat residual varicosities.

Thermal Ablation Therapy

This includes laser and RFA. Many of the principles are common to either technique as are many of the complications.

Laser Therapy

Laser Equipment

- Diode laser of at least 15 watts power and emitting in the range 810–980 nm wavelength or Nd/YAG laser (1064 or 1340 nm wavelength).
- Laser fiber: 3 m bare-ended glass fiber of appropriate notional aperture (NA) and with appropriate fitting for the laser. Normally 600 μm but can use 400 μm or even 200 μm diameter especially for small veins.

Access

- Plan according to duplex ultrasound findings.
- Access vein just below the last significant varicose branch using 19G needle or cannula or micropuncture set.
- Guide needle into vein lumen using ultrasound in a longitudinal scanning plane.

Treatment Technique

- Advance guidewire to the proximal site of reflux (usually the SFJ or SPJ).
- Position the sheath to at least 2 cm beyond the junction within the deep vein.
- Advance laser fiber to tip of sheath.
- Withdraw sheath 2 cm to expose 2 cm of the fiber.
- Fix fiber to sheath using a Tuohy Borst adapter or sterile sticky tape.
- Inject tumescent anesthesia solution (Fig. 45.4),using ultrasound guidance and a spinal needle, around the whole length of the vein ensuring that there is a good volume of fluid around the whole circumference of the vein. This usually requires about 400 ml per meter of vein.

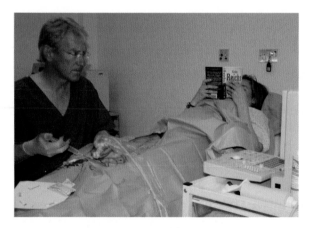

Fig. 45.4 Ultrasound-guided injection of tumescent analgesia. Note the set-up of the room with the ultrasound clearly visible to the operator

- Withdraw the sheath under ultrasound guidance until the tip of the laser fiber is at least 2 cm away from the deep veins.
- Fire laser and withdraw fibre/sheath at a rate of about 2 mm per second achieving at least 70 J energy per cm.
- Stop firing the laser at least 1 cm from skin puncture.
- Repeat with further veins as necessary.
- Apply dressings and compression stockings.

Technical tips. In difficult cases:

- Try hydrophilic wire and catheter techniques.
- Use ultrasound and external pressure to direct tip of catheter through tortuous segments.
- Consider fluoroscopic guidance with contrast injection.
- If severe spasm prevents visualization of vein try
  - o Waiting for 15 minutes
  - o Getting patient to walk around
  - o Elevating head of bed

Radiofrequency Ablation Therapy

Radiofrequency Devices

- RF generator
- RF catheter supplied by generator manufacturer
- RF SEPS needles for perforators

Technique

- Essentially similar to laser technique.
- But use conventional 7F vascular sheath.
- No need for guidewire in most cases; just advance RF catheter through sheath to the proximal portion of the vein to be treated.
- Apply pressure over the tip of the catheter during energy deposition.
- Follow manufacturer's instructions regarding withdrawal rate. The withdrawal rate is typically significantly slower than the laser withdrawal rate.
- If difficulty use a 0.25″ guidewire through the catheter or first place a long 7Fr sheath along whole length of vein using techniques above.

Foam Sclerotherapy

- Most practitioners do not recommend this as a primary means of closing a truncal vein as there is a high recanalization rate compared to laser or RF.
- Insert 18G cannula below the origin of the last significant varicosity.

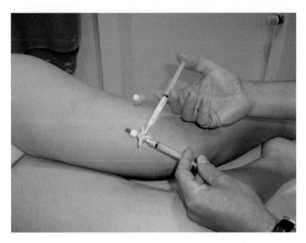

Fig. 45.5 Tessari technique for mixing STD foam using two luer lock syringes and a three-way tap

- Mix 3% sodium tetradecyl sulphate (STD) with air/CO_2 (1 ml STD: 3 ml air/CO_2) ratio into foam by rapidly squirting from one syringe to another via a three-way tap (Tessari method) (Fig. 45.5).
- Elevate leg to empty veins.
- Inject foam: the foam is easily recognized on ultrasound due to the reflective nature of the trapped air.
- Watch progress of foam up the vein on ultrasound until the foam has reached the proximal part of the vein to be treated.
- Apply pressure at this point to prevent passage of foam into deep veins.
- Actively exercise foot to stimulate flow in deep veins.
- Repeat injection as per operator's preference. The ultrasound probe can be used to milk the foam up and down the vein.

Clinical Scenarios

Gonadal/internal iliac veins. If duplex ultrasound or clinical history/examination suggests significant contribution from the pelvis, then undertake venography and embolization as necessary (see Chapter 44).

Truncal vein ablation. This is most commonly the great or small saphenous vein but can be the anterolateral thigh tributary or the Giacomini vein or other variants. Although some operators use foam sclerosant for this purpose, most use a thermal method as it is more reliable and quicker.

Perforating veins. Incompetent perforators from the deep to the superficial veins are an important but often overlooked cause of varicosities. These are especially important as a source of high-pressure venous blood beneath ulcers. Some will occlude after the truncal vein they feed is ablated, but many will remain a problem and lead to a varicosity requiring treatment.

- The perforating vein is punctured under ultrasound guidance and a guidewire passed into the deep venous system. The technique is then as for laser or RFA. AS ALWAYS BE CAREFUL NOT TO APPLY HEAT INTO THE DEEP VEINS (Fig. 45.2).

Varicosities

- Varicosities can be dealt with at the time of initial treatment or more commonly at follow-up after 6 weeks.
- Immediate treatment is more convenient for the patient but may not be possible due to spasm induced by the first treatment or due to the dose of local anesthetic administered.
- Delayed treatment often reveals that the varicosities have disappeared to the patients' satisfaction and require no further treatment.

  Two main methods are used and are as follows:

Foam Sclerotherapy

- The varicosities are needled either by direct vision/palpation or using ultrasound and injected with 3%, 1%, or 0.5% STD foam one-fourth sclerosant/air ratio. The strength depends on vein size with most veins requiring 1%.

Avulsions

- Varicosities are marked pre-operatively with the patient standing.
- Patient placed supine and tumescent local anesthetic injected.
- 19G needle used to puncture skin every 2–4 cm over the varicosities.
- Vein hook inserted through needle puncture and the vein wall hooked and withdrawn through the skin.
- Vein teased out grabbing it with mosquito forceps. Pulled until one end tears off.
- Hook inserted into next puncture point and vein again teased out. Try to remove long lengths of vein rather than small fragments.
- Repeat until all marked varicosities removed.

Prominent Veins in Other Sites

Varicose veins usually occur on the legs but prominent and unsightly veins can occur in other sites.

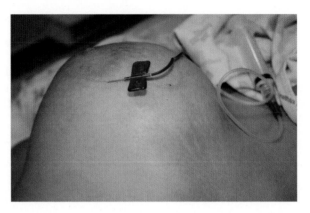

Fig. 45.6 Foam sclerotherapy injection in prominent breast veins

- *Periorbital*. Do not use chemicals in this region. Treated with avulsions. Best left to a specialist.
- *Breast*. Especially after breast augmentation. Treated by injection of 0.5% STD foam. No compression necessary (Fig. 45.6).
- *Genitalia*. Usually due to pelvic reflux. Treat by embolization of the pelvic source with coils or STD foam. Dislodgement of coils and travel to lung reported especially with internal iliac embolization.
- *Hands*. Often cosmetically unappealing especially for women. Treated using foam injections or avulsions.

Aftercare

- Discuss pain control with the patient and ensure that they have a supply of analgesics.
- Explain difference between superficial thrombophlebitis and deep vein thrombosis and instruct patient to return immediately if any sign of DVT.
- Explain care of compression bandaging and make arrangements for removal in 1 week followed by compression hosiery.
- The patient may be discharged as soon as they are comfortable.

Follow-Up

- Follow-up is essential if only truncal veins are treated.
- Recommend clinical follow-up at 6 weeks.
- At this stage, any residual varicosities can be treated with foam sclerotherapy or avulsions. Duplex ultrasound is normally performed to check truncal vein closure but rarely reveals persistent flow.

- Follow-up can be at patients discretion if foam sclerotherapy or avulsions were performed at the initial treatment session.

Keypoints

- Varicose veins are typically a benign condition.
- Most patients with venous reflux disease can be managed without surgery.
- Listen to patients and understand what they want from the treatment.
- Carefully establishing the sources/causes of reflux is essential for successful treatment planning and execution.
- Treatment should abolish all sources of reflux starting with the most central.
- Abolishing reflux will usually be sufficient to relieve itching and aching but may leave prominent varicosities.

Safety

- Get properly trained to use new technology!
- Take care in patients with procoagulant conditions.
- Avoid heating the deep veins.
- Warn patients of the small risk of DVT and encourage them to return if they develop suggestive symptoms.
- Warn patients regarding visual effects of STD foam.

Suggested Reading

A. Cavezzi, N. Labropoulos, H. Partsch, S. Ricci, A. Caggiati, K. Myers, A. Nicolaides and P.C. Smith. Duplex Ultrasound Investigation of the Veins in Chronic Venous Disease of the Lower Limbs – UIP Consensus Document. Part II. Anatomy. European Journal of Vascular and Endovascular Surgery 2006;31:288–299

P. Coleridge-Smith, N. Labropoulos, H. Partsch, K. Myers, A. Nicolaides and A. Cavezzi. Duplex Ultrasound Investigation of the Veins in Chronic Venous Disease of the Lower Limbs – UIP Consensus Document. Part I. Basic Principles. European Journal of Vascular and Endovascular Surgery 2006;31:83–92

B Eklöf, R Rutherford,J Bergan, P Carpentier, P Gloviczki, R Kistner , M Meissner, G Moneta, K Myers, F Padberg. Revision of the CEAP Classification for Chronic Venous Disorders: Consensus Statement. Journal of Vascular Surgery 2004;40(6):1248–1252.

R Muller. Ambulatory phlebectomy [article in German]. Ther Umsch 1992;49(7):447–450. Describes the technique of avulsion therapy

"Miscellaneous Embolic Agents: Laser and Radiofrequency"   Chapter 6   in this book Miscellaneous agents and tools

Chapter 46
Lymphatic Malformations: Sclerotherapy

Richard J.T. Owen

Clinical Features and Presentation

Etiology: lymphatic malformations (LM) are part of the spectrum of congenital vascular malformations. LMs are developmental abnormalities related to the failure of normal differentiation of mesenchymal lymphatic tissue.

- LMs are usually isolated but may coexist as part of lymphatico-venous or lymphatico-arterial malformations, such as Proteus or Klippel-Trenaunay syndromes.
- Histologically appearances vary, but enlarged lymphatic channels and spaces with septae composed of fibrous tissue unconnected to lymphatic channels are universally seen.
- Lumen usually contains lymphatic fluid, but proteinaceous material and erythrocytes may be present.
- Lymhangioma contents may be clear, serosanguineous, or greenish fluid. Fresh or altered blood may be present following recent swelling or injury.

Occurrence

- Roughly half of all LM are detected at or before birth, with an incidence of 1:6,000–16,000 live births.
- 80–90% detected by the age of 2 years.
- The majority are seen in the head and neck, but can be widely distributed elsewhere in the body (Fig. 46.1).
- Often present with cosmetic or functional difficulties.
- Adult LMs are rare and development is linked to predisposing factors such as trauma, infection, tumor growth, or iatrogenic stimuli.

Transcatheter Embolization and Therapy,
Techniques in Interventional Radiology, DOI 10.1007/978-1-84800-897-7_46,
© Springer-Verlag London Limited 2010

Classification

- LM should be classified according to their radiological and pathological appearances into micro or macrocystic lesions. These differences to some extent predict treatment response.
- Macrocystic LMs contain one or more cystic spaces greater than 2 cm in diameter, whereas microcystic LMs contain multiple small cavities (Fig. 46.1).
- Macrocystic and microcystic types commonly coexist within the same lesion. Lesions often show a progression from macrocystic to microcystic, and this may occur with treatment.
- Historical classifications into capillary LM, cavernous LM, and cystic hygroma are to be discouraged.

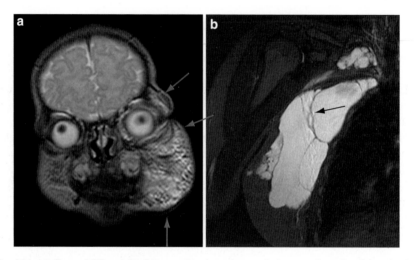

Fig. 46.1 (a) Coronal T2-weighted image showing microcystic lympangioma involving the face and orbit. (b) T2 FS coronal image of the chest wall of a 12-year-old girl with a recurrent multicystic LM following three treatments with OK 432. The internal septae are clearly seen. The lesion showed complete resolution after two treatments of doxycycline

Manifestations

Lesions may be solitary or multifocal; well circumscribed or deeply infiltrative; remain unchanged in size, enlarge slowly, or rarely involute.

- Size varies, but in general lesions continue to grow in proportion to the patient.
- When seen in the head and neck, LM may be diffusely infiltrative or discrete. Depending on the anatomic location, proptosis or other manifestations may be present.
- During episodes of hemorrhage or infection, adjacent vital structures may become compressed.

- Overlying skin changes may be present and vary from abnormal pigmentation to lymphedema and hyperkeratosis.
- Lymphangioma circumscriptum is the terminology used to describe the intradermal form of LM, where thin-walled vascular channels lined by a single layer of endothelium are seen in the papillary dermis. These are characterized by translucent papulovesicles that may demonstrate evidence of intravesicular bleeding. These changes may overlie the macrocystic form of LM.
- Patients often give a history of intermittent swelling, erythema, and pain.
- Intralesional hemorrhage may occur spontaneously or as a result of trauma (Fig. 46.2) and may predispose to infection.
- Cellulitis is common and may present with rapid expansion, erythema, fever, and tenderness, and there may be a lengthy clinical course.

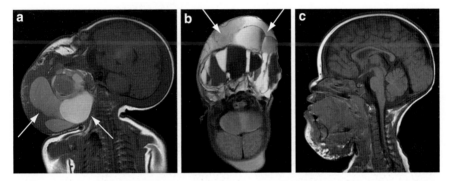

Fig. 46.2 (**a** and **b**) Large LM detected at birth, which resulted in tilting of the head. (**a**) Coronal and (**b**) axial T1-weighted images show a loculated transfacial multicystic mass with multiple fluid levels of different signal intensity that represent intracystic hemorrhage. Lesion measures 10.4 × 10.6 × 9.7 cm, approximately the same volume as the cranial cavity. (**c**) Marked shrinkage and predominantly microcycstic appearance following treatment

Diagnostic Evaluation

- Thorough clinical evaluation of the anatomical site, cosmetic deformity, adjacent structures involved or potentially at risk from injury (direct or indirect), is required prior to treatment considerations.
- Requires a multidisciplinary approach involving pediatricians, plastic surgeons, interventional radiologists, maxillofacial surgery, and ophthalmic surgeons. These lesions are often complex, requiring multiple treatments, and may require surgery.
- Lengthy consultation may be required to outline the goals and expectations of treatment to patients and parents.

Laboratory

- Clinical and radiological diagnoses are usually adequate.
- Biopsy of the more superficial microcystic lesions may reveal the classic histological features, particularly in the case of lymphangioma circumscription.
- Aspiration of lesions is discouraged as it may predispose to infection. Avoid "diagnostic aspiration" in emergency departments!

Imaging

Ultrasound: initial diagnosis is usually suggested on ultrasound.

- Macrocystic LM
  - Show septa separating anechoic cavities that can contain debris (Fig. 46.3a).
  - Flow is absent.
  - There may only be a single cavity *(Fig. 46.3b)*.
  - In some cases, although a multiloculated lesion is suspected, this may represent a single interconnecting cavity. This can often be demonstrated during treatment when small air bubbles trapped in the sclerosing fluid show clearly which cysts have been injected and if communication exists between cysts.
- Microcystic LMs have small cavities resulting in innumerable reflective interfaces and a hyperechoic appearance.

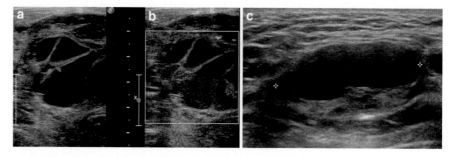

Fig. 46.3 (**a** and **b**) Ultrasound of macrocystic LN showing septae and debris within the cysts. There is absence of flow in the lesion on color flow (**c**) Unilocular cyst

MRI

- MRI is generally required prior to treatment to establish the extent of the lesion. Although often considered localized and superficial, these lesions extend into adjacent structures and are much larger than suspected on ultrasound.

- Where there is a history of trauma or recent swelling, hemorrhage may be present with lesions showing a progression through fresh hemorrhage, old blood, solidification, and sometimes spontaneous resolution.
- *Macrocystic LM*
  - o Usually demonstrate iso- or hypointense signal on T1-weighted sequences and high signal on T2 sequences.
  - o Proteinaceous fluid, hemorrhage, or fluid–fluid levels can cause a more heterogeneous appearance. No vascular signal voids are present (Fig. 46.2).
  - o Do not usually contrast enhance, although mild enhancement may be seen within the walls particularly after surgery or sclerotherapy.
- Microcystic LM
  - o Individual cystic spaces are often too small to be discernible by MRI.
  - o The overall more homogeneous appearance is hypointense on T1-weighted imaging and hyperintense on T2-weighted imaging (Fig. 46.1).

CT

LM may also be seen on CT.

- Low-attenuating fluid-filled non-enhancing mass.
- CT does not usually demonstrate the cyst walls (Fig. 46.4).

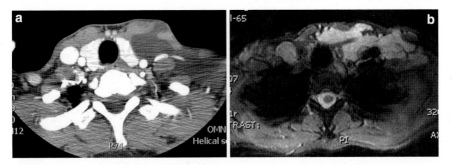

Fig. 46.4 Lymhangioma in the neck and chest. (**a**) CT shows low attenuation without enhancement. (**b**) T2 FS MRI shows the true complexity of the cysts

Other Cystic Lesions in the Head and Neck

Differentiation of LMs from other cystic lesions in the head and neck may pose some difficulties, and CT and/or MRI are required to differentiate between a lymphangioma and other entities such as the following:

- Ranula: ranulas retain tapered communication with the sublingual space and are homogeneous, thin-walled, anatomically defined, fluid-containing masses.

- Branchial cleft cysts.
- Thyroglossal duct cysts.
- Other cystic spaces in the neck.
- Of interest is that both pediatric plunging ranulas and branchial cysts have been treated with sclerotherapy using (OK 432) to good effect.

Treatment Options

- Sclerotherapy is now widely regarded as the first-line treatment, although the traditional approach has been surgical excision.
- Surgery is often complex and prolongued procedure with the potential for poor cosmesis and morbidity.
- Complete excision is only possible in a third of cases.
- Surgery remains an option when
  - Percutaneous sclerotherapy is proving ineffective
  - The lesion is predominantly microcystic
  - A combined approach has been planned, e.g., surgical excision of residual LM following sclerotherapy

Contraindications to Treatment and Specific Complications of Treatment

These relate to the following:

- The site and size of the lesion.
- Associated abnormalities.
- Related structures: airway compression may require ventilation; nerve palsy may take many months to recover.
- The agents used:
  - Fatal bleomycin-induced pulmonary fibrosis has been reported.
  - Fever, pain, and erythema have been reported with all agents.

Evidence for Sclerotherapy

Acevedo et al. reviewed 289 treatments published in 22 articles. The two most commonly used agents were OK 432 and bleomycin. When used as first-line therapy

- Complete regression (inability to detect the lesion radiologically or clinically) was seen in 43%.
- Good response (50% or greater decrease in size of the lesion) was seen in 23%.
- 87.5% of patients exhibited a response of some sort.
- Only 12% required salvage surgery.

- A trend towards OK 432 being more efficacious was observed and this is supported by other publications.
- Complications appeared less serious with OK 432 but no significant differences were seen.
- The majority of recent literature refers to OK 432, although there are several series demonstrating the efficacy of bleomycin.

Anatomy

- Clearly this depends on the location of the lesion.
- Review of pre-procedure imaging will identify the extent of the lesion and allow treatment planning.
- It is crucial to have a thorough understanding of the local anatomy and to consider any adjacent structures that might be at risk.

Equipment

Catheters

- 23- or 24-gauge butterfly needle
- 6-French pigtail drainage catheter
- Basic angiography tray

Embolic agents: these are all sclerosant agents and are not commonly used elsewhere.
  OK432 (*Picibanil*; Chugai Pharmaceutical Co., Tokyo, Japan)

- Lipophilized preparation of *Streptococcus pyogenes* incubated with penicillin, acts as a biological response modifier drug for the treatment of lymphangiomata.
- Promotes the neoangiogenesis of lymphatic channels into the tumor.
- Not widely available and is imported on a named-doctor basis in the United States and Canada.
- *Dosage*—0.1–0.3 mg (1–3 vials, 0.1 mg/vial) per treatment, according to lesion size.

Bleomycin

- Anticancer drug.
- Scleroses lymphatic endothelium via a non-specific inflammatory reaction.
- *Side effects*
  o Local swelling and inflammation.

- *Pulmonary fibrosis.* This is very severe and often fatal side effect is usually limited to patients receiving greater than 300 mg. Bleomycin is absorbed systemically, even if administered locally, and is suspected in the development of fatal pulmonary fibrosis even in low doses.
- *Dosage*—0.5–1 mg/kg body weight, at intervals of greater than 2 weeks, injected into lesions.
- Total permissible dose <6 mg/kg.
- Strict adherence to dosing and interval treatment is required to reduce the risk of the severe side effect of pulmonary fibrosis.
- Treatment not recommended in pregnancy.

Doxycycline

- A tetracycline with sclerosant properties.
- Alternative agent, anecdotally may be effective when first-line agent has failed.
- *Side effects*: use with caution in young children. May cause dental enamel staining.
- *Dosage*—100 or 200 mg, mix into 10 or 20 ml saline.

Medication

- *Pain control*: often not required, may need simple analgesics, such as acetominophen (± codeine) or anti-inflammatory drugs, such as ibuprofen.
- *Infection control:* strict aseptic technique, avoid treating lesions that are weeping or showing signs of infection.
- *Admission:* admit young children if the lesion is near the airway, as the degree of post-treatment swelling is unpredictable

Treatment Plan and Technique

- Initial referral should be followed by clinic/multidisciplinary team assessment.
- Treatment options must be discussed with patient/parents.
- The treatment plan should be explained including the following
  - Complications
  - Expected outcomes
    - Multiple treatments may be required.
    - Lesions may recur months and years later requiring further treatment.

Children

- The majority of cases present in the first 2 years of life. These patients require general anesthetic for comfort and safety.

Adults

- The procedure is generally not painful when OK 432 is used and can be carried out under local anesthetic.
- When complex lesion is in the deep cervical and face/orbital region, general anesthetic is sometimes advantageous to help protect the airway.
- Bleomycin and doxycycline are more painful and may require IV sedation and analgesia.

Technique

- Strict aseptic technique should be used during procedure.
- Ultrasound-directed insertion of a 21–25G needle into the anechoic cystic portion of the lesion.
- Confirm position by aspiration of lymphatic or serosanguinous fluid.
- Aspirate as much of the cyst contents as possible. A small pigtail drainage catheter maybe used in large lesions.
- Contrast can be injected to assess size and distribution of the lesion and show any communications with other cysts or other draining channels (Fig. 46.5).
- The sclerosant is injected in aliquots depending on the size and multiplicity of the cysts.

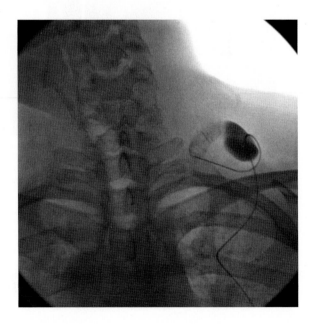

Fig. 46.5 Contrast injected through a 21-gauge butterfly needle under fluoroscopic imaging demonstrates a unilocular cyst in this case

Post-embolization

- Keep puncture sites clean.
- Lesions may show significant increase in size within the first few days post-treatment. This may herald a good response.
- Swelling usually resolves spontaneously; however, pressure effects may be seen on adjacent structures and should be taken into account when considering treatment options (Fig. 46.6). This is particularly important when lesion is near the airway.
- Advise patients that swelling is to be expected and to seek advice from the performing physician rather than attend emergency/casualty departments.
- In extreme swelling drainage may be needed, particularly if adjacent structures are at risk or to relieve excessive discomfort.
- If drainage is necessary
    - o OK 432 usually demonstrate turbid fluid with high monocyte count.
    - o Doxycycline and bleomycin may demonstrate intralesional hemorrhage.
    - o Culture should be negative.

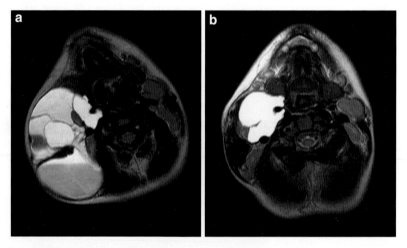

Fig. 46.6 (**a**) Demonstrates a multiloculated LM with fluid levels in the neck of a 17-month-old boy (axial T2 FLAIR MRI). (**b**) Axial FLAIR MRI in the same patient 4 months after initial treatment with intralesional OK 432. There is a marked reduction in size of the lesion

Follow-Up

Repeat procedure at 6 week intervals until resolution, no further progress, or failure of treatment. Six treatments are usually the maximum offered.

Keypoints

- Most commonly congenital and involves the head and neck in children under 2.
- Multidisciplinary teams should be involved in patient care.
- Ensure adequate imaging assessment prior to initiation of treatment.
- Classification according to cyst size is most useful. Macrocystic lesions have the best prognosis.
- Multiple treatments may be required.
- Lesions may recur months and years later, requiring further treatment.
- First-line agents OK 432 and bleomycin; second-line agent doxycycline.

Safety

- Thorough assessment of lesion extent and adjacent structure involvement prior to sclerotherapy, identifying structures at risk.
- Provision for hospital stay if airway is at risk.
- Strict aseptic technique to avoid infection.

Recommended Further Reading

Acevedo J, Shah R, Brietzke S. Nonsurgical therapies for lymphangiomas: A systematic review. Otolaryngology – head Neck Surg 2007;134(4): 418–424

Legiehn BM, Heran MKS. Advances in Musculoskeletal Imaging – Classification, Diagnosis, and Interventional Radiologic Management of Vascular Malforma-tions. Orthopedic Clin North Am. 2006; 37(3): 435–474

Woo EK, Connor SE. Computed tomography and magnetic resonance imaging appearances of cystic lesions in the suprahyoid neck: a pictorial review. Dentomaxillofac Radiol. 2007 Dec;36(8):451–458

Chapter 47
Thoracic Duct Embolization

Jess Campagna and Raj Jain

Clinical Features—Chylothorax

- Chylothorax results from lymphatic leakage containing chylomicrons and triglycerides in the pleural cavity following damage to the thoracic duct along its intrathoracic route.
- Lymphatic flow (1.5–2.5 L/day) varies with diet; ingesting fats, especially long chain fatty acids (>16 carbons) and water increase lymphatic flow while starvation decreases it.
- Etiology of chylothroax is varied:
  - 50% due to neoplasm (especially lymphoma and bronchogenic carcinoma).
  - 25% due to surgery (especially esophagectomy, coronary artery bypass, congenital heart disease repair, lung or mediastinal surgery, radical neck dissection, aortic coarctation repair) or trauma (shearing action of the right crus of the diaphragm on the thoracic duct—seen with spine hyperextension, deceleration injury, weight lifting, severe coughing or vomiting, vigorous stretching while yawning).
  - Congenital (birth trauma, Noonan and Down syndromes, H-type trachealesophageal fistula, lymphangiectasia, thoracic duct hypoplasia).
  - Idiopathic (congestive heart failure, tuberculosis, histoplasmosis, filariasis, sarcoid, mediastinal fibrosis, yellow nail syndrome, Kaposi sarcoma, lymphangioleiomyomatosis)
  - Miscellaneous (radiation-induced mediastinal fibrosis, subclavian or superior vena cava obstruction secondary to an indwelling catheter, lumbar aortography, esophageal sclerotherapy, sequelae of chylous ascites).
  - These relative incidences are changing as the numbers of thoracic procedures increase.
- Patients present with shortness of breath, cough, and chest discomfort.
- Chylothorax should always be suspected when a pleural effusion develops in a patient who has had a thoracic procedure, especially with a high thoracostomy tube output; however, overall incidence is less than 1% after all thoracic procedures.
- In patients with a pleural drain in place after thoracic surgery, chylothorax will often manifest itself on resumption of eating with the drain output becoming

Transcatheter Embolization and Therapy,
Techniques in Interventional Radiology, DOI 10.1007/978-1-84800-897-7_47,
© Springer-Verlag London Limited 2010

turbid; confirmation can be done by feeding the patient cream which will result in the drainage turning from serous to opalescent.
- Unremitting chylothorax can have a mortality between 25 and 50%, despite conservative treatment, due to loss of plasma proteins, triglycerides, electrolytes, intravascular volume, lymphocytes (mostly T cells), and fat-soluble vitamins. This results in patients progressing to an immunocompromized, malnourished, and hypovolemic state, often with respiratory and cardiac dysfunction.

Diagnostic Evaluation/Laboratory

- A thoracentesis is necessary to make the definitive diagnosis; chylous effusions are odorless, exudative, and bacteriostatic, with predominate lymphocytes.
- Diagnosis is made by the presence of one or more of the following criteria:
   o A pleural fluid triglyceride level of 110 mg/dL or greater.
   o The presence of chylomicrons in the pleural effusion.
   o A chylous leak into the pleural cavity documented on lymphangiography or during surgery.
- Chyle has a high content of albumin (30 g/L) and fat (30 g/L) which is why its loss results in dramatic nutritional impact.

Imaging

- A chest X-ray is the first step in order to document the presence of a pleural effusion.
- Upon making the diagnosis of a chylothorax in non-surgical cases, a computerized tomography scan of the chest and abdomen should be performed to evaluate the mediastinum and intra-abdominal para-aortic lymph nodes to rule out lymphoma (Fig. 47.1).
- Ultrasound can also be attempted to try and localize the cisterna chyli.
- Pedal lymphangiography is also used to identify the site of lymphatic leakage or obstruction.
   o In stable patients, provocative steps can be taken to increase the sensitivity of lymphangiography (stop the total parental nutrition (TPN), ensure that the chylothorax is well drained, and give a high-fat diet).
   o Lymphangiography itself can help abate a lymphatic leak in greater than 50% of cases as the opacifying agent (lipiodol) is also a mild sclerosant.

Indications

- There are no randomized control studies led to help direct management, likely due to the low incidence of disease.

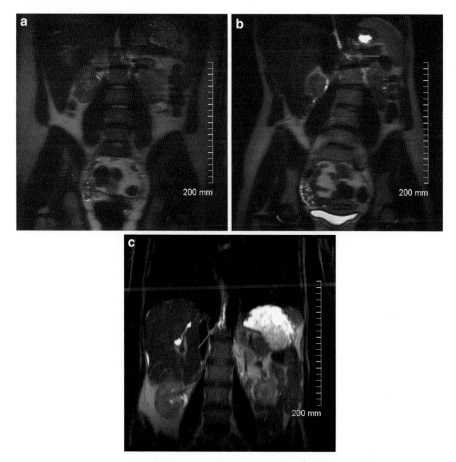

Fig. 47.1 Magnetic resonance imaging (T2 HASTE) of the thoracolumbar region is useful to identify the presence and location of the cisterna chyli (*arrows*) as a suitable target of access, as well as to assess adjacent structures that may affect a percutaneous approach (aorta, inferior vena cava, right renal artery)

- Operative intervention is typically indicated only when conservative management fails.
- Numerically, surgical intervention is indicated if the average daily chyle loss exceeds 1500 mL in adults (or 100 mL per year of age in children) over a 5-day period or persistent chyle loss of 200 mL per day despite 2 weeks of conservative management.
- There is some disagreement in the literature as some authors believe that early operative intervention prevents nutritional demise and decreases morbidity and mortality, (especially in already nutritionally depleted patients), and prevents pleural adhesions and infections which may complicate operative intervention.

Alternative Therapies

- Operative interventions include thoracotomy or video-assisted thorascopic surgery to clip the thoracic duct, talc or fibrin glue pleurodesis, or pleuroperitoneal shunting.
- Initial approach to conservative therapy is to decompress the pleural space with a thoracostomy tube, which allows measurement of the rate of leakage and may facilitate pleural surface apposition to the thoracic duct fistula to accelerate healing.
- Need to try and avoid nutritional deficiency and immunodeficiency by monitoring weight and repleting albumin and electrolytes as needed.
- Dietary modification with the medium-chain triglyceride (MCT) diet has a 50% success rate.
    o MCTs are absorbed directly into the portal system as opposed to the intestinal lacteal vessels like long-chain fatty acids.
    o MCT diet helps to minimize flow in the thoracic duct, which may promote leak healing.
- If leakage does not decrease in response to the MCT diet, oral intake should cease since this may stimulate lymphatic flow. In the setting of cessation of oral intake, the patient should be placed on intravenous total parenteral nutrition.
- Treatment of the underlying etiology may result in resolution of the chylothorax (e.g., radiation therapy or chemotherapy for lymphoma).

Medical Therapies

- These have been reported to be useful adjuncts in patients already being managed with MCT diet or TPN.
    —*Somatastatin/Octreotide* (synthetic analog): inhibits gastrointestinal secretions (gastric acid, pancreatic enzymes, bile, colonic fluids) and reduces intestinal absorption of fats by inhibiting the gut-wall transport process, lowering splanchnic blood flow, and decreasing gastrointestinal motility.
    o Somatastatin is given as an intravenous infusion at 6 mg/day for ~4 days. Once chyle output ceases, the rate is cut in half for 2 days and then stopped to prevent rebound effect. Dosing for the pediatric population starts at 0.5 mcg/kg/hr.
    o Blood glucose needs to be monitored every 6 h as somatastatin modulates the blood glucose regulatory system.
    o Side effects: abdominal cramping, nausea, diarrhea, fatty stools, flatulence, liver dysfunction, and blood glucose dysregulation.
    o Octreotide is advantageous in that it is a subcutaneous injection (rather than intravenous like somatastatin) given every 8 h (50–500 μg) for 7–14 days.
    —*Etilefrine*: α- and β-adrenergic sympathomimetic drug, used to treat postural hypotension and priapism, which causes smooth muscle (known to be present in

the thoracic duct) contraction, resulting in decreased diameter of the lymphatic vessels.

- o Given as an intravenous infusion at 5 mg/hr for 4–7 days. Once chyle output ceases, the rate is cut in half for 2 days and then stopped.
- o Side effects: headache, tachycardia, flushing, hypertension.
- o Use with caution with patients taking halogenic and imipraminic drugs.
- Local injection of tetracycline hydrochloride has been described to treat cervical thoracic duct leaks.

Contraindications

- Nutritional and performance status of the patient may make a return or primary trip to the operating room not feasible in certain populations, which would favor percutaneous intervention.
- Laboratory values that increase the risk of bleeding (INR >1.5, platelets <50,000/dL) should be corrected prior to percutaneous intervention.

Specific Complications

- There are no significant risks from a percutaneous approach, which should be attempted prior to surgical intervention when conservative management fails or perhaps even as soon as the diagnosis of chylothorax is made.
- Technical failure: lack of suitable retroperitoneal ducts for catheterization (seen with prior abdominal surgery, trauma, chronic aortic dissection) or failure to visualize the chyle leak on lymphangiography.
- Damage to surrounding anatomic structures depending on path of needle approach (intra-abdominal hemorrhage, peritonitis, chylous ascites).
- Thoracic duct rupture or misplaced microcoils.
- Contrast dye allergy or pulmonary dysfunction from lipiodol embolization.
- Pedal incision infection or chronic foot pain from lipiodol extravasation from pedal lymphangiography.

Anatomy

- Anatomy of the retroperitoneal lymph vessels can be highly variable. A successful procedure requires a large lymphatic trunk at least 2 mm in diameter or opacification of the cisterna chyli.

Normal Anatomy

- The thoracic duct arises from the cisterna chyli in the upper abdomen and empties either directly or through multiple branches into the left jugular or left subclavian vein.
- It traverses the diaphragm at the aortic aperture and ascends in the posterior mediastinum between the descending thoracic aorta (to its left) and azygos vein (to its right).
- The thoracic duct has multiple valves and is typically 2–6 mm in diameter.
- The cisterna chyli is a sac of variable shape and length that ranges from 2 to 16 mm in diameter. It is visualized on 64–80% of pedal lymphangiograms.

Anatomic Variation

- The thoracic duct is usually a single duct at the level of the eighth thoracic vertebra, but frequently splits above this level into two to three parallel branches that typically rejoin the main duct more cephalad.
- A second thoracic duct may occasionally be noted coursing in the left mediastinum.
- It is fairly common (in up to 40% of cases) for the retroperitoneal lymphatic trunks to be replaced by numerous small collateral vessels. This may be congenital or related to collateral formation in response to lymphatic occlusion or disruption by diseased lymph nodes, lymphoma, previous retroperitoneal surgery, or trauma.

Equipment

- Long micropuncture set with J-tip guidewire.
- 10-F peel-away sheath.
- 3-cm bulbous-tip stiff 8-F malleable cannula.
- Coaxial 20–25 cm flexible 21–22-gauge needle.
- 0.018 inch hydromer-coated microscopic guidewire.
- 3-French microcatheter.

Embolic Agents

- Complex platinum microcoils, 5 cm long, and 3–6 mm in diameter.
- 1–1.5 ml of glue and Ethiodol diluted in a 1:1 or 1:2 ratio or 500–710 μm of PVA.
- Other agents may include absolute ethanol, cyanoacrylate adhesive, or gelfoam.

Medication

- Broad-spectrum antibiotic at start of procedure.
- Local anesthesia for the pedal lymphogram, abdominal puncture site, and puncture of the opacified cisterna chyli.
- Sedation and analgesia with fentanyl and midazolam are helpful in most cases.

Procedure

Preparation

- When possible, administer one to two cups of barium the night before procedure to opacify transverse colon.
- Administer barium milkshake just before procedure to stimulate lymphatic flow.

Pedal Lymphography

- Used to assess the presence of cisterna chyli or large retroperitoneal lymph trunks that can be catheterized in the upper abdomen to the right of the aorta.
- Methylene blue dye is injected into the interdigital web spaces so that a suitable lymphatic vessel can be visualized.
- After 1–2 h, a cut down is performed over a methylene-blue-stained lymphatic duct over the dorsum of the foot.
- A 30-g angiocatheter is gently placed into the dye-stained lymphatic duct (magnifying devices are helpful).
- Usually inject 8–12 ml (no more that 20 ml) of iodinated oil (lipiodol) into a right foot lymphatic vessel at a rate of 8–10 ml/hr using a 27–30 gauge needle. A special lymphangiogram injector is used for this step.
- Bipedal lymphography only used if there is inadequate opacification of the lymphatic vessels with the unilateral approach.
- Flow of iodinated oil is then followed fluoroscopically until the retroperitoneal lymph trunks and/or cisterna chyli are opacified. These large trunks are typically located between L3 and T12 and take approximately 2–5 h to opacify.

Access

- Midline skin puncture is made with a micropuncture set 5–10 cm below the xiphoid, cephalad to the transverse colon. In order to avoid vital organs, ultrasound can be used to evaluate the tract from the skin to the cisterna chyli.
- A J-tip guidewire is then threaded into the peritoneal cavity through the sheath of the micropuncture set to allow for insertion of a 10-Fr peel-away sheath.

- A 13-cm bulbous-tip stiff 8-Fr malleable cannula is introduced through the sheath into the peritoneal cavity. This provides accurate guidance of a coaxial 20–25 cm flexible 21–22-gauge needle, which is used to puncture the lymphatic trunk.
- Typically at the level of the first lumbar vertebra, a 0.018-inch hydrophilic guidewire is threaded through the needle into the thoracic duct via the cisterna chyli or a large retroperitoneal lymph trunk.
- A 3-French microcatheter is inserted and advanced into the chest.
- 5–10 ml of non-ionic contrast is injected to opacify the complete length of the thoracic duct, assess branch pattern (i.e., parallel lymph ducts), and evaluate for the site of leakage.

Treatment Plan and Technique

- When the thoracic duct is successfully cannulated, treatment proceeds with embolization. In patients in whom lymphatic trunks cannot be catheterized and who have no opacification of the cisterna chyli, disruption of the small retroperitoneal lymphatic vessels can be attempted.

Embolization

- Three to eight overlapping complex platinum microcoils, 5 cm long, and 3–6 mm in diameter, are packed in a row to occlude the proximal thoracic duct above the diaphragm and below the suspected leak.
- If the coils are not completely occlusive after injection of contrast, either 500–710 μm of PVA or 1–1.5 ml of cyanoacrylate glue and ethiodol diluted in a 1:1 or 1:2 ratio may be injected into the thoracic duct.

Disruption of Lymph Channels

- Typically only used when lymphatic trunks cannot be catheterized and when there is no opacification of the cisterna chyli.
- In this situation, typically there are a variable number of tiny retroperitoneal lymphatic collaterals, which feed the thoracic duct via a few uninterrupted channels or indirectly via a complex ductal meshwork.
- Attempts can be made to directly mechanically occlude these vessels by using rotary and back-and-forth motions with a 21–22-gauged needle in the region of these vessels.

Case Example (Fig. 47.2)

Follow-Up

- No specific follow-up is necessary and will be symptom driven, i.e., recurrent cough, shortness of breath, etc.

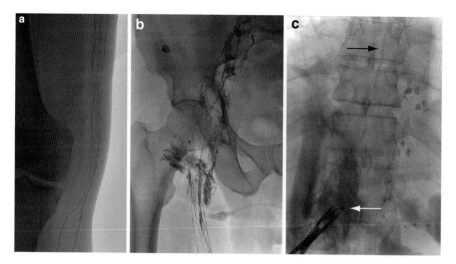

Fig. 47.2 Sixty-one-year-old male who underwent an esophagectomy with gastric pull-through for distal esophageal adenocarcinoma complicated by a high-output chylothorax (3L/day) failed conservative management. Lymphangiography demonstrates opacification of the medial lymphatics in the knee and the progression of lipiodol through the pelvis. The inferior portion of the thoracic duct (*white arrow*) was percutaneously accessed from an anterior transabdominal approach with a Chiba needle, with subsequent opacification of the thoracic duct (*black arrows*) following the injection of Omnipaque 300. Opacified lymph nodes can also be seen. Embolization of the thoracic duct was successfully carried out with a combination of 3 cc of absolute ethanol, 2 cc of cyanoacrylate glue in 4 cc of lipiodol, followed by gelfoam through the Chiba needle. The thoracostomy tube output subsequently decreased to <100 cc/day immediately after the percutaneous procedure

- If embolization is successful, thoracostomy tube outputs will decrease almost immediately.

Keypoints

- Chylothorax from disruption of the thoracic duct carries a significant mortality with continued chyle loss leading to life-threatening weakness, dehydration, edema, emaciation, and hemodynamic distress due to hypoproteinemia, hyponatremia, lymphopenia, and pulmonary compression.
- Conservative treatment includes thoracostomy tube drainage, MCT diet, TPN, somatastatin (octreotide), and etilefrine.
- Percutaneous approach is advantageous compared to surgical intervention due to the use of local anesthesia and conscious sedation versus general

endotracheal anesthesia and lung decompression, especially in this often
critically ill population.

- Percutaneous intervention can be attempted immediately following the
  diagnosis of chylothorax to help avoid long-term complications and costs
  associated with conservative management with initial success rates around
  70% with lower morbidity and mortality compared to surgical intervention
  (<5% versus 25–40%).

- The most time-consuming aspect of the percutaneous approach is pedal
  lymphangiography.

Suggested Reading

Binkert, C. Percutaneous Management of High-Output Chylothorax with Embolization or Needle
  Disruption Technique. J Vasc Interv Radiol. 2005; 16:1257–1262.

Cope, C. Management of Unremitting Chylothorax by Percutaneous Embolization and Blockage of
  Retroperitoneal Lymphatic Vessels in 42 Patients. J Vasc Interv Radiol. 2002;13(11):1139–48.

Doerr, C. Etiology of Chylothorax in 203 Patients. Mayo Clin Proc. 2005; 80(7):867–870.

Nair, S. Aetiology and Management of Chylothorax in Adults. Eur J Cardiothorac Surg. 2007;
  32(2):362–369.

Syed, L. Lymphangiography: A Case Study. Semin Intervent Radiol 2007; 24:106–110.

Valentine, V. The Management of Chylothorax. Chest 1992;10: 586–591.

Chapter 48
Post-partum Hemorrhage: Embolization and Endovascular Management

P. Anondo Stangl

Clinical Features

- Post-partum hemorrhage (PPH) is the most common cause of maternal mortality world-wide.
- PPH is defined as greater than 500 ml blood loss for vaginal deliveries or greater than 1000 ml for cesarean deliveries.
- PPH generally occurs in the immediate peri-partum period.
- Most common etiology is uterine atony (occurs in 5% of deliveries).
- Other etiologies: genital tract lacerations, episiotomy, retained products of conception, abnormal placentation, intra-uterine pseudoaneurysm or arteriovenous fistula.

Diagnostic Evaluation

- Diagnosis is made clinically.
- Blood product requirement is variable.
- In severe cases, patients may be hemodynamic instability and/or DIC.

Imaging

- Imaging prior to intervention is not generally indicated for acute PPH.
- In cases of known abnormal placentation (placenta accreta, increta, percreta), ultrasound and/or MRI have generally been performed. Delivery is often by elective cesarean section.
- Patients with delayed PPH who are stable may benefit from pelvic ultrasound, CTA or MRA prior to intervention to assess for retained products of conception, pseudoaneurysm or AVF.

Transcatheter Embolization and Therapy,
Techniques in Interventional Radiology, DOI 10.1007/978-1-84800-897-7_48,
© Springer-Verlag London Limited 2010

Indications for Intervention/Embolization

- Prevention of PPH: prophylactic placement of internal iliac artery IIA catheters or occlusion balloons prior to cesarean delivery is indicated in high-risk cases (especially abnormal placentation).
- First-line treatment of PPH.
  - o Induce uterine contraction: uterine massage, IV oxytocin, or prostaglandin.
  - o Resuscitation: transfusion of blood and fluid products.
- Second-line treatment of PPH.
  - o Protocols vary regarding management of PPH depending on local expertise.
  - o Exploration for and repair of genital tract tears are standard prior to angiography and embolization.
  - o Embolization is appropriate as the initial intervention or following unsuccessful surgical therapy (IIA ligation or hysterectomy).

Contraindications to Intervention/Embolization

- None. PPH should be considered a life-threatening emergency; intervention should not be delayed for correction of coagulopathy or transfusion requirements.

Anatomy

- Uterine arteries arise from the anterior division of the IIAs and have rich collateral networks across the midline.
- Ovarian arteries may contribute to PPH. They arise from the juxtarenal aorta and often will not be visualized with standard pelvic arteriography.
- Hemorrhage from genital tract lacerations may involve other IIA branches including vaginal, cervical, internal pudendal, and obturator arteries.

Equipment

- Non-selective catheters: straight flush, pigtail, or omni flush 4–5 Fr.
- Selective catheters: hydrophilic cobra 4–5 Fr, Roberts uterine catheter 5 Fr. High-flow microcatheters may be necessary for selective embolization.
- Prophylactic cases: 4–5 Fr selective end-hole catheters or occlusion balloons (e.g., 5.3 Fr flow directed over the wire occlusion balloons) placed in both IIAs.

Embolic Agents

- Gelfoam pledgets or slurry (empiric or selective embolization).
  - o Large majority of the reported cases use gelfoam primarily, with other agents as an adjunct in fewer cases.

- Polyvinyl alcohol (PVA) or tris-acryl gelatin particles 700–900 or 900–1200 μm (empiric or selective embolization).
- Microcoils with or without gelfoam (localized extravasation/arterial injury).
  - Coils are generally avoided due to the permanence of the occlusion and the inability to re-embolize (in case of recurrent bleeding).

Procedure

Therapeutic Embolization for Acute PPH

Access

- Common femoral artery access (unilateral or bilateral).
- "Up-and-over" selection of contralateral proximal IIA and branches.
- Reverse curve catheter for ipsilateral IIA selection.
- Brachial or axillary access may be preferable in the operating room (OR) when patient is draped.
- Microcatheters generally not needed unless superselective catheterization is necessary.

Angiography

- According to operator preference, flush pelvic arteriogram with catheter at the level of the renal arteries may be performed initially or following initial embolization.
- Bilateral IIA angiograms should include pelvic floor and perineum in field of view for evaluation of genital tract lacerations.
- Uterine hypervascularity without extravasation or focal abnormality is most common angiographic appearance.
- Extravasation may occur into uterine cavity, peritoneum, or extra-peritoneal pelvis.
- Distinct arterial injuries should be further evaluated with more selective arteriograms, particularly if extra-uterine.

Embolization (See Fig. 48.1)

- Surgical ligation of IIAs is ineffective at controlling hemorrhage in over half of cases due to bleeding from retrograde feeding vessels. The goal of embolization is to provide a more distal occlusion.
- Uterine hemorrhage should be treated with bilateral embolization; however, genital tract lacerations may require only unilateral embolization.
- In the absence of localized pathology, bilateral IIA anterior divisions or uterine arteries are empirically embolized to stasis with gelfoam or particles.
- Identifiable sites of hemorrhage (e.g., genital tract lacerations) may benefit from coil embolization as significant recanalization and recurrent hemorrhage have been reported.

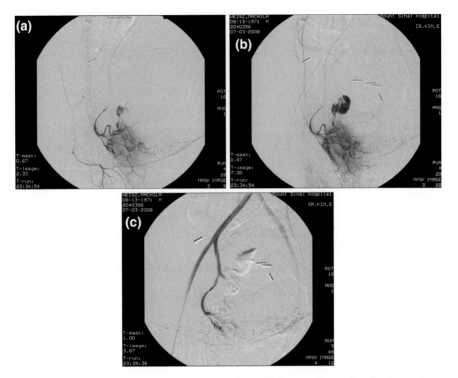

Fig. 48.1 (**a**) Unstable patient post-cesarean section with hypotension and active hemorrhage. Digital subtraction angiogram, early arterial phase, demonstrates early bleeding site. (**b**) Same patient as Fig. 48.1a. Late arterial phase angiography further demonstrates active contrast extravasation. (**c**) Same patient as prior figures, post-embolization with polyvinyl alcohol particles. There is truncation of the embolized vessels, and no further contrast extravasation is noted

- Empiric embolization (performed in the absence of identifiable bleeding source) with coils is to be avoided since occlusion may be too proximal to be effective and can preclude sufficiently selective interventions.
- Embolization (empiric or selective) is >90% effective in clinically controlling PPH; the remainder of patients require surgery or repeat interventions.
- If possible, the posterior divisions of IIAs are spared in order to reduce post-procedural pain. True ischemic complications from unilateral or bilateral IIA embolization are rare.

Prophylactic Interventions

Prophylactic placement of catheters for planned cesarean delivery in high-risk patients may be performed in OR compatible IR suites, in the OR with C-arm fluoroscopy, or in IR prior to transport to the OR for delivery. The patient should have a urinary catheter and any epidural anaesthesia in place before arterial access is obtained to avoid dislodgement of arterial catheters.

Access

- Bilateral common femoral access is preferred (catheter stability, rapid intervention possible).
- Brachial or axillary access can be used (may reduce radiation to pelvis, clear from operative field and drapes), although there is increased concern for catheter migration and access site complications
- Any arterial access must be secured (e.g., sutured), connected to pressurized drips, and monitored by IR personnel during transport to OR and during delivery.

Angiography

- Placement of catheters or occlusion balloons into IIAs or anterior divisions prior to cesarean delivery.
- To decrease the fetal radiation exposure, minimize fluoroscopy time, use pulsed fluoroscopy and use tight collimation. Avoid angiographic runs if possible.
- Diagnostic angiography is not necessary prior to delivery.
- If hemorrhage is not fully controlled with empiric embolization or balloon occlusion, diagnostic arteriography should be performed to assess the bleeding source and the need for further embolization.
- Remember the incision: injury to abdominal wall vessels (e.g., inferior epigastric artery) can occur and may not be evident upon IIA injections.

Embolization

- If significant hemorrhage occurs following delivery, empiric embolization is immediately performed with Gelfoam slurry.
- If using occlusion balloons, these are inflated empirically as soon as the umbilical cord is severed.
- Balloon occlusion of the IIAs or anterior divisions is often too proximal to provide adequate control of hemorrhage
- If initial embolization or occlusion balloons do not provide adequate hemostasis, additional or more selective embolization should be performed

Arterial Puncture Site

- Clinical condition of the patient will determine management.
- Arterial sheaths should be retained in unstable patients with severe hemorrhage to allow blood pressure monitoring and rapid arterial access if further intervention is needed.
- Patients with large transfusion requirements are often coagulopathic.
- Use closure devices with caution: young, female patients with small vessels (exacerbated by hypovolemia) may be prone to complications.

Follow-Up

- Clinical observation for ongoing hemorrhage.
- Imaging typically not necessary.
- Hemorrhage related to retained products of conception may require dilatation and curettage as definitive therapy.
- Normal menses and fertility can be expected in most cases after several months.
- Multiple cases of successful pregnancy and delivery following embolization for PPH have been reported.
- Recurrence rates of PPH with subsequent deliveries are likely higher than the incidence in the general population.

Alternative Therapies

- Surgical treatment typically involves ligation of both IIAs.
- Patients with persistent hemorrhage proceed to hysterectomy.
- Surgery can usually be avoided where there are clear protocols in place for the management of PPH.
- Case selection and utilization of endovascular therapy vary widely across institutions.

Specific Complications

- Unsuccessful embolizations—minority of cases require repeat embolization, and failures requiring surgery are rare.
- Non-target embolization resulting in symptomatic lower extremity ischemia has been described; standard techniques of careful embolization under fluoroscopy should prevent most instances of non-target embolization.
- Ischemic complications in the distribution of the anterior division of the IIA have been reported in 3–7% of patients. Such complications include uterine necrosis, transient ovarian failure, bladder necrosis, vaginal fistulae, muscle pain, and neurological damage.
- Use of temporary embolic agents (gelfoam) or larger particles should minimize ischemic complications.
- Theoretical concerns about radiation and embolization impacting fertility have largely been allayed (the alternative, hysterectomy, has a clear impact on fertility).

Keypoints

- Work with the labor and delivery team to develop a strategy and written protocol.

- Embolization for PPH is an established therapy, safe, and effective.
- Negative angiographic findings do NOT contraindicate embolization.
- Embolization is appropriate before, during, after, or instead of surgery.
- Bilateral embolization is necessary for uterine bleeding unless a specific bleeding source is identified.

Suggested Reading

Banovac F, Lin R, Shah, D, White A, Pelage JP, Spies J. Angiographic and Interventional Options in Obstetric and Gynecologic Emergencies. *Obstetric and Gynecologic Clinics of North America* 2007;34(3):599–616

Eriksson LG, Mulic-Lutvica A, Jangland L, Nyman R. Massive Postpartum Hemorrhage Treated with Transcatheter Arterial Embolization: Technical Aspects and Long-Term Effects on Fertility and Menstrual Cycle. *Acta Radiologica* 2007;48(6):635–642

Mitty HA, Sterling KM, Alvarez M, Gendler R. Obstetric Hemorrhage: Prophylactic and Emergency Arterial Catheterization and Embolotherapy. *Radiology* 1993;188(1):183–187

Index